MATE CHOICE

MATE CHOICE

Edited by

PATRICK BATESON

Reader in Animal Behaviour and
Director of the Sub-Department of Animal Behaviour
Department of Zoology, University of Cambridge

CAMBRIDGE UNIVERSITY PRESS
Cambridge
London   New York   New Rochelle
Melbourne   Sydney

Published by the Press Syndicate of the University of Cambridge
The Pitt Building, Trumpington Street, Cambridge CB2 1RP
32 East 57th Street, New York, NY 10022, USA
296 Beaconsfield Parade, Middle Park, Melbourne 3206, Australia

© Cambridge University Press 1983

First published 1983

Printed in Great Britain by the University Press, Cambridge

Library of Congress catalogue card number: 82–14669

British Library Cataloguing in Publication Data
Mate choice.
1. Sexual behavior in animals – Congresses
I. Bateson, Patrick
596′.0562   QL761

ISBN 0 521 25112 5
ISBN 0 521 27207 6 Pbk

UP

CONTENTS

List of contributors vii
Preface by Patrick Bateson ix

I Introduction
1 T. R. HALLIDAY The study of mate choice   3
2 WOLFGANG WICKLER AND UTA SEIBT Monogamy: an
   ambiguous concept   33

II Characteristics of sexual selection
3 PETER O'DONALD Sexual selection by female choice   53
4 STEVAN J. ARNOLD Sexual selection: the interface of theory
   and empiricism   67
5 JACK W. BRADBURY AND ROBERT M. GIBSON Leks and
   mate choice   109

III Sex differences in choosiness
6 G. A. PARKER Mate quality and mating decisions   141
7 MARION PETRIE Mate choice in role-reversed species   167
8 ANTHONY ARAK Male–male competition and mate choice in
   anuran amphibians   181
9 DIANA J. BELL Mate choice in the European Rabbit   211

IV Non-random mating
10 LINDA PARTRIDGE Non-random mating and offspring
    fitness   227
11 PATRICK BATESON Optimal outbreeding   257
12 F. COOKE AND J. C. DAVIES Assortative mating, mate choice
    and reproductive fitness in Snow Geese   279
13 DIANE M. WILLIAMS Mate choice in the Mallard   297
14 BRUNO D'UDINE AND ENRICO ALLEVA Early experience
    and sexual preferences in rodents   311

V Compatibility of mates
15 IAN ROWLEY Re-mating in birds   331
16 J. C. COULSON AND C. S. THOMAS Mate choice in the
    Kittiwake Gull   361

17 STEVE DUCK AND DOROTHY MIELL   Mate choice in humans as an interpersonal process   377

VI **Hormonal mechanisms**
18 J. B. HUTCHISON AND R. E. HUTCHISON   Hormonal mechanisms of mate choice in birds   389
19 ERIC B. KEVERNE   Endocrine determinants and constraints on sexual behaviour in monkeys   407

VII **Decision rules**
20 R. I. M. DUNBAR   Life history tactics and alternative strategies of reproduction   423
21 JAMES F. WITTENBERGER   Tactics of mate choice   435

Index   449

CONTRIBUTORS

Enrico Alleva, *Consiglio Nazionale delle Ricerche, Laboratorio di Psicobiologia e Psicofarmacologia, Via Reno, 1, 00198 Roma, Italy*

Anthony Arak, *Department of Zoology, Downing Street, Cambridge CB2 3EJ, UK*

Stevan J. Arnold, *Department of Biology, University of Chicago, 1103 East 57th Street, Chicago, Illinois 60637, USA*

Patrick Bateson, *Sub-Department of Animal Behaviour, High Street, Madingley, Cambridge, CB3 8AA, UK*

Diana J. Bell, *School of Biological Sciences, University of East Anglia, Norwich NR4 7TJ, UK*

Jack W. Bradbury, *Department of Biology, C-016, University of California, La Jolla, California 92093, USA*

F. Cooke, *Department of Biology, Queen's University, Kingston, Canada K7L 3N6*

J. C. Coulson, *Department of Zoology, University of Durham, Science Laboratories, South Road, Durham DH1 3LE, UK*

J. C. Davies, *Department of Biology, Queen's University, Kingston, Canada K7L 3N6*

Steve Duck, *Department of Psychology, Fylde College, Bailrigg, Lancaster LA1 4YF, UK*

Bruno D'Udine, *Consiglio Nazionale delle Ricerche, Laboratorio di Psicobiologia e Psicofarmacologia, Via Reno, 1, 00198 Roma, Italy*

R. I. M. Dunbar, *Sub-Department of Animal Behaviour, High Street, Madingley, Cambridge CB3 8AA, UK*

Robert M. Gibson, *Department of Biology, C-016, University of California, La Jolla, California 92093, USA*

T. R. Halliday, *Department of Biology, The Open University, Walton Hall, Milton Keynes MK7 6AA, UK*

J. B. Hutchison, *M.R.C. Unit on The Development and Integration of Behaviour. Sub-Department of Animal Behaviour, High Street, Madingley, Cambridge CB3 8AA, UK*

R. E. Hutchison, *Sub-Department of Animal Behaviour, High Street, Madingley, Cambridge CB3 8AA, UK*

Eric B. Keverne, *Department of Anatomy, Downing Street, Cambridge CB2 3DY, UK*

Dorothy Miell, *Department of Psychology, Fylde College, Bailrigg, Lancaster LA1 4YF, UK*

Peter O'Donald, *Department of Genetics, Downing Street, Cambridge CB2 3EH, UK*

G. A. Parker, *Department of Zoology, University of Liverpool, Brownlow Street, P.O. Box 147, Liverpool L69 3BX, UK*

Linda Partridge, *Department of Zoology, University of Edinburgh, West Mains Road, Edinburgh EH9 3JT, UK*

Marion Petrie, *School of Biological Sciences, University of East Anglia, Norwich NR4 7TJ, UK*

Ian Rowley, *CSIRO, Division of Wildlife, Clayton Road, Helena Valley, via Midland, Western Australia 6056*

Uta Seibt, *Max-Planck-Institut für Verhaltenphysiologie, D-8131, Seewiesen, W. Germany*

C. S. Thomas, *Department of Zoology, University of Durham, Science Laboratories, South Road, Durham DH1 3LE, UK*

Wolfgang Wickler, *Max-Planck-Institut für Verhaltenphysiologie, D-8131, Seewiesen, W. Germany*

Diane M. Williams, *156 Queens Road, Yardley, Birmingham B26 2AJ, UK*

James F. Wittenburger, *Department of Zoology NJ-15, University of Washington, Seattle, Washington, 98195, USA*

PREFACE

This book arose from a conference held by the Association for the Study of Animal Behaviour in Cambridge in July 1981. However, the book is emphatically not a set of conference proceedings. Some chapters were specially commissioned and contributors to both conference and book re-wrote their papers as surveys rather than as presentations of new data. The attempt has been to give a clear picture of the current state of the subject. Furthermore, wherever it was possible (and relevant), the chapters have been linked together so that, even when authors disagree, the reader will be aware of the areas of overlap.

The growing interest in mating preferences in animals has been generated in part by the renewed vitality of evolutionary biology. A characteristic that successfully attracts a member of the opposite sex might become increasingly common in the population simply because it is likely to be transmitted to offspring which in turn may be better than others at winning mates. This evolutionary process, which is a part of what is called sexual selection, could be an important source of genetic change. Even though sexual selection is uppermost in many minds, what animals actually do must not be confused with the hypothetical evolutionary process. When the term 'mate selection' is used for what animals do, it can quickly lead to unconscious punning and the assumption that a preference for a particular kind of mate necessarily has implications for sexual selection. As will become plain, the assumption is false. For these reasons, the immediate outcome of an animal's mating preference is consistently referred to in this book as 'mate choice', 'sexual selection' is used for an evolutionary process and 'mate selection' is dropped.

Anybody who is at all unfamiliar with the subject would do well to start reading the book at the beginning. In Chapter 1 Halliday provides an essential curtain-raiser for what follows. He reviews the major issues which recur throughout the book and points to both the possibilities and the difficulties of testing some of the current theories about mate choice. As in many rapidly expanding subjects, the concepts have been inadequately defined and are liable to generate considerable confusion. The trouble has arisen in part because interests in mate choice and mating systems have converged from a number of quite different directions. The point is brought out well by Wickler & Seibt who, in Chapter 2, show how 'monogamy' had quite different origins in the social sciences, evolutionary biology and population genetics. Much muddle, disagreement and inconsistency could be avoided if the different meanings were clearly recognised.

The second part of the book is devoted to the evolutionary process of sexual selection and how it might work. In Chapter 3 O'Donald summarises succinctly the results of his computer simulations and recent thinking. He criticises the widely held view derived from R. A. Fisher that sexual selection has a runaway character to it. In other words, he does not believe that once a choosy female mates preferentially with a male bearing a particular character, that character must necessarily grow in size or conspicuousness in subsequent generations at a geometric rate. The view of another modern theorist, Lande, is summarised and made understandable to a non-mathematical audience by Arnold in Chapter 4. Lande's modelling approach is very different from O'Donald's and leads him to re-affirm that Fisher's runaway evolutionary process could have occurred sometimes. However, Lande's work also suggests that under certain conditions, equilibria are to be expected. If and when they occur, the frequency of females with a preference for a particular kind of male and the frequency of that type of male have both stabilised.

All the evolutionary theorists are concerned about the interplay between sexual and natural selection pressures. In the second part of his chapter Arnold provides a method for distinguishing between current pressures due to sexual selection and those due to natural selection. This method does not provide any solution to the problem of what has happened in the past in a particular case, but could provide an indication as to what will happen in the future. The need to provide good ways of distinguishing between rival hypotheses is the major message of Bradbury & Gibson's contribution in Chapter 5. They consider the phenomena of leks which are assemblies of adult males visited by females solely for the purpose of copulation. Leks have been treated as classic examples of male competition and female choice. Bradbury & Gibson see the promise of using leks for testing controversial ideas about males being chosen on the basis of cues that indicate the adaptedness of the male. However, they point to the many factors that can complicate the interpretation of such tests.

The third part of the book on sex differences in choosiness is closely linked to the second and many of the contributors start from the position which is commonly held in the sexual selection literature, that males compete with each other for opportunities to mate with females, and females choose their mates. In Chapter 6 Parker presents several theoretical grounds for doubting the generality of this conclusion, and shows that a variety of possibilities is evolutionarily stable. He also argues strongly against the notion that choice by either sex is made on the basis of qualities that are likely to be transmitted genetically to offspring. Petrie takes a different view in Chapter 7, suggesting a number of circumstances in which female choice of mates on the basis of genetically transmitted quality could be maintained in the population. She goes on to consider the conditions in which the male might become the choosy sex, but agrees with one of Parker's points when she notes that male choosiness is not exclusively found in polyandrous species.

The next two chapters are more empirical in character and review what is known to happen during the mating of respectively anuran amphibians and rabbits. The frogs and toads have proved a particularly rich source of material for studies of mate choice. Arak's survey in Chapter 8 provides ample evidence for major differences between the sexes in terms of competition and choosiness. However, he also underscores the point that many pressures have probably contributed to the evolution of the observed behaviour and, like Bradbury & Gibson, he argues against squeezing everything into the framework of a theory about sexual selection. A very similar point emerges from Bell's survey of mate choice in the rabbit in Chapter 9. She notes that while female 'choice' in this species is primarily determined by intrasexual competition for warren littering sites, females do nonetheless prefer the odour of socially dominant males in laboratory tests.

Part III of the book is concerned with non-random mating and the evolutionary and developmental processes that lead to preferences for particular kinds of mates. These chapters provide direct evidence for mating preferences in both sexes. They also provide examples of mating preferences, such as those for non-siblings, that are very unlikely to facilitate sexual selection and may sometimes oppose it. In Chapter 10 Partridge leads off with a general discussion of the ways in which offspring fitness can be enhanced by non-random mating. Many of her examples are taken from studies of the fruitfly, but her points can be usefully generalised to other species. She stresses the advantage of avoiding inbreeding and also points to the value of assortative mating where it maintains local adaptations. I take up this point on the balance between inbreeding and outbreeding in Chapter 11 and suggest a sharply-tuned preference might be required. I go on to ask how an animal might be able to recognise an optimally related mate and conclude that early experience with close kin is frequently essential for developing mating preferences for individuals that are related by an optimal amount. Cooke & Davies provide support for part of this conclusion from their long-term study of the polymorphic Snow Goose in Chapter 12. The geese generally mate with the morphs which have the same colour as themselves but can be fooled when reared by foster-parents of a different colour. However, Cooke & Davies fail to find any reduction of fitness in the offspring when different morphs mate with each other. Even so, they do not altogether rule out the possibility that fine tuning of its preference could enable a bird to choose the partner that would maximise its reproductive success.

Williams reviews the evidence from another wildfowl species, the Mallard, in Chapter 13. Here again, early experience plays an important role in influencing the mating preference – but only in the male. The females' preferences for males are much less obviously influenced by learning in ontogeny and are strongly influenced during courtship by the condition of the male plumage, a point which ties her chapter in with Parker's and Petrie's discussions of mate quality. The important influence of early experience emerges once more in the review of rodents' sexual preferences by D'Udine & Alleva in Chapter 14. The evidence also indicates the subtle and complex interactions which can occur between learning and other ontogenetic processes that influence sexual preferences. As with evolutionary processes, a question about developmental influences on mate choice does not reduce conveniently to a single answer.

Learning about close kin and choosing mates that are a bit different provides a way of obtaining the best genetic mix for the offspring. However, compatibility between mates also operates at a behavioural level, particularly in monogamous species in which both sexes care for the young. In such cases, successful behavioural meshing of mates can crucially influence whether or not the young are adequately looked after. Part V raises some of these issues of compatibility. Long-term monogamous pair-bonds are particularly common in birds. Rowley provides, in Chapter 15, a thorough review of this phenomenon and of what precedes and follows the break-up of a pair-bond. A pair often becomes separated outside the breeding season, but Rowley argues that there is usually considerable value in re-mating with the same individual. However, a new partner may be sought if the old one was incompatible. Some of the evidence for this view comes from the long-term studies of Coulson and his co-workers on the Kittiwake, summarised in Chapter 16. They find that 'divorce' is correlated with failure to breed successfully in the previous year which, in turn, is likely to be associated with incompatibility of the pairs particularly during incubation of their eggs. Coulson & Thomas also find that breeding success increases in birds that retain their mate for the previous year. This suggests that, in some long-lived species at least, the achievement of compatibility is not just a matter of initial choice but is also a consequence of experience with a partner.

Chapter 17 by Duck & Miell is the only one written explicitly about humans, and is the only one written by non-biologists. They are concerned to show that friendships, sexual as well as non-sexual, are not simply determined by initial attraction. The level at which judgements are made about whether or not a person is or is not a friend, deepens as he or she becomes more familiar. This occurs as a result of the transactions taking place with that person. Although it is easy to be glib about such comparisons, there does seem to be considerable value in linking Duck & Miell's conclusions to those of Rowley and Coulson & Thomas.

The two chapters in Part VI are markedly different in character from all the others in the book in as much as they deal with the internal control of mate choice. While this book is primarily concerned with behaviour and not with underlying mechanisms, it seemed important that something should be included about the role of sex hormones. These play a fundamental role both in inducing the development of sexual behaviour and also as integrating agents that hold the sexual repertoire together. In their chapter, the Hutchisons show that androgen in adult male birds is directly involved with the expression of a learnt preference for a particular type of female. They go on to argue that changing levels of androgen and its metabolites during courtship facilitate the processes of assessment and synchronisation during courtship. In Chapter 19 Keverne deals with the involvement of sex and stress hormones in the mating behaviour of monkeys. He considers the ways in which hormonal levels and social status interact. Both play their part in influencing the sexual attractiveness of males and females. For the would-be reductionist, Keverne's analysis is salutary because what might seem an obvious index of mating quality (testosterone in the case of males and oestrogen in the case of females) cannot be used on its own.

A final change of direction occurs in the last part of the book. This part deals with the kinds of decisions an animal must take in relation both to the long-term mating strategy that it should adopt in the environmental and social conditions in which it finds itself, and to short-term tactics. Should it plump for the member of the opposite sex in front of it or wait for another which might prove even more satisfactory? Dunbar considers alternative mating strategies in Chapter 20. He develops points alluded to by both Bradbury & Gibson and Arak earlier in the book. It is particularly obvious in leks that it is not only the vigorously displaying males that copulate successfully. Other males adopt a very different mode of behaviour, quietly sneaking copulations without any explicit competitions with other males. Since reproductive success is determined by many components, an individual can trade losses on one component such as rate of mating against gains on another such as length of reproductive life which may be greater in uncompetitive males. Dunbar makes the point that alternative reproductive strategies that yield comparable net gains are possible.

Wittenberger in Chapter 21, concludes the book by considering the tactics of mate choice. Ideally, a mate should be maximally attractive, optimally related, highly fertile or fecund, a holder of valuable resources, and so forth. In practice, he or she is unlikely to combine all these qualities. Even in the simplest situation where all the likely potential mates are available, the chooser must be equipped with rules for deciding on the relative weight that should be given to each independent set of characteristics, such as a set based on kinship and a set based on physical well-being. The problem becomes more complex when the potential mates are not available simultaneously and mating with one reduces the likelihood of mating with another. It is a familiar enough human dilemma. A better possibility (pub, picnic site or petrol pump) might be found round the next corner. Fortunately it is not a problem which defies solution and Wittenberger points the way to how animals might solve it in the case of choosing a mate.

While many people are interested in mate choice because of its relevance to sexual selection, it will be obvious from the contents of the book that interest in the subject has also arisen for quite other reasons. For instance, the problems of how particular preferences develop in an individual's lifetime are logically distinct from the evolutionary issues. Nonetheless, it becomes apparent that when a coherent topic like mate choice is examined in different ways, the various approaches to it can help each other. The value of evolutionary theory as a cohesive force, even in areas of biology that are not directly concerned with problems of evolution, is well known.

But the evolutionary biologist can also benefit from contact with people working on problems of development and control. A familiar criticism directed at theories of evolution is that they are not amenable to testing because history cannot be replayed. Some of this criticism is scientifically illiterate since the theories and the comparative approach they encourage have certainly brought order to the existing material in all its astonishing diversity.

Furthermore, even in a non-experimental subject, theory can offer guidance on where to gather fresh evidence and, quite properly, can be embarrassed by the collecting of such evidence. It is in this respect that contact with other biologists can be helpful to the evolutionary theorists. The relevant and sometimes embarrassing evidence may have already been collected. More importantly, different perspectives contributed by each specialist inevitably provide a more complete picture of the requirements of the whole animal than is obtained by any one view.

My sense is that the various approaches to mate choice are combining in important and valuable ways. As a result, the face of the subject is changing rapidly and, as with a developing embryo, its various features are more easily distinguished. If this book contributes to these processes of growth and differentiation, it will have served its purpose.

Patrick Bateson
Cambridge, May 1982

I : INTRODUCTION

1

The study of mate choice

T. R. HALLIDAY

There are compelling reasons for believing that animals should not mate indiscriminately, but should choose their mates. Since individuals vary in their quality as potential mates, we would expect natural selection to have favoured mechanisms that ensure that mating occurs with partners of the highest possible quality. The word 'quality' is used here to cover a wide variety of properties of individual animals, including resources that they actually or potentially hold, their abilities as parents, and their genotype. Another reason why mate choice is a topic of considerable interest is that it is the behavioural mechanism that is central to the theory of intersexual selection as first propounded by Darwin (1871) and elaborated subsequently by Fisher (1930) and others (Halliday 1978*b*; Arnold, this volume, O'Donald, this volume).

The inherent plausibility of the hypothesis that mate choice is a common feature of the sexual behaviour of animals should make us especially cautious and critical in our evaluation of attempts to demonstrate its occurrence in nature. There is a danger that we may accept evidence of a standard that we would reject if it was presented in support of a more contentious hypothesis, for example, that birds use olfaction in orientation.

The principal aim of this chapter is to review some of the evidence for mate choice in animals and to discuss a number of conceptual and methodological problems that arise from studies of mate choice. A particularly important issue is the relationship between mate choice and mating competition which, since Darwin (1871) differentiated between inter- and intra-sexual selection, have typically been discussed as distinct and mutually exclusive processes. First, it is necessary to define what is meant by mate choice.

3

The definition of mate choice

Mate choice may be operationally defined as any pattern of behaviour, shown by members of one sex, that leads to their being more likely to mate with certain members of the opposite sex than with others. It is important to note that this definition is in terms of observable behaviour and contains no reference to concepts that relate to the internal state of an animal, such as 'preference', as used in everyday language. The definition covers a variety of phenomena, some of which, in a human context, we would generally not call choice. For example, Ryan (1980) has shown that males of the frog *Physalaemus pustulosus* are more successful in attracting females if they produce complex calls consisting of a basic 'whine' followed by one or more 'chucks', than if they produce simple calls consisting only of a whine. Evidence that this does not represent a preference, in the usual sense of the word, on the part of females for complex calls, but is due to the fact that complex calls are more easily located, is provided by the observation that certain predatory bats, who use the males' calls to locate their prey, are more likely to take those males that produce complex calls (Ryan, Tuttle & Taft, 1981).

This example raises a difficult issue. What we may observe, at a behavioural level, is selective responsiveness by animals to particular stimuli. The mechanism by which the nervous system brings about such selectivity may involve sensory processing at the sense organ level, matching against a centrally-located template, or a preference developed through learning. However, for the purposes of understanding the dynamics of mating systems, the precise mechanism involved is irrelevant.

What is important in terms of the possible evolutionary consequences of mate choice is not whether a true preference is involved, but whether variations in the behaviour of members of one sex are correlated with variations in their mating success. The production of more complex calls by male *Physalaemus pustulosus* will be favoured by sexual selection, because they are more easily located by females, just as surely as they would be if females preferred them.

The benefits and criteria on which mate choice is based

There are many different kinds of benefit that animals may derive by choosing certain mates rather than others; these benefits may be realised more or less immediately. When choosing a mate, an animal may use as its criterion of mate quality, either the benefit itself, or some feature of the behaviour or appearance of prospective mates that is a predictor of the benefits that they offer.

Choice for high fecundity or fertility

In many animals, though less dramatically so in most birds and mammals, females continue to grow after reaching sexual maturity and become capable of producing larger numbers of progeny, or more viable progeny, as their body size increases. Male choice for larger, more fecund females has been described for the isopod *Asellus aquaticus* (Manning, 1975), the mormon cricket (*Anabrus simplex*) (Gwynne, 1981), and the mottled sculpin (*Cottus bairdi*) (Downhower & Brown, 1981). Males of the checkered white butterfly (*Pieris protodice*) exhibit choice on two criteria, preferring larger females and those that are young and, therefore, more likely to be virgins (Rutowski, 1982).

Female choice for males with high fertility may operate quite simply by females responding selectively to those males that court them most vigorously, provided that a male's display rate is correlated with his sperm supply (Halliday, 1978b). Such a correlation has been shown for smooth newts (*Triturus vulgaris*) (Halliday, 1976, 1978a) and for checkered white butterflies (Rutowski, 1979). Female newts, having responded positively to a male's display, also favour the most fertile males by being more likely to pick up each successive spermatophore that a male deposits (see below). In *Drosophila melanogaster*, yellow mutant males show lower courtship rates than normal males and, as a result, have reduced success in fertilising normal females (Bastock, 1956).

Choice for immediate gains and parental abilities

In a variety of species, males give females a gift of food as a necessary prelude to mating. Courtship feeding has been studied in the hanging fly, *Hylobittacus apicalis*, by Thornhill (1976, 1980). Females tend to accept only those males carrying insect prey larger than a certain size. Thornhill suggests that females may benefit from such a preference in three possible ways. First, since large insects take longer to eat and since the male mates while the female eats, large meals lead to longer copulations which, in turn, lead to accelerated oviposition. Secondly, the more food females get from males, the less they have to find for themselves and the lower the risk they run of being caught in a spider's web when searching for food. Thirdly, Thornhill has argued that males that bring large prey to females may be genetically of higher quality. However, the first two, immediate benefits are so substantial that the third, rather tenuous hypothesis seems to be redundant.

Among birds, food given to the female by the male during courtship may make an important contribution to her reproductive success, although it may fulfil other functions, such as strengthening of the pair bond and appeasement of the female (Smith, 1980). Nisbet (1977) has shown that food provided during courtship feeding by male common terns (*Sterna hirundo*) contributes to a female's fecundity, and there is some evidence that females do not associate for long with males who feed them at a low rate (Nisbet, 1973). In the red-billed gull (*Larus novaehollandiae scopulinus*), females who are well fed by their males during one breeding season tend to remain with them in the next, whereas those which are inadequately fed seek new mates (Tasker & Mills, 1981).

In species in which males carry out some or all of the parental care of the young, females may choose males on the basis of their capacity to do so. Female mottled sculpins prefer larger males, who are more effective egg guardians, partly because they are less often absent from their nest than small males (Brown, 1981). Ridley & Rechten (1981) have shown that female sticklebacks (*Gasterosteus aculeatus*) are more likely to lay their eggs in male nests that already contain eggs than in empty nests. One of the advantages of this preference may be a simple dilution effect; the more eggs there are in a nest, the lower the chance that any one batch will be eaten by a conspecific or heterospecific predator. Another possible advantage relates to the fact that males keep other fish away from their nests more assiduously during the parental phase than during the courtship phase. Females who lay their eggs in full nests are more likely to be mating with a male who will soon enter the parental phase. Nisbet (1973) presents evidence that female common terns (*Sterna hirundo*) choose their mates on the basis of the quantity of fish brought to them by males during courtship feeding, using this as a predictor of their performance when later they feed the young. A male's courtship feeding performance is positively correlated with the total weight of the clutch that he subsequently fathers and cares for. Petrie (this volume) suggests that female moorhen (*Gallinula chloropus*) choose small fat males, who make the most effective incubators of eggs.

Choice for resources and for high male status

Where one sex holds resources that make an important contribution to the reproductive success of a mating pair, individuals of the other sex are expected to show preferences based on the quality of the resources held by prospective mates (Davies, 1978). Females of the wrasse, *Pseudolabrus celidotus*, show a tendency to choose males with territories in deeper water, where their eggs are most safe from predators (Jones, 1981). Female green frogs (*Rana clamitans*) choose those male territories that contain dense vegetation in which to lay their eggs (Wells, 1977). Female bullfrogs (*Rana catesbeiana*) choose those males that hold territories whose water temperature ensures an optimum rate of egg development and in which predatory leeches are scarce (Howard, 1978). Female lark buntings (*Calamospiza melanocorys*) choose males holding territories in which there is good cover, ensuring that their eggs will be shaded from the sun (Pleszczynska, 1978). In the polygamous long-billed marsh wren (*Telmatodytes palustris*), the number of females that a male attracts is influenced by the amount of food available in his territory (Verner & Engelsen, 1970). Lenington (1980) reports that female red-winged blackbirds (*Agelaius phoeniceus*) choose males holding territories on which the number of young fledged per nest is highest. However, predation rates on preferred territories are such that females choosing them do not have the highest reproductive success.

In species in which males establish dominance relationships with one another, it may be to a female's benefit to mate preferentially with a male of high status. The advantage she gains may be immediate, in terms of being able to mate without interruption by other males, or longer-term, if her progeny benefit from their father's high status through greater paternal care and protection. There may also be a genetic advantage, provided that an animal's ability to assume high status has some genetic basis.

In cockroaches (*Nauphoeta cinerea*), dominant males mate more often than expected on a random basis than subordinate males (Breed, Smith & Gall, 1980). This is partly due to the fact that dominant males are more active, and therefore encounter females more frequently, but is also attributable to females being able to discriminate between dominant and subordinate males on the basis of their odour.

Among primates, there is considerable variation, within and between species, in the extent to which high-ranking males obtain a majority of matings (Bernstein, 1976). One reason why dominant males may obtain fewer matings than expected is that females may develop preferences for particular, sub-dominant individuals (e.g. Packer, 1979). The importance of male dominance as a determinant of reproductive success in primates has probably been overemphasised (Hausfater, 1975). Bernstein (1976) suggests that what may be important in many primates is not the immediate choice that a female makes when she mates, but the establishment of long-term alliances between males and females which promote the survival of immature animals.

Choice for mate complementarity

The reproductive success of a mating pair may be affected not only by their various qualities as individuals, but also by the extent to which their genotypes and their capacities to expend reproductive effort, especially in parental care, complement one another.

An example of mate choice for genetic complementarity is provided by the assortative mating among ecotypes of the three-spined stickleback (*Gasterosteus aculeatus*) in Canada (Hay & McPhail, 1975). There are two forms; one is exclusively freshwater, the other is andaromous and lives mostly in the sea but returns to freshwater to breed. In choice experiments, 62% of females chose a male of their own type. Offspring of parents belonging to different ecotypes will be less well adapted to either habitat than pure-bred offspring.

Another aspect of genetic complementarity between mates is the degree of relatedness between them (Bateson, this volume; Partridge, this volume). Female chimpanzees tend to associate closely with their siblings until their first oestrus, when they abruptly start to avoid them (Pusey, 1980). At this time females commonly move to other groups, either permanently or temporarily, apparently attracted to unfamiliar males. Differential dispersal from their natal area by male and female birds tends to reduce the incidence of matings with close kin (Greenwood, Harvey & Perrins, 1978; Greenwood, 1980).

While it is generally argued that it will be adaptive for animals to avoid inbreeding, because of its harmful genetic consequences, some authors have suggested that it may be advantageous to mate with kin of a certain degree of relatedness (Bateson, 1980; Shields, 1983). While a cost of inbreeding is that it leads to a high level of homozygosity, and consequent expression of deleterious recessive alleles, a benefit is that it means that favourable gene combinations tend to be preserved. Bateson (1980) has argued for a mechanism ensuring an optimum level of breeding in Japanese Quail (*Coturnix coturnix*), which tend to avoid mating with very familiar individuals, who are likely to be siblings, but prefer birds similar to those with which they are reared to totally unfamiliar individuals. These preferred birds are likely to be kin with a coefficient of relatedness less than that of siblings (Bateson, 1982).

Complementarity in the reproductive behaviour of paired animals is especially important in species in which the pair bond is maintained over several breeding seasons. In Kittiwakes (*Rissa tridactyla*), pairs that stay together tend to show enhanced reproductive success as a result of their accumulated breeding experience. However, if a newly-formed pair have low breeding success, they tend to split up and seek new mates (Coulson, 1966).

Choice for good physical condition

Whereas it may clearly be to the benefit of females to mate with males possessing 'good' genes, the criterion for such choice could never be the genes themselves, but would have to be some phenotypic expression of them. This expression might be in the form of general physical well-being (see Williams, this volume).

The question of whether animals can choose their mates on the basis of the quality of their genotypes is the most controversial issue in the mate choice literature. Two, very different problems are involved. The first concerns how animals might detect variations in the genetic quality of potential mates. The second is the more basic question of the heritability of fitness; to what extent are variations in fitness passed on to progeny? This second question is beyond the scope of this chapter but is discussed by Partridge elsewhere in this volume.

A point which I have alluded to in a number of the examples I have discussed earlier is that it is often not necessary to invoke a good gene argument to explain the adaptive value of mate choice. Where choice is directed towards short-term gains, such as resources, parental ability or fecundity, the benefits gained by animals that choose well may be so substantial that it is irrelevant whether or not the attributes chosen have a genetic basis that can be passed on to progeny.

Another important point is that mechanisms of mate choice will generally involve costs, as well as benefits. For a female to discriminate between males on the basis of their genotypes may be such a costly process, in terms of time spent or exposure to risks, that she may do better to choose a male at random. As discussed below, the pay-off from mating reliably with a member of the correct species may be much greater than that to be gained by discriminating between conspecifics (Gerhardt, 1982).

The handicap principle (Zahavi, 1975) proposes a mechanism by which females may detect the fitness of males. This theory has been much criticised (Maynard-Smith, 1976; Davis & O'Donald, 1976; Halliday, 1978b) and, if the handicap principle can work at all, it is probably only under certain, very limited conditions (Bell, 1978). A crucial point about the handicap principle is that it expressly discounts a basic function of male courtship displays, that they stimulate females, and that males will vary in their ability to attract females. If this effect is accepted, then it would seem that the logic of Fisher's (1930) 'sexy son' hypothesis is irrefutable and the handicap argument becomes redundant.

In conclusion, the concept of mate choice for good genes is fraught with problems and must be regarded as an open question. Perhaps the only instances where it is tenable, on the basis of existing studies, are those where there is evidence that females choose older males, whose ability to survive may have a heritable basis.

Choice for the most effective courtship displays

If males vary in the vigour of their sexual displays, then, assuming that the effect of such displays is to increase female sexual motivation, females will be more likely to mate with the most vigorous males. Whether one chooses to interpret such an effect in terms of female choice or as a function of female motivation is a moot point, whose resolution depends on whether there is good reason to believe that the vigour of a male's display is a correlate of some measure of male quality, other than his fertility (see above). At present, there seems to be no convincing demonstration that this is so.

Given a choice of red and non-red males, female Three-spined Sticklebacks (*Gasterosteus aculeatus*) from Lake Wapato, Washington, show a significant preference for the rarer red form (Semler, 1971). This appears to be because red males are sexually more stimulating. However, the rarity of the red morph in this population (only 14% of males are red) suggests that it is at a severe selective disadvantage, probably through predation by trout. Male Pacific Treefrogs (*Hyla regilla*) form choruses which call in bouts, separated by silent periods (Whitney & Krebs, 1975). Females tend to pair with those males, called bout leaders, who call for longer, louder and at a faster rate than others in a chorus. Whitney & Krebs could find no convincing reason for believing that bout leaders are of higher quality than other males and suggest that, because they usually begin and end bouts of calling, and therefore call for some time on their own, they are easier for females to locate. Locatability of males has also been suggested as the basis of discrimination among males by female frogs (*Physalaemus pustulosus*), who are more likely to be attracted to males producing complex calls than to those producing simpler ones (Ryan, 1980).

Female choice for the most effective male displays provides the basis of Darwin's theory of intersexual selection, in which it is argued that selection will favour those characters that make males more attractive to females. Such characters, often referred to as epigamic characters, include such morphological features as elaborate plumage and bright colours, as well as courtship displays. The evidence that females choose those males with the most highly developed epigamic characters is virtually non-existent, though Williams (this volume) has shown that female Mallard (*Anas platyrhynchos*) choose males with bright plumage. In fact, as discussed below, there is good reason to be sceptical about the role of female choice in the evolution of a number of male characters that are widely assumed to be epigamic.

Mate choice and mating competition

Darwin (1871) made a clear distinction between intrasexual selection, in which members of one sex compete directly with one another for mating opportunities, and intersexual selection, in which mating success depends on an individual's ability to attract members of the opposite sex. Whereas intrasexual selection has been widely accepted as the evolutionary process that has led to such male characters as large size, horns and antlers, intersexual selection has been the subject of considerable debate (Halliday, 1978*b*). The principal issue has been the concept that females may mate preferentially with certain males, simply because they find those males more attractive. Such apparently arbitrary, even whimsical, behaviour is in sharp contrast to the intensely utilitarian emphasis of the theory of natural selection. The question of what adaptive benefit females may gain by choosing certain males rather than others has been discussed above. In this section I wish to question the utility of the dichotomy between intrasexual and intersexual selection.

The mating rookeries of Elephant Seals (*Mirounga angustirostris*) have been described as an expression of 'rampant machismo'. Elephant seals provide one of the clearest examples of the behavioural basis and the evolutionary consequences of intense intrasexual selection. However, studies by Cox & Le Boeuf (1977) and Cox (1981) have shown that, despite the prevalence of male aggression, female elephant seals can exercise effective choice of mates. Females frequently protest when mounted by males, and are more likely to do so if a male attempting to mount them is of low status. The effect of a female's protests is to attract the attention of another male, who attacks the mounting male and makes it impossible for him to mate successfully. In effect, female elephant seals exercise choice in favour of high-status males. What this example shows is that intense competition among members of one sex does not preclude the expression of mate choice by the other sex.

It is also possible for mate choice and mating competition to be important behaviour within the same sex. Although this possibility has not expressly been discounted, there is a temptation to regard female choice and inter-male competition as alternative processes leading to variation in male mating success. The degree to which both processes will occur in the same sex will depend largely on the extent to which members of one sex show a 'consensus' in terms of their choice of mates. A high level of consensus describes the situation in which all or most individuals of one sex choose the same individual, or a limited number of individuals, of the opposite sex. If it is not possible, or not adaptive, because of the dynamics of the particular mating system, for there to be a high level of polygamy, then members of the choosing sex may have to compete with one another in order to exercise their choice. Such behaviour may be called competitive mate choice (Altmann, Wagner & Lenington, 1977). In lek species, where male parental effort is limited to fertilising eggs, there may be little or no limit on an individual male's capacity to fertilise many females. Consequently, females will not incur significant costs if they all choose and mate with the same male. Conversely, in polygynous systems in which males hold important resources, a male's capacity to apportion parental effort to the offspring of a particular female will be reduced in proportion to the number of females that he acquires. Thus, we would expect females to compete with one another for exclusive access to the resources held by a male.

A number of studies provide evidence for competitive female choice. In Red-winged Blackbirds (*Agelaius phoeniceus*), those male territories most preferred by females, assessed in terms of the order in which females moved into them, do not contain the largest harems (Lenington, 1980). This appears to be due to resident females actively excluding those females that arrive later. Male Mormon Crickets (*Anabrus simplex*) produce large spermatophores that are rich in proteins (Gwynne, 1981). These proteins are eaten by females after mating and make an important contribution to females' reproductive effort. Females compete with one another for access to males, who call from elevated vegetation. Female Moorhens (*Gallinula chloropus*) frequently fight with one another, sometimes for males. The heaviest females tend to be most successful in fighting and also tend to pair with those males who are in the best condition, defined in terms of weight of fat reserves per unit body weight (Petrie, this volume). The small, fat males apparently chosen by females are probably the most effective at incubating eggs, a predominantly male activity, because of the reduced time that they will have to devote to foraging for food.

The conditions that favour competitive female choice may also make it possible for males to exercise mate choice. A female Mormon Cricket who successfully competes for access to the plant stem on which a male is calling does not necessarily mate with him. Males reject all but the largest, most fecund females (Gwynne, 1981). Female Mottled Sculpins (*Cottus bairdi*) can increase their reproductive success significantly by mating preferentially with larger males, who are more effective guardians of eggs than small males (Brown, 1981). As a result of female choice for larger males, there is high variance in male mating success, with the largest males receiving as many as thirteen egg clumps. However, the advantage that a female gains by choosing a large male can be entirely lost if she is the last female to mate with him, since last egg masses have very low hatching success. The pressure to avoid spawning late has resulted in highly synchronised spawning among females (Downhower & Brown, 1981). This commonly results in more than one female approaching a male's burrow at the same time. In this situation, a male will generally court the largest, most fecund female rather than smaller ones.

The extent to which only one sex exercises mate choice, or whether both sexes choose, is likely to depend on the extent to which they make comparable investment in parental care. When both sexes make substantial parental investment, the reproductive success of each will depend on the quality of parental care performed by their partner. We would thus expect both partners to exercise choice. As the ratio of male to female parental investment departs from unity, mate choice should increasingly be more apparent in the behaviour of the higher-investing sex. This is a corollary of Trivers' (1972) principle that the intensity of competition within one sex depends on the extent to which it invests in parental care; mating competition should be most intense in the lower-investing sex.

What these examples show is that mate choice and mating competition are not alternative ways by which variance in mating success may come about. Within the mating system of a species, there may be competition among one sex and choice among the other, as in Elephant Seals, or choice and competition within the same sex, as in female Red-winged Blackbirds, Mormon Crickets and Moorhens, or both choice and competition may occur, to varying degrees, in both sexes, as in Mottled Sculpins.

That intrasexual and intersexual selection may be acting together in various ways within a single mating system does not invalidate Darwin's original dichotomy. These two concepts have considerable heuristic value in the analysis of the selection pressures that have produced sexually dimorphic characters. However, we should be extremely cautious about attributing any single character exclusively to one or other form of sexual selection. More important to the theme of this chapter, attempts to demonstrate the occurrence of mate choice within a particular mating system may be made much more difficult by the simultaneous involvement of some form of mating competition.

Some classic epigamic characters revisited

Throughout the literature on evolution in general and on sexual selection in particular, it is commonplace for the results of intersexual selection to be exemplified by the peacock, birds of paradise and the ruff. The evidence that females actually choose their mates in these species is slight or non-existent. Indeed, some recent studies suggest that elaborate male plumage in these birds may be the evolutionary consequence of inter-male competition rather than female choice.

The mating system of birds of paradise has been investigated by Le Croy and co-workers (Le Croy, Kulupi & Peckover, 1980; Le Croy, 1981). In *Paradisaea decora*, only some males have elaborate plumes. Mating occurs in a small area, akin to a lek, consisting of a small group of tall trees. Each tree is occupied by two plumed males who are visited frequently by other plumed and unplumed males. The resident males display to one another, perform loud, duetting songs, and chase other males away. When the female visits a tree, the resident pair of males switch to performing silent displays to her. At this stage, any plumed males in the tree start to leave, though unplumed males remain. The display sequence reaches its peak when one of the resident pair of males moves aside, leaving his partner to display alone. The attending unplumed males then all copulate briefly with the female before the remaining plumed male starts a prolonged bout of copulation with her. Le Croy found no evidence that the identity of the males that females mated with was the result of any choice exerted by them. Within a tree, the same male performed all the final copulations that occurred, and was clearly dominant over his resident partner and over other males that visited the tree. The male dominance hierarchy is the result of display interactions between males that occur throughout the year.

These observations of the sexual behaviour of birds of paradise do not entirely preclude a role for female choice in the evolution of the males' elaborate plumage. Visual displays appear to be important in the sexual stimulation of the females, although male vocal displays are probably more important in the initial attraction of females to display trees. However, since the same display structures are used in interactions with other males, as well as with females, and since mating success seems to be determined primarily by male competition, it is most likely that the plumes of birds of paradise are more the result of intrasexual than of intersexual selection.

It may be a feature of many lekking species that male competition is more important than female choice in determining male mating success (but see Bradbury & Gibson, this volume). This will be true where female choice is directed towards males holding particular territories, usually central ones, and where possession of those territories is the product of male competition. There is evidence from studies of manakins (Lill, 1974), sage grouse (Wiley, 1973) and Uganda kob (Buechner & Schloeth, 1965) that females choose particular positions in leks rather than particular males. Leks typically occur in traditional sites, and it may be that, by choosing arbitrary positions, such as the centre, within a lek females force males to compete for those positions so that they can then mate selectively with the most competitive males (Davies, 1978).

For the European Ruff (*Philomachus pugnax*) interactions between males are a major factor in determining the distribution of matings among the males on a lek. Males of the dark morph establish territories by fighting and displaying to one another, but show varying degrees of tolerance to intrusions by the pale, non-aggressive satellite males (van Rhijn, 1973). The presence of satellites on a resident male's territory increases the number of females that visit him, but tends to reduce his copulation frequency. There is thus a trade-off between the costs and benefits of being tolerant to satellites and, when the rate of female visits is high, resident males tend to be more aggressive towards satellite males (van Rhijn, 1973). Shepard (1975) suggests that the mating choices shown by female ruff are based on some combination of three factors. Females exhibit choice for central territories, for males who display at a high rate, and for territories that contain satellite males. Only one of these factors, male display rate, directly involves female choice for a male characteristic. The other two, central position and presence of satellites, are products of inter-male competition.

Moyles & Boag (1981) have investigated how males establish territories within a lek in the Sharp-tailed Grouse (*Pedioecetus phasianellus*). Males are present at a lek for the greater part of the year and for much of that time no females are present. Male mortality is high and, as territories fall vacant, individual males tend to move centripetally into them. This process involves male displays and some fighting, and males in adult plumage have a competitive advantage over immature males. Clearly, direct competition between males is a major component of lekking behaviour.

In the Black Grouse (*Lyrurus tetrix*), females show a strong tendency to choose males holding central territories but, within the central group of territories, males who court in particularly attractive ways achieve high mating success (Kruijt & Hogan, 1967). The ability to adopt successful courtship 'tactics' appears to be dependent on experience, and older males are more successful than younger ones.

The evolutionary pressures that brought about the peacock's tail are something of a mystery because no field studies have been made of peacocks (Ridley, 1981). However, Davison (1981) has studied a related, and equally striking species, the Argus Pheasant (*Argusianus argus*) in its forest habitat. Some males hold display sites which they largely clear of foliage; other adult and sub-adult males are non-territorial and move around widely. Davison found no evidence that females sample several males and exercise choice on the basis of their plumage, but suggests that they only mate with males that hold territories.

The tail of an argus pheasant takes several years to become fully developed. Its length and the number of ocelli on it are thus an indicator of a male's age (Davison, 1981). The same is true of male Lyrebirds (*Menura superba*), whose tails do not reach full development until they are seven or eight years old (Smith, 1965). In species in which a male's only contribution is his sperm, it can be argued that females will benefit by mating with older males, since they have a proven capacity to survive which, if it has a genetic basis, may be passed on to their progeny (Halliday, 1978b). The degree of development of male epigamic characters may, in species in which they take a long time to grow, be used by females as a means of identifying older males. This hypothesis is not incompatible with that which suggests that the better-developed adornments of older males are more effective at stimulating females (Ridley, 1981). However, the fact that, in argus pheasants, it is older, fully-plumed males who hold display territories suggests that male plumage development may be an important factor in competition between males.

Such field studies as have been carried out on species in which the evolution of elaborate male plumage has classically been attributed to female choice clearly cast doubt on that assumption. Not only is there no evidence that females sample several males in a way that intersexual selection theory would predict, but there is considerable evidence that the distribution of matings among males is largely determined by inter-male competition. Where female choice has been described, it plays an ancillary, and probably less significant, role than competition between males. Thus, the conclusion is the same as in the previous section; we must be very cautious about how the distinction between intrasexual and intersexual selection is used.

Modelling mate choice

In setting out to investigate mate choice it may be helpful to detach oneself from the detailed analysis of how animals actually behave to consider how they might be expected to behave. This can be done by a modelling approach, in which one first defines the problems faced by an animal that has to choose a mate and then seeks the optimal solution to those problems. This kind of approach is discussed elsewhere in this volume by Wittenberger.

Janetos (1980) has developed a series of simple models of female choice. Among the female strategies that Janetos considers are:

(i) Mating with a random male.

(ii) Mating only with a male whose quality exceeds a pre-determined threshold value. A variant of this model allows a female to mate with a sub-threshold male if she has failed to meet one who exceeds her criterion within a certain time period.

(iii) A one-step decision process, in which females initially have a high criterion which is gradually relaxed as they run out of time.

(iv) Sampling n males and mating with the best of them. This is the only model in which females return to a male that they have met earlier.

Of these models, random mating yields the worst return to females, in terms of the fitness of their mates. The best of n males model gives the highest return, followed by the one-step decision model, followed by the fixed threshold model (Fig. 1.1). This is true whatever assumption is made about the shape of the male fitness distribution curve.

Fig. 1.1. The average expected fitness (E(W)) of males chosen by hypothetical females employing different choice strategies, as a function of n, the number of males sampled. From Janetos (1980).

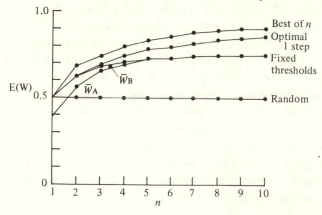

The validity of the predictions of such models depends on the extent to which the models' assumptions are an accurate reflection of the natural situation. All the models assume that females mate only once, which is not true of many species, and that a male's fitness is not reduced as he accumulates matings, which will generally not be true in mating systems based on male defence of resources. It is also assumed that males are essentially passive, being randomly distributed in space and not interacting with one another in ways that influence their chances of mating. As emphasised earlier, mating competition is a widespread phenomenon which cannot be separated from mate choice in a simple way. Janetos counters this objection, not very convincingly, by asserting that female behaviour should be adapted to neutralise the effects of male competition.

Despite the fact that such assumptions are probably not appropriate to many natural situations, Janetos' approach has considerable value. As with many biological models, it forces one to be explicit about assumptions and mechanisms. For example, Janetos lists three constraints on a female's behaviour; time, mobility and memory. Time and mobility affect a female's ability to sample large numbers of males. The best of n model can only be effective if females accurately remember the characteristics of males they have sampled. This model, which yields the best results from a female's point of view, also requires that females have a lot of time and the opportunity to return to any male that they have sampled. Such conditions are probably rather rare in natural mating systems.

An important result that emerges from Janetos' study is that, as shown in Fig. 1.1, all models, except random mating, produce negatively accelerating curves as the number of males sampled by a female increases. In other words, the more males a female has sampled, the smaller is the expected pay-off from sampling one more male. Thus, whatever system of choice females employ, they need only sample a few males to ensure that they mate with a male whose fitness is well above average.

The value of Janetos' modelling approach is not that it provides models that can be directly applied to living species. Its assumptions are such that natural situations will, at best, only approximate to those envisaged in the models. What is of value is the emphasis on identifying constraints on female behaviour. In most mating systems, females are constrained in a variety of ways and, as a result, only certain kinds of choice will be open to them. However, these models suggest that very simple forms of female choice can yield large benefits to females, and that the ability to obtain good quality mates does not necessarily require females to have unrealistically high perceptual capacities.

Perhaps the most important conclusion to emerge from Janetos' models is that females obtain fitter mates if they assess on a relative, as opposed to an absolute, criterion. A relative criterion appears to be used by female mottled sculpins (*Cottus bairdi*) (Brown, 1981). The observed pairing behaviour of females fits very closely that predicted by a model in which each female samples a series of males and pairs with the first who is larger than the last one she met. The larger a male, the more effectively he defends eggs.

Demonstrating mate choice – some methodological problems

In this section I discuss a number of factors which may make the collection and interpretation of data on mate choice difficult. All the examples I use are of choice exercised by females.

(1) *Mate choice may assume a very subtle form*

In a majority of animals, males adopt the more active role in courtship and have a repertoire of ritualised, often very conspicuous displays. This makes the collection of data on male behaviour a relatively simple matter, and variations in male sexual responsiveness can usually be easily detected and quantified. By contrast, female courtship behaviour is often not in the form of stereotyped displays, but simply involves the adoption or non-adoption of receptive postures or movements. When a female is courted by more than one male at a time, she may exercise choice simply by moving towards a particular male. However, the observer may not be able to tell whether such a movement represents a positive female response, or whether she was moving in that direction for other reasons. This problem is very apparent in some species of lekking birds, where, as discussed earlier, the high mating success of certain males may be due, more to their topographical position within a lek than to any aspect of their behaviour directed towards females. A further complication is that, if a female approaches one of two males that are available to her, this may be wholly or partly due to behaviour shown towards her by that male, which may or may not be detected by the observer. This problem, as it relates to experimental studies of mate choice, is discussed by Bateson in this volume.

Variations in the behaviour of female Smooth Newts (*Triturus vulgaris*) may be interpreted as a very subtle form of mate choice. In newts, sperm is transferred by means of a spermatophore, and, in the course of a single courtship encounter, a male usually deposits a number of spermatophores on the substrate, each deposition being the culmination of a ritualised courtship sequence (Halliday, 1974). The probability with which females pick spermatophores up increases with each successive sequence (Fig. 1.2). As a result, females are more likely to be inseminated by males who put down several spermatophores during a courtship encounter than by those who produce only one or two. These variations in female newt behaviour, which satisfy the definition of mate choice given earlier, are essentially a statistical effect which only becomes apparent when many observations of newt behaviour are analysed.

(2) *Mate choice may be masked by mating competition*

As discussed in previous sections, mate choice and mating competition may both be important determinants of the distribution of matings among individuals within a particular mating system. In elephant seals, fighting between males is spectacular and has such an obvious influence on male mating success, that the variations in female behaviour towards males of different rank, described by Cox & le Boeuf (1977) might easily have been overlooked. This, and other examples of the interaction between mate choice and mating competition were discussed in a previous section.

(3) *The scope for animals to choose mates may be constrained by other factors*

The Soldier Beetle (*Chauliognathus pennsylvanicus*) tends to aggregate on certain food plants, where mating also takes place. The same food plants are used by four species of wasp, which compete aggressively with the beetles for feeding space (McClain, 1981). When no wasps are present, female soldier beetles show a tendency to pair preferentially with larger males. However, on plants where wasps are present, females show no preferences and will even pair with males before their ova have fully developed. As a result, the proportion of beetles engaged in mating is higher on plants where there are also wasps than on those where they are absent. The explanation for this effect is that wasps are less aggressive to paired beetles than to single ones, so that female beetles are probably able to feed more efficiently when paired. Thus, in the presence of wasps, female Soldier Beetles becomes less punctilious in their choice of males and thereby benefit in terms of feeding efficiency. In this example, the extent to which mate choice can be demonstrated will depend on the ecological circumstances in which observations are made.

Fig. 1.2. Variation in female response to spermatophores in the Smooth Newt (*Triturus vulgaris*). Upper figure: the proportion of spermatophores picked up in relation to their order within a courtship encounter and to the total number deposited during an encounter. Lower figure: the proportion of encounters that are successful, i.e. at least one spermatophore is picked up, in relation to the number of spermatophores deposited during an encounter. Data from Halliday (1974).

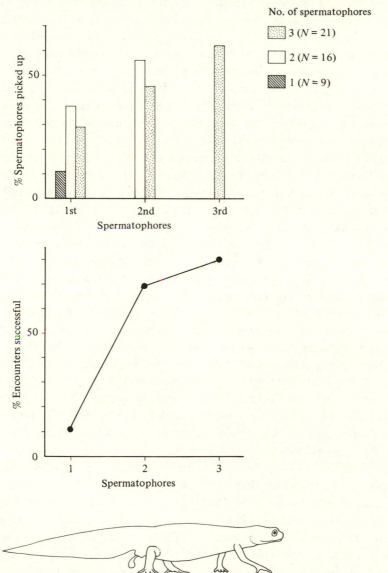

(4) *Experiments on mate choice may be based on false assumptions*

The European Newts (*Triturus*) are unusual among tailed amphibians in being highly sexually dimorphic, males bearing bright colours and pronounced dorsal crests (Halliday, 1975, 1977). Since males show no kind of direct competition (with the possible exception of one species), it seems reasonable to assume that these male characters are the result of intersexual selection. However, the usual response of a female newt when simultaneously courted by two males is to swim vigorously away (P. A. Verrell, personal communication). They appear to avoid a situation in which they might compare the appearance of different males. Variations in female response to males seem to be entirely a matter of their response to spermatophores (Fig. 1.2), not to males' obvious physical characteristics, whose significance remains enigmatic.

Gerhardt (1982) has tested the responses of female Green Treefrogs (*Hyla cinerea*) to male calls of various frequencies. In this species, as in many anurans, the low frequency peak of a male's call is negatively correlated with his body size, so that larger males produce a lower-pitched sound. The range of values for the low frequency peak in *Hyla cinerea* is 700 to 1250 Hz. Using synthetic calls, Gerhardt tested the responses of females when given a choice between a call of 900 Hz, representing the middle of the species range, and calls of higher or lower frequency. In both two-way and four-way choice experiments, females showed a clear tendency to avoid calls near either the upper or the lower end of the frequency range in favour of those of intermediate frequency. *Hyla cinerea* frequently breeds in the same ponds as two closely related species, the Barking Treefrog (*Hyla gratiosa*) and the Squirrel Treefrog (*Hyla squirella*). The low frequency peak of the male call varies between 400 and 500 Hz in *Hyla gratiosa*, and between 1000 and 1400 Hz in *Hyla squirella*. Thus, the calls of these two species fall either side, and slightly overlap with the range of *Hyla cinerea* calls. Gerhardt interprets the preference of female Green Treefrogs for male calls in the middle of the species range as an adaptation that reduces the risk of engaging in hybrid mating with males of either of the other two species that share their breeding pond.

A number of authors (Licht, 1976; Davies & Halliday, 1977; Wilbur, Rubenstein & Fairchild, 1978) have suggested that, for many female anurans, it will be adaptive to mate with the largest available males, since these will tend to be the oldest, and therefore to have proven survival capabilities. However, for Green Treefrogs such a preference would carry considerable risk of engaging in a hybrid mating. The gain that a female may derive by mating with a particular conspecific male who is of higher quality than another will be much smaller than the cost she will incur from a hybrid mating. Females appear to avoid actively those males who, on *a priori* grounds, appear to be the most desirable mates.

(5) *Mate choice may be masked or confounded by motivational effects*

The behavioural criterion that female choice has occurred will often be whether or not a female responds positively to a male's courtship behaviour. However, a female's responsiveness to males at any given moment is also a function of her sexual motivation. Thus, when a female fails to respond to a male, we can interpret this either as her rejecting him as a suitable mate, or as her having low sexual receptivity. Conversely, if a female responds positively to a male, this may not necessarily represent a positive choice from among several males, because she may be so strongly motivated that she is responding to the first male that displays to her. The following examples illustrate the complex interaction between female choice and sexual motivation.

The North American Red-spotted Newt (*Notophthalmus viridescens*) has alternative modes of courtship (Fig. 1.3) (Verrell, 1982). When a male first approaches a female, she commonly swims away; the male pursues

Fig. 1.3. Alternative forms of courtship in the Red-spotted Newt, *Notophthalmus viridescens*. The male is shown in black. Based on Verrell (1982).

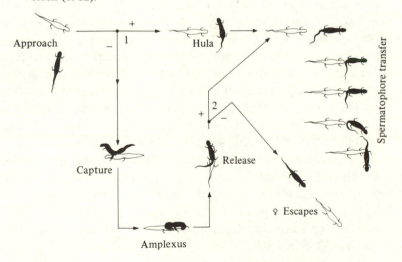

her and attempts to clasp her round the neck with his hindlimbs. If he succeeds, there follows a prolonged period of amplexus, which may last for as long as three hours, during which he stimulates the female by rubbing glands on his cheeks against her snout and by beating his tail. Amplexus ends when the male releases the female and slips in front of her. If she is responsive, she follows him, and the male initiates spermatophore transfer behaviour; if she is unresponsive, she swims away. A much quicker sequence occurs when the female is initially responsive to the male. If she does not swim away when first approached, the male performs a 'hula' display, in which he waggles his body and tail. If she then approaches him, he turns and begins the spermatophore transfer phase. This quick courtship mode, in which there is no amplexus, takes only a few minutes. In both courtship modes, the male usually deposits several spermatophores during the spermatophore transfer phase.

There are at least two points in a sequence when a female may or may not respond positively to a male (see Fig. 1.3). Point 1 is when the male first approaches her, point 2 is when the male releases her at the end of amplexus. Point 2 is only reached if her response at point 1 was negative. A third point at which a female may be regarded as exercising some sort of choice is when she picks up, or fails to pick up a spermatophore, though red-spotted newts do not show the order effect shown by smooth newts, illustrated in Fig. 1.2 (Verrell, 1982).

The fact that most females (71%) who are unresponsive when first approached by a male have become responsive after capture and amplexus, suggests that the function of the male's cheek-rubbing and tail-beating during amplexus is to raise her sexual receptivity. The corollary of this is that females who do respond positively when first approached are so highly motivated that they require no stimulation from males. If females are exercising some kind of choice, those who are initially responsive must make only a minimal assessment of a male, whereas those who go through capture and amplexus appear to have ample opportunity to assess males on the basis of their courtship. Females who escape when released by the male at the end of amplexus have either rejected them as unsuitable mates, or have not been sufficiently stimulated by male courtship.

A curious feature of this dual pattern of courtship is that those females who respond immediately to males and go through the quick courtship sequence are less likely to be inseminated than those who go through the longer, amplexus sequence. Following quick courtship, only 26.2% of spermatophores are picked up, whereas 62.2% are picked up following amplexus (Verrell, 1982).

It is important to remember that courtship behaviour fulfils a variety of functions, which Tinbergen (1953) summarised as orientation, persuasion, synchronisation and reproductive isolation. We should not allow our preoccupation with interpreting male courtship as a means by which females may assess males to lead us to ignore these other important functions. The word 'persuasion' refers to the role of displays by one partner, usually the male, in increasing the sexual motivation of the other partner. In some species, male displays play a vital role in bringing females into full reproductive condition. Female Green Anoles (*Anolis carolinensis*) will only complete their ovarian development, to the extent of producing shelled eggs, if they are exposed to sexually active males (Crews, 1980). For female Ring Doves (*Streptopelia risoria*), exposure to courting males is essential for secretion of oestrogen and progesterone to reach effective levels. Females exposed to castrated males show significantly reduced follicular size, oviduct weight and ovulation frequency, in comparison to those exposed to intact, sexually active males (Erickson & Lehrman, 1964; Erickson, 1970). In animals such as these, females may solicit courtship from several males but fail to respond positively to most of them. However, it would be misleading to infer that they have rejected them as suitable mates. Failure to respond to a male may more often be a function of a female's motivational state than of her assessment of males as suitable mating partners. While we may be able to interpret a positive female response in terms of choice for a certain male, we cannot make such an inference about negative responses.

In the pomacentrid fish *Chromis cyanea* females visit and are courted by territorial males (de Boer, 1981). It appears that when a female mates with a particular male, it is not the result of any critical aspect of his behaviour, but of the cumulative effect of all the male courtship that she has received. It seems that she must be subjected to a certain amount of courtship before she is ready to spawn. A few males, each displaying for a long time, have a comparable effect to many males, each displaying for a short time.

The same problem of interpretation arises in species in which the 'normal' sex roles are reversed and the female plays an active role in courtship. In the butterfly *Pieris protodice*, females frequently chase conspecific males and solicit matings (Rutowski, 1980). Female solicitation is shown most strongly by females who are virgins or who are carrying spermatophores that are significantly smaller than average. Thus when a female solicits a mating from a male, it appears that her behaviour is motivated by the need to maintain a good supply of sperm, not by a preference based on male quality.

In a laboratory study of sexual behaviour in Rhesus Monkeys (*Macaca mulatta*), Michael and co-workers have directly assessed the motivational state of females by means of an operant procedure (Michael & Bonsall, 1977). To gain access to a male, a female must press a lever 250 times. The time that she takes to do this is a measure of her sexual motivation and changes in a characteristic way over the course of the menstrual cycle (Fig. 1.4). Females gain access to males most quickly near mid-cycle, when ovulation occurs. Bonsall, Zumpe & Michael (1978) compared the behaviour of females working to gain access to males for whom they showed a preference, with their behaviour towards non-preferred males. Before and after the few days around ovulation, females worked considerably harder to reach preferred than non-preferred males, but this difference is less marked around ovulation (Fig. 1.4). Thus a female's preference for a particular male is much more apparent when her sexual motivation is relatively low than when it is very high.

A related complication is that females may express different choices at different times, according to their physiological state. Some days away from ovulation, a female baboon may consort·with a subordinate male, but, at the time of ovulation, she may switch her attention to a dominant male (see Keverne, this volume).

All these examples illustrate that a female's motivational state and her expression of mate choice interact in a complex way. Consequently, we

Fig. 1.4. Changes in the sexual motivation of captive female Rhesus Monkeys in an experiment in which they had to press a bar 250 times to gain access to a male. Closed circles, responses to preferred males; open circles, responses to non-preferred males. (From Bonsall *et al.* (1978). Copyright (1978) by the American Psychological Association. Reprinted by permission of the authors.)

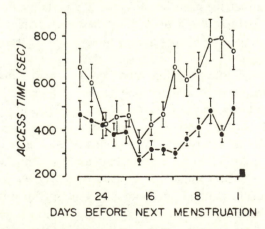

should be extremely cautious about interpreting individual positive or negative responses by females to males as expressions of mating choices. Such interpretations are only valid if we have a clear picture of the female's motivational state at the moment she makes each response.

(6) *Individuals may mate with several partners*

In some mating systems, females mate with several males, but this does not necessarily mean that they do not exercise some sort of mate choice. A female may ensure that a particular male fathers her progeny by mating exclusively with him at the point in her reproductive cycle when she is most likely to conceive, and by mating with non-preferred males at other times. Reviewing the literature on male dominance hierarchies and reproductive success in primate societies, Bernstein (1976) points out that the relationship between a male's rank and his reproductive success is often not as clear-cut as many authors have suggested. Hausfater (1975) found that, among wild baboons (*Papio cynocephalus*), high-ranking males achieved fewer, and low-ranking males more, copulations than expected on the basis of a simple priority-of-access model, which assumes that a male's ability to gain matings is solely determined by his rank. However, Hausfater's data do not permit analysis of which matings were successful in terms of conception. Such an analysis has been made in a study of captive Rhesus Monkeys by Duvall, Bernstein & Gordon (1976), who tested the paternity of offspring and found that male rank was rather a poor correlate of the distribution of successful matings. Packer (1979) has listed several factors that may lead to male mating success not being correlated with male status in olive baboons (*Papio anubis*); one of these is female choice. In many social primates, females may mate with several males, but it is quite possible that they choose the fathers of their progeny by consorting with certain males at critical times in their reproductive cycle.

The role of mate choice by females who mate with several males may be even more complex in species that show sperm competition. Sperm competition of the type described for insects by Parker (1970), in which ejaculates from different males compete for access to a female's eggs, is usually regarded as a form of inter-male competition. However, as Walker (1980) has pointed out, because the form that sperm competition takes depends on the anatomy, physiology and behaviour of females, it is important that we should consider it as an adaptive aspect of female reproductive biology. For example, it is possible that a female could use that form of sperm competition in which the last male's ejaculate has precedence over the ejaculates of previous males, to ensure that her eggs are fertilised by a male of the highest possible quality, in the following way. If she mates with the first male she meets, she can guarantee that her eggs will be fertilised. Thereafter, she can sample further males and, by mating only with males of higher quality than the first, she can maximise the quality of her progeny. Such a mechanism is entirely speculative, but it demonstrates that multiple mating by females need not imply that they do not exercise mate choice.

If females do engage in several matings, then the only reliable evidence that mate choice has occurred is that obtained by testing the paternity of their offspring. At present, data on paternity are very scarce, but, in the future, such studies may be of great importance in providing conclusive evidence for mate choice.

Summary

That animals choose their mates, as opposed to mating indiscriminately, is an attractive and evolutionarily important hypothesis. There are many different kinds of benefit that animals may derive by choosing a particular mate, ranging from the immediate gain provided by courtship feeding to the long-term advantage of mating with an individual of high genetic quality. There is abundant evidence for mate choice that yields short-term benefits, such as resources that support breeding effort. However, the evidence for long-term benefits relating to the genotype of a chosen mate is very weak, and this is an area that requires considerable theoretical and empirical investigation.

Mate choice is only one of many factors that may determine the distribution of matings among individuals in a breeding population. Most important of these is mating competition. There are strong theoretical reasons for supposing that mate choice and mating competition will often occur together and interact within a single mating system, and this view is confirmed by a number of studies.

The long-accepted role of female choice in the evolution of male epigamic characters is challenged by recent studies of certain sexually-dimorphic species, notably birds of paradise and lekking species. These studies suggest that competition between males is a more potent force in these species than female choice.

A number of methodological problems involved in the collection and interpretation of data on mate choice are discussed. Among these is the fact that other processes, notably mating competition, are at work in many mating systems. A general conclusion is that, in seeking to demonstrate mate choice, we may overlook other important biological functions of sexual behaviour, such as the role of displays in stimulating males, and in ensuring reproductive isolation. A modelling approach may facilitate the investigation of mate choice by encouraging the comparison of alternative hypotheses and a greater rigour in the formulation of assumptions about behavioural mechanisms.

I should like to thank Patrick Bateson and Paul Verrell for their comments on a draft of the chapter.

References

Altmann, S. A., Wagner, S. S. & Lenington, S. (1977). Two models for the evolution of polygyny. *Behavioural Ecology and Sociobiology*, **2**, 397–410.

Bastock, M. (1956). A gene mutation which changes a behaviour pattern. *Evolution*, **10**, 421–39.

Bateson, P. (1980). Optimal outbreeding and the development of sexual preferences in Japanese quail. *Zeitschrift für Tierpsychologie*, **53**, 231–44.

Bateson, P. (1982). Preferences for cousins in Japanese quail. *Nature*, **295**, 236–7.

Bell, G. (1978). The handicap principle in sexual selection. *Evolution*, **32**, 872–85.

Bernstein, I. S. (1976). Dominance, aggression and reproduction in primate societies. *Journal of Theoretical Biology*, **60**, 493–7.

Bonsall, R. W., Zumpe, D. & Michael, R. P. (1978). Menstrual cycle influences on operant behaviour of female rhesus monkeys. *Journal of Comparative and Physiological Psychology*, **92**, 846–55.

Breed, M. D., Smith, S. K. & Gall, B. G. (1980). Systems of mate selection in a cockroach species with male dominance hierarchies. *Animal Behaviour*, **28**, 130–4.

Brown, L. (1981). Patterns of female choice in mottled sculpins (Cottidae, Teleostei). *Animal Behaviour*, **29**, 375–82.

Buechner, H. K. & Schloeth, R. (1965). Ceremonial mating behaviour in Uganda kob (*Adenota kob thomasi* Neumann). *Zeitschrift für Tierpsychologie*, **22**, 209–25.

Coulson, J. C. (1966). The influence of the pair-bond and age on the breeding biology of the kittiwake gull *Rissa tridactyla*. *Journal of Animal Ecology*, **35**, 269–79.

Cox, C. R. (1981). Agonistic encounters among male elephant seals: frequency, context and the role of female preference. *American Zoologist*, **21**, 197–209.

Cox, C. R. & Le Boeuf, B. J. (1977). Female incitation of male competition: a mechanism of sexual selection. *American Naturalist*, **111**, 317–35.

Crews, D. (1980). Studies in squamate sexuality. *Bioscience*, **30**, 835–8.

Darwin, C. (1871). *The Descent of Man, and Selection in Relation to Sex*. John Murray: London.

Davies, N. B. (1978). Ecological questions about territorial behaviour. In *Behavioural Ecology. An Evolutionary Approach*, ed. J. R. Krebs & N. B. Davies, pp. 317–50. Blackwell Scientific Publications: Oxford.

Davies, N. B. & Halliday, T. R. (1977). Optimal mate selection in the toad *Bufo bufo*. *Nature*, **269**, 56–8.

Davis, J. W. F. & O'Donald, P. (1976). Sexual selection for a handicap, a critical analysis of Zahavi's model. *Journal of Theoretical Biology*, **57**, 345–54.

Davison, G. W. H. (1981). Sexual selection and the mating system of *Argusianus argus* (Aves: Phasianidae). *Biological Journal of the Linnean Society*, **15**, 91–104.

de Boer, B. A. (1981). Influence of population density on the territorial, courting and spawning behaviour of male *Chromis cyanea*. *Behaviour*, **77**, 99–120.

Downhower, J. F. & Brown, L. (1981). The timing of reproduction and its behavioural consequences for mottled sculpins, *Cottus bairdi*. In *Natural Selection and Social Behaviour*, ed. R. D. Alexander & D. W. Tinkle, pp. 78–95. New York: Chiron Press.

Duvall, S. W., Bernstein, I. S. & Gordon, T. P. (1976). Paternity and status in a rhesus monkey group. *Journal of Reproduction and Fertility*, **47**, 25–31.

Erickson, C. J. (1970). Induction of ovarian activity in female ring doves by androgen treatment of castrated males. *Journal of Comparative and Physiological Psychology*, **71**, 210–15.

Erickson, C. J. & Lehrman, D. S. (1964). Effect of castration of male ring doves upon ovarian activity of females. *Journal of Comparative and Physiological Psychology*, **58**, 164–6.

Fisher, R. A. (1930). *The Genetical Theory of Natural Selection*. The Clarendon Press: Oxford.

Gerhardt, H. C. (1982). Sound pattern recognition in some North American treefrogs (Anura: Hylidae): implications for mate choice. *American Zoologist*, **22**, 581–95.

Greenwood, P. J. (1980). Mating systems, philopatry and dispersal in birds and mammals. *Animal Behaviour*, **28**, 1140–62.

Greenwood, P. J., Harvey, P. H. & Perrins, C. M. (1978). Inbreeding and dispersal in the great tit. *Nature*, **271**, 52–4.

Gwynne, D. T. (1981). Sexual difference theory: mormon crickets show role reversal in mate choice. *Science*, **213**, 779–80.

Halliday, T. R. (1974). Sexual behaviour of the smooth newt, *Triturus vulgaris* (Urodela: Salamandridae). *Journal of Herpetology*, **8**, 277–92.

Halliday, T. R. (1975). On the biological significance of certain morphological characters in males of the smooth newt *Triturus vulgaris* and of the palmate newt *Triturus helveticus* (Urodela; Salamandridae). *Zoological Journal of the Linnean Society*, **56**, 291–300.

Halliday, T. R. (1976). The libidinous newt. An analysis of variations in the sexual behaviour of the male smooth newt, *Triturus vulgaris*. *Animal Behaviour*, **24**, 398–414.

Halliday, T. R. (1977). The courtship of European newts: an evolutionary perspective. In *Reproductive Biology of Amphibians*, ed. D. H. Taylor & S. I. Guttman, pp. 185–232. Plenum Press: New York.

Halliday, T. R. (1978a). The newt as an honest salesman. *Animal Behaviour*, **26**, 1273–4.

Halliday, T. R. (1978b). Sexual selection and mate choice. In *Behavioural Ecology. An Evolutionary Approach*, ed. J. R. Krebs & N. B. Davies, pp. 180–213. Blackwell Scientific Publications: Oxford.

Hausfater, G. (1975). Dominance and reproduction in baboons (*Papio cynocephalus*). *contributions in Primatology*, No. 7.

Hay, D. E. & McPhail, J. D. (1975). Mate selection in threespined sticklebacks. *Canadian Journal of Zoology*, **53**, 441–50.

Howard, R. D. (1978). The influence of male-defended oviposition sites on early embryo mortality in bullfrogs. *Ecology*, **59**, 789–98.

Janetos, A. C. (1980). Strategies of female choice: a theoretical analysis. *Behavioural Ecology and Sociobiology*, **7**, 107–12.

Jones, G. P. (1981). Spawning-site choice by female *Pseudolabrus celidotus* (Pisces: Labridae) and its influence on the mating system. *Behavioural Ecology and Sociobiology*, **8**, 129–42.

Kruijt, J. P. & Hogan, J. A. (1967). Social behaviour on the lek in black grouse, *Lyrurus tetrix tetrix*. *Ardea*, **55**, 203–40.

Le Croy, M. (1981). The genus *Paradisaea* – display and evolution. *American Museum Novitates*, No. 2714, 52 pp.

Le Croy, M., Kulupi, A. & Peckover, W. S. (1980). Goldie's bird of paradise: display, natural history and traditional relationships of people to the bird. *Wilson Bulletin*, **92**, 289–301.

Lenington, S. (1980). Female choice and polygyny in redwinged blackbirds. *Animal Behaviour*, **28**, 347–61.

Licht, L. E. (1976). Sexual selection in toads (*Bufo americanus*). *Canadian Journal of Zoology*, **54**, 1277–84.

Lill, A. (1974). Social organisation and space utilisation in the lek-forming white-bearded manakin, *M. manacus trinitatis* Hortert. *Zeitschrift für Tierpsychologie*, **36**, 513–30.

Manning, J. T. (1975). Male discrimination and investment in *Asellus aquaticus* (L.) and *A. meridianus* Racovitsza (Crustacea: Isopoda). *Behaviour*, **55**, 1–14.

Maynard Smith, J. (1976). Sexual selection and the handicap principle. *Journal of Theoretical Biology*, **57**, 239–42.

McClain, D. K. (1981). Interspecific interference competition and mate choice in the soldier beetle *Chauliognathus pennsylvanicus*. *Behavioural Ecology and Sociobiology*, **9**, 65–6.

Michael, R. P. & Bonsall, R. W. (1977). Periovulatory synchronisation of behaviour in male and female rhesus monkeys. *Nature*, **265**, 463–4.

Moyles, D. L. J. & Boag, D. A. (1981). Where, when and how male sharp-tailed grouse establish territories on arenas. *Canadian Journal of Zoology*, **59**, 1576–81.

Nisbet, I. C. T. (1973). Courtship-feeding, egg-size and breeding success in common terns. *Nature*, **241**, 141–2.

Nisbet, I. C. T. (1977). Courtship-feeding and clutch size in common terns, *Sterna hirundo*. In *Evolutionary Ecology*, ed. B. Stonehouse & C. Perrins, pp. 101–9. Macmillan: London.

Packer, C. (1979). Male dominance and reproductive activity in *Papio anubis*. *Animal Behaviour*, **27**, 37–45.

Parker, G. A. (1970). Sperm competition and its evolutionary consequences in insects. *Biological Reviews*, **45**, 525–67.

Pleszczynska, W. K. (1978). Microgeographic prediction of polygyny in the lark bunting. *Science*, **201**, 935–6.

Pusey, A. E. (1980). Inbreeding avoidance in chimpanzees. *Animal Behaviour*, **28**, 543–52.

van Rhijn, J. G. (1973). Behavioural dimorphism in male ruffs, *Philomachus pugnax* (L.). *Behaviour*, **47**, 153–229.

Ridley, M. (1981). How the peacock got his tail. *New Scientist*, **91**, 398–401.

Ridley, M. & Rechten, C. (1981). Female sticklebacks prefer to spawn with males whose nests contain eggs. *Behaviour*, **76**, 152–61.

Rutowski, R. L. (1979). The butterfly as an honest salesman. *Animal Behaviour*, **27**, 1269–70.

Rutowski, R. L. (1980). Courtship solicitation by females of the checkered white butterfly, *Pieris protodice*. *Behavioural Ecology and Sociobiology*, **7**, 113–17.

Rutowski, R. L. (1982). Epigamic selection by males as evidenced by courtship partner preferences in the checkered white butterfly (*Pieris protodice*). *Animal Behaviour*, **30**, 108–12.

Ryan, M. J. (1980). Female mate choice in a neotropical frog. *Science*, **209**, 523–5.

Ryan, M. J., Tuttle, M. D. & Taft, L. K. (1981). The costs and benefits of frog chorusing behaviour. *Behavioural Ecology and Sociobiology*, **8**, 273–8.

Semler, D. E. (1971). Some aspects of adaptation in a polymorphism for breeding colours in the threespine stickleback (*Gasterosteus aculeatus*). *Journal of Zoology, London*, **165**, 291–302.

Shepard, J. M. (1975). Factors influencing female choice in the lek mating system of the ruff. *Living Bird*, **14**, 87–111.

Shields, W. M. (1983). Optimal inbreeding and the evolution of philopatry. In *The Ecology of Animal Movement*, ed. I. R. Swingland & P. J. Greenwood, pp. 132–59. Oxford University Press: Oxford.

Smith, L. H. (1965). Changes in the tail feathers of the adolescent lyrebird. *Science*, **147**, 510–13.

Smith, S. M. (1980). Demand behaviour: a new interpretation of courtship feeding. *Condor*, **82**, 291–5.

Tasker, C. R. & Mills, J. A. (1981). A functional analysis of courtship feeding in the red-billed gull (*Larus novaehollandiae scopulinus*). *Behaviour*, **77**, 222–41.

Thornhill, R. (1976). Sexual selection and nuptial feeding behaviour in *Bittacus apicalis* (Insecta: Mecoptera). *American Naturalist*, **110**, 529–48.

Thornhill, R. (1980). Mate choice in *Hylobittacus apicalis* (Insecta: Mecoptera) and its relation to some models of female choice. *Evolution*, **34**, 519–38.

Tinbergen, N. (1953). *Social Behaviour in Animals*. Methuen: London.

Trivers, R. L. (1972). Parental investment and sexual selection. In *Sexual Selection and the Descent of Man*, ed. B. Campbell, pp. 136–79. Heinemann: London.

Verner, J. & Engelsen, G. H. (1970). Territories, multiple nest building and polygamy in the long-billed marsh wren. *The Auk*, **87**, 557–67.

Verrell, P. A. (1982). The sexual behaviour of the red-spotted newt, *Notophthalmus viridescens* (Amphibia: Urodela: Salamandridae). *Animal Behaviour*, **30**, 1224–6.

Walker, W. F. (1980). Sperm utilisation strategies in nonsocial insects. *American Naturalist*, **115**, 780–99.

Wells, K. D. (1977). Territoriality and male mating success in the green frog (*Rana clamitans*). *Ecology*, **58**, 750–62.

Whitney, C. L. & Krebs, J. R. (1975). Mate selection in Pacific tree frogs. *Nature*, **255**, 325–6.

Wilbur, H. M., Rubenstein, D. I. & Fairchild, L. (1978). Sexual selection in toads: the roles of female choice and male body size. *Evolution*, **32**, 264–70.

Wiley, R. H. (1973). Territoriality and non-random mating in the sage grouse *Centrocercus urophasianus*. *Animal Behaviour Monographs*, **6**, 87–169.

Zahavi, A. (1975). Mate selection – a selection for a handicap. *Journal of Theoretical Biology*, **53**, 205–14.

2

Monogamy: an ambiguous concept

WOLFGANG WICKLER AND UTA SEIBT

Interest in a systematic survey of animal societies dates back to the beginning of sociology in the nineteenth century, as can be seen from writings of A. Compte, A. Espinas, and H. Spencer (see Crook, 1970). A first comprehensive list of social organisation types in animals is that by the German P. Deegener (1918). Thirty years later, in November 1948, American zoologists and ethologists, aiming at a comparative sociology of all living species, founded a theoretical interdisciplinary science which they called Sociobiology (Scott, 1950). They did not refer to the earlier comparative sociologists. Another 25 years later, sociobiology started to become one of the most attractive branches in evolutionary zoology, mainly through E. O. Wilson's new synthesis (1975). Again Wilson did not refer to the earlier sociobiologists. This unfortunate lack of historical continuity in the researchers' minds, coupled with a shift of interest from descriptive sociography towards evolutionary sociobiology resulted in a double set of scientific meanings for popular words like Monogamy or Polygamy. Today it is common, although unjustified, to infer socio-biological and evolutionary conclusions from demographic descriptions, indicating that the ambiguity of concepts still goes largely unnoticed.

Three monogamy concepts

Much attention has been drawn to monogamy, for two reasons: First it had been declared Man's ideal family structure, so that any similar system in the animal kingdom was of special interest. Second, virtually all animal species are anisogamous, and since males produce a surplus of gametes, monogamy should from the standpoint of evolutionary theory be expected to be counterselected in males. This second line of reasoning treats monogamy as part of a mating system and refers to the reproductive

33

consequences, to the fitness of the monogamously mated individual. From the original comparative sociological point of view, however, monogamy refers to the social characteristics of a relationship: e.g. that two individuals spend a disproportionately large amount of time together, or share a disproportionately large amount of activities. Here, monogamy means a social unit, based on a bond between two individuals. Mixing the two concepts, social systems versus mating systems, has confused the terminology and devalues generalisations up to the present day, simply because 'mating exclusivity has genetic consequences, whereas an emotional bond (or lack of bond) does not' (Kleiman, 1977).

Both concepts are in use to define human monogamy as well. Encyclopaedia Britannica (1974) lists monogamy as a contract between two individuals, legally married to only one spouse at a time. This clearly means a social grouping; marriage is a social event, the marital stage needs acknowledgement by the society. Webster's New World Dictionary (1966) defines monogamy as the 'habit of having only one mate', thus referring to the individuals' mating (and reproductive) tactic. This tactic may be different in males and females. In a stable polygynic harem as seen in the Steppe Zebra, *Equus quagga* (Klingel, 1967), every female is monogamous, having only one mate, while the male is polygamous. If continuity over time is taken into account, the two concepts lead to contradictory statements.

In many species adult individuals are typically seen in heterosexual pairs but nevertheless change mates between breeding periods. This is sociographically described as 'successive (or serial) monogamy', a special case of monogamy. It means that an individual through time has several mates. These multiple monogamic engagements are therefore, as a reproductive strategy, called 'successive polygamy', that is a special case of polygamy. Serial monogamy is indistinguishable from successive polygyny in the classification of Wittenberger (1979); it is explicitly likened to serial polygamy by Brown (1975), here in contrast to 'simultaneous polygamy' as a social unit of more than two adults (and both sexes represented). Sociographically, 'successive polygamy' would suggest that a male changes its entire harem between breeding periods without ever forming a monogamous pair.

There are further discrepancies. Animals that are typically found as single individuals within a defended territory are classified – with respect to their social organisation – as 'solitary'. They may nevertheless exhibit a monogamous mating system, if the individuals over successive breeding periods mate exclusively with one particular partner. This is the case in several marine fish species such as the Jawfish *Opistognathus aurifrons* (Colin, 1972). True solitary reproduction is possible in hermaphrodites with self fertilization, as for example in the fishes *Rivulus marmoratus* (Harrington, 1961) and *Serranus subligarius* (Hastings & Bortone, 1980). Thus, the terms solitary, monogamous, and polygamous may indicate social units, in line with other units like peer groups, or bachelor herds; or, alternatively, they may indicate mating systems and reproductive tactics. As another inconsistency, the tactic may be ascribed to the breeding unit *or* to the individual, even by the same author: Selander (1972) describes long term monogamy as a breeding unit, 'a relationship involving one male and one female', but short term monogamy, or monobrachygamy, as an individual mating tactic, 'one individual mating with one other individual'.

Promiscuity is understood by Pianca (1978) as an idealised mating system (or rather lack of system), 'in which each organism has an equal probability of mating with every other organism', reflecting the population biologists' myth of panmixia. Brown (1975) uses 'promiscuity' for a meshed polygynous–polyandrous mating system within a multi-male–multi-female group. In addition, the term 'promiscuous' connotes a lack of discrimination in choice of partners (Selander, 1972). But selectivity is independent from the resulting social or mating system, and often it is sex specific, females generally being more selective than males in their choice of mates.

Finally, there exists a third definition of the term 'monogamy', referring to the essential competitive nature of many evolutionary aspects of mating interactions between the sexes. Verner & Willson (1966) and Orians (1969) have argued that any mating pattern will usually be more advantageous for one individual than for another. Different mating systems are understood as alternative adaptive tactics; monogamy- and polygamy-thresholds are defined with respect to habitat quality as a decisive factor. A good example is given by Pleszczynska (1978) for monogamy and polygamy in the Lark Bunting, *Calamospiza melanocorys*. Again it is individual fitness that interests. However, Gowaty (1981) elaborating on an idea from Wiley (1974), defines mating systems by 'the gametic contribution ratio, the ratio of individual males to individual females who contribute gametes to zygotes in any mating season'. Admittedly, 'this definition implies nothing about the duration or quality of the pair bond'. But it says that 'monogamy occurs when equal numbers of individual males and individual females contribute gametes to zygotes in any mating season'. Of course, this condition could be fulfilled by x males with x females, if each female is going to lay x eggs and every male fertilises one egg of every female. This would be the idealised equal probability of mating that constitutes promiscuity according to Pianca (see above). Since these definitions for promiscuity and monogamy are easily muddled, 'promiscuity, by definition, is excluded from consideration' by Gowaty.

The pair bond
Most confusions basically originate from the difficulty to ascertain gene flow from the individuals' overt behaviour, even if it lends itself to be interpreted in terms of a pair bond.

Pair bond equivalents
Similar social systems as well as mating systems may result from quite different proximate causes. Sociologists, basically interested in how and why an individual establishes relationships and integrates in social groupings, normally consider separate and independent individuals. The zoologist, however, has to take into account any equivalents of a pair bond (Wickler, 1970) that lead to preferential matings. Thus, *Diplozoon* undoubtedly is a monogamous fluke, since one male and one female are morphologically united; *Ceratias*, a deep-sea angler fish, forms polyandric units, since several small males attach and fuse histologically with a female. Some marine shrimps are forced into permanent monogamy because they are enclosed pairwise in *Euplectella* sponges (the famous Venus's flower basket). Such cases normally remain excluded from the sociologists' view, obviously because long term monogamy here results from a lack of alternatives. Sociologists and sociobiologists are interested in the individual's decision taking. Therefore, they concentrate on cases where a permanent togetherness of individuals is less self-evident. Partner fidelity is more challenging to our understanding, if more decisions by the individual are necessary to maintain the pair stability. We assume that separate unconfined individuals have more chances to part than individuals that have grown together, are encaged or otherwise mechanically hindered from changing partners – although in fact developing a strong attachment (like imprinting or falling in love) may fixate an individual to one particular partner as strongly as if they were glued together. Being bound together is, after all, yet another limit on freedom of action.

The motivational aspect

Monogamy may help to maximise fitness in various ways. Correspondingly different behaviour performances will be involved, reflecting different underlying motivational systems. Partner fidelity may be a side effect of philopatric site attachment (Fricke, 1975); whether an individual is 'mated' to its partner or to a locality shared by its partner is often difficult to decide, and both factors are not mutually exclusive (see Fernald, 1973, for the Barbet Bird *Trachyphonus d'arnaudii*, and Seibt, 1980, for the monogamous shrimp *Hymenocera*). Different 'attachment drives' have evolved convergently in different animal species, like shrimps, cichlid fish, budgerigars, or Greylag Goose (Wickler & Seibt, 1972; Wickler, 1973, 1976). Several partner-specific behaviours, each indicative of monogamous mate attachments, may be present in the same species, appearing in several different motivational connections, thus ruling out one single cause (see Trillmich, 1976, for the Budgerigar, *Melopsittacus undulatus*). And the continuity of partner fidelity through courtship, spawning, brood-care and non-breeding phases may result from different behaviour mechanisms and attachments, replacing each other in time (see Lamprecht, 1973, for the cichlid *Tilapia mariae*, and Scott, 1980, for swans).

In several bird species stable pairs are formed long before sexual maturity; there are even special moulting patterns to ensure sexual identification while the individuals are still juveniles (Nicolai, 1968). In the Bullfinch, *Pyrrhula pyrrhula*, lacking such aids, siblings of the same nest form heterosexual as well as homosexual pairs. Though pair-specific behaviour patterns (except copulation) are performed, a new mate is invariably sought sooner or later (even if the sibling pair had been heterosexual), and only then is a final monogamous relationship established (Nicolai, 1956).

These facts are mentioned here to point out the difficulties that arise from the common practice of inferring sexual mate relationships from non-copulatory social behaviour patterns.

Reference behaviour suggestive of monogamy

Monogamy as a mating system means exclusivity of copulation or of its functional equivalents. According to the evolutionary tenet of natural selection operating at the level of the individual genome (Emlen & Oring, 1977), this exclusivity basically refers to a given individual, that copulates and produces offspring with only one partner of the other sex.

Some authors call for mutual exclusivity: Monogamy is an 'exclusive relationship involving one male and one female' (Selander, 1972); 'each breeding adult is mated to one member of the opposite sex' (Brown, 1975); 'a given male and female will mate only with each other' (Kleiman, 1977). But regardless of whether or not mutual exclusivity results because both partners choose monogamy as their best tactic, be it for different reasons, the research worker has to confirm and understand each individual's own monogamy tendency beforehand.

Exclusivity in mating is normally inferred from indirect evidence rather than observed directly. Following Kleimann (1977), sources of inference are: repeated sightings or trappings of the same individuals together (suggestive for their continual close proximity), mating preferences, an absence of adult unrelated conspecifics on the pair's home range or territory, and breeding by only one adult pair in a group. The breeding pair in a group clearly is an example of monogamous mating in a non-monogamous social unit; Rothe (1975) therefore concludes that marmosets are not monogamous. All such characteristics result from preferences or degrees of exclusiveness with which particular behaviours of an individual are directed towards, or performed in the presence of, a specific other individual or a given locality; maintaining proximity is one of these behaviour patterns (Wickler, 1976). It is with absolute frequencies in mind, that Kleimann says 'monogamy does not imply anything concerning the frequency of social or sexual interactions between mates'; but it must imply relative frequency. There must be a difference in occurrence or omission of at least one behaviour pattern with respect to the pair mate relative to other conspecifics, or else the pair would not be recognisable. The often-mentioned emotional bond or attachment as a requirement for monogamy (Rothe, 1975) is a hypothetical construct (like 'drive'), to be inferred from observed behaviour. However, an individual does restrict different behaviour patterns to different individuals indicating different attachments and dependencies in a group. Thus, the reliability of deducing mating preference from other preferences depends upon the correlation between sexual behaviour and the other observed behaviour.

Again, sociography and sociobiology differ markedly with respect to the data they look for. Sociography, interested in individual groupings in a society, usually recognises and defines a pair by behaviour variables other than sexual behaviour itself. A stable pair is often quite obvious although sexual behaviour may be either not partner-restricted, or completely absent. Even with human laws in mind there is no agreement as to which behaviour has to be partner-specific for married human couples. From the sociographic point of view, social relationships and responsibilities outweigh genetics: step-children do not call for a specific family structure; and for the Roman Catholic Church godparents are deliberately equated (rather than confused) with true parents insofar as this spiritual parenthood constitutes an impediment to marriage, comparable to the parents–offspring incest taboo. But for the evolutionary and sociobiological question of how allele frequencies are connected to mating systems, monogamy is best ascertained by its outcome, that is by the degree of genetic variation in the litters of a population (where parental genes could have been spread). This can be tested by electrophoretic protein analysis, as done by Foltz (1981) for the monogamous rodent *Peromyscus polionotus*; it does not require that the parent individuals live together and build up a family unit.

Monogamy and brood care

Monogamous systems within a given animal taxon are likely to have characteristics that are side-effects rather than pre-requisites for monogamy. A typical biased deduction resulting from non-representative sampling is the widespread assumption that male-female bonding is necessary and expected in those species where both the father and the mother care for the brood (Trivers, 1972; Tinbergen, 1973), implying that biparental brood care was an important step towards monogamy: 'The phylogenetic prototype of the personal bond and of group formation is the attachment between two partners which together tend their young' (Lorenz, 1963, p. 167). Specifically, Brown (1975) argues that in mammals 'monogamy occurs mainly in the few species in which the male brings food to the female and to the young', and 'in birds, the male may be important in the care and feeding of the young, and monogamy is the general rule'; therefore, 'since parental care of the young by the male is rare in most invertebrates and lower vertebrates, monogamy is correspondingly rare' (p. 168). Maynard Smith (1978), discussing mammals and birds, states that 'in monogamous species it is common for both parents to contribute to the care of the young' (p. 183), although Kleimann (1977) in her review of mammalian monogamy points out that 'monogamy does not imply anything about the degree of paternal investment'. Finally, Wilson (1975) explicitly defines monogamy as 'the condition in which one male and one female join to rear at least a single brood' (p. 589). And this has been phrased as an evolutionary plausibility by Bischof (1980, p. 37): 'It is typical for monogamy that the male's parental investment nearly equals that of the female. This becomes unavoidable in all cases where the female alone is simply unable to rear the young. Whenever this occurs, selection operates against those males that desert their females' (our translation).

Coupling paternal brood care to monogamy, however, omits some well known facts:

(1) Chaetodonts, a large family of marine fish, typically form hetero-sexual pairs which are stable over many years (Fricke, 1973), yet exhibit neither male nor female brood care. Chaetodonts are not included in any review of vertebrate mating systems. Stable male–female pairs without paternal brood care occur in other animals as well. Evolution has proceeded toward monogamy in some cases starting from pre-copulatory mate guarding (if there is precedence of the first male's sperm; or if the female allows only one copulation), or from post-copulatory mate guarding (if through sperm displacement selection favours males that are the last to mate with any given female). This has happened already in lower animals like beetles (Mason, 1980) and Crustacea (Wickler & Seibt, 1981).

(2) If the female alone can rear only about half of each brood, selection would operate against a male that stays with his family if he had the alternative of getting two or more females and deserting each brood. From this alternative he would gain at least two half-broods without brood-care efforts. If he helps to rear one brood, he still would gain by any young he sired with other females, leaving them alone with brood care or even cuckolding their male mates. Examples are male Bank Swallows, *Riparia riparia*, that form monogamous pair bonds with females with whom they will share parental duties, but in addition go on to seek copulations with other females (Beecher & Beecher, 1979). A mammalian parallel is the Hoary Marmot, *Marmota caligata*, studied by Barash (1981).

(3) Even if males participate in caring for the brood, they will be selected to stay with the brood, not necessarily with the female. This has been shown by Lamprecht (1973) for the cichlid fish *Tilapia mariae*. In some cichlid species (*Apistogramma*, see Burchard, 1965; *Tilapia galilaea*, see Apfelbach, 1966), as well as in the Marsh Warbler, *Acrocephalus palustris*, among birds (Dowsett-Lemaire, 1979), each parent may care for part of the brood without the parents staying together.

(4) Wilson's definition of monogamy (one male and one female join to rear a brood) includes a special type of helper system. In Coke's Hartebeest, *Alcelaphus cokii*, an African antelope, a female with calf can be seen together with her sexually mature son who helps to protect her youngest calf, which is his youngest sibling (Gosling, 1969). In general, a son joining his deserted mother to rear full siblings would functionally and genetically

be equivalent to the sibling's true father and would, following Wilsons's criterion, constitute an effective mother-son monogamy, though without copulation.

Producing offspring and caring for offspring obviously are two different things, and monogamy does not generally include co-operation of two parents in rearing offspring. This has been explicitly stated already by Deegener (1918), who clearly distinguished between 'Monogamium' (as a 'connubium complex' = pairing of conspecific Metazoa) and 'monogamous patrogynopaedium' (= male–female–family, grown from a monogamium). Monogamy may be maintained through the brood-care period if the reduced success of females rearing young without male assistance is accompanied by brevity of breeding season reducing male alternatives (as in the savannah sparrow *Passerculus sandwichensis*; Weatherhead, 1979) and/or male competition over paternity (as in the desert woodlouse *Hemilepistus*; Linsenmair, 1979) and/or other factors (Wickler & Seibt, 1981).

Continuity over time

'The duration of the male–female bonding (if any) is the other key variable in describing mating systems' (Tutin, 1979). Brown (1975) distinguishes between perennial (permanent) monogamy, where mates are together even in the non-breeding season, and seasonal monogamy, where mates separate during the non-breeding season and re-pair in successive seasons, with the continuity of the pair as an identifiable social unit being the difference. For cases where the pairbond is very brief ('an hour or so at most, or absent'), Selander (1972) coined the term 'brachygamy' (monobrachygamy: an individual mating with one individual in a breeding season; polybrachygamy: an individual mating with two or more individuals in a breeding season).

Unfortunately, there is a tendency towards linear classification of mating systems, even to the extent of switching from 'continuity' to 'number of mates' as the key variable. Brown (1975, p. 152) offers an example. Next to seasonal monogamy he lists 'serial monogamy'; again there is no pair bond during the non-breeding season, but here individuals mate with different partners for successive broods or breeding seasons, though with only one at a time. This, he says, is identical to serial polygamy, and he then goes on to simultaneous polygamy and finally to promiscuity, without noticing that he has confused the *sociographic aspect of continuity* and the *sociobiological viewpoint of exclusivity*, each of which serves to define one of his extremes. For perennial monogamy 'at least some sort of loose association between sexes in the pair is maintained even in the nonbreeding season'; but in promiscuity 'no one individual has exclusive rights over any individual of the opposite sex' (p. 153). He seems unaware of the fact that recognisability of a pair as a subunit within a population, and exclusivity of mating between individuals, are two independent variables. Consequently, he misses perennial polygamy, be it one male with several females as in the Steppe Zebra, or one female with several males as in the deep-sea angler fish of the genus *Ceratias*, or several males with several females as in the African lion. None of these cases is in his list.

Duration of the individual relationship is often measured against lifetime, but usually without making a clear distinction between lifetime of the relationship and lifetime of the individual. The statement that two individuals have paired for life normally refers to their post-pubertal sexual lifetime only; 'for life' excludes the individual's lifetime prior to pair formation. A more serious difficulty is evident from Kleimann's statement that 'monogamy need not imply a lifetime relationship since, if one member of a pair dies, the remaining may develop a bond with a new conspecific individual' (1977, p. 39). One should expect that any relationship between two individuals ends if one partner dies. But, curiously enough, the pair bond is often judged against the lifetime of the surviving partner, implying that sexual fidelity or any other bonding behaviour continues beyond the partner's death. This seems to originate in anthropomorphic thinking. It is (or was) in fact a romantic wish of many human pair partners to die together, or else to be assured of the surviving partner's fidelity. Everlasting fidelity as a characteristic of ideal monogamy has explicitly been claimed for Greylag Geese by Heinroth (1911) and Lorenz (1963), though without any attempt towards a biological explanation of such continuing preference for a no-longer-existing partner. (Such a mechanism might even lead to a fixation on a never-existing 'ideal partner in mind'.)

But indeed, superfaithfulness may arise from the very real and biologically relevant problem for an individual to differentiate between reversible and irreversible mate absence. (For humans who believe in eternal life even death may constitute a reversible separation of mates). Unavoidably, pair members will have to spend part of their time separated from each other, due to alternation in parental roles, or to migratory separation of sexes between breeding seasons, etc. To be, or not to be, faithful to the absent mate and to reject, or not reject, alternative partners, is part of a time-investment strategy as outlined by Parker (1974). When an individual should stop waiting for the absent mate will follow from the same rules that Parker discussed for courtship persistence. This waiting time varies considerably between species, depending upon the partners' normal return interval, which in incubating Emperor Penguin is up to three months, but only a few minutes in brooding cichlid fish. (The temporal organisation of brood relief in fishes and birds has been discussed by Rechten, 1980.)

The individual's decision is further influenced by available alternatives: the latent pair bond survives 70 days of separation in budgerigars if partners are in unisexual groups during that time; in heterosexual groups new pairs are formed within 20 days. The pair bond increases (non-linearly) with time spent together interacting; it weakens during periods of separation (indicated by increasing probability for change of partners, and decreased selectivity for courtship feeding and beak touching). If a new pair bond is formed during long absence of the first partner, the outcome of competition between old and new partner depends upon the relative strengths of the newly-grown and the weakened old pair bond (Trillmich, 1976a). While brooding or tending young, pair bonds and parental bonds are interfering; deserting the brood may depend upon the parents' foraging efficiency (see Fisher, 1967, for the Laysan Albatross; Nelson, 1969, for Redfooted Boobies), and mate deserting may correlate with breeding failure (Coulson, 1980, and chapter 16 for Kittiwake Gulls).

The following four situations seem especially relevant with respect to partner fidelity and latent pairbond:

(1a) Partner present, but unresponsive as when sleeping or dead. (We had an Emperor Goose, *Anser canagicus*, staying for days next to its dead mate, finally with the mate's head only, after the rest of the corpse had been removed. A comparable situation is that of primate mothers which go on carrying their dead babies for many days.)

(1b) Partner present and alive, but aversive. (Unsuccessful breeding may lead to mate switching; see Coulson & Thomas, this volume.)

(2a) Partner absent, no alternative available. (A latent pair bond survives several months of non-breeding partner separation in Ring Doves (Morris & Erickson, 1971), budgerigars (Trillmich, 1976a), or Desert Woodlice (Linsenmair & Linsenmair, 1971). Persistence of memory may be the only relevant factor here.)

(2b) Partner absent, and alternative(s) available. (Common situation; decision taking is an optimisation process.) The decision to retain or to reject a former mate, and to reject or accept a new partner, may be entirely a consequence of extinction, forgetfulness or retention of memory (e.g. in the monogamous Desert Woodlouse, Linsenmair & Linsenmair, 1971). In such cases the physiology of memory may be assumed to be adapted to the normal biological situation of the species. In higher animals where memory serves several functions, the mating decision process seems to be separable from memory processes. Seemingly unadaptive faithfulness should not be idealised, but rather seen as resulting from the animal's normal behaviour performed in a rare abnormal situation.

Monogamy – a matter of degree

The term 'monogamous' has been attributed to temporal coalitions between individuals, to a single individual's life strategy, and to the typical social or mating system of a species (or population).

In either case the degree of monogamy depends on the following considerations:

(a) How long does a monogamous relationship continue with respect to an individual's lifetime? This obviously depends upon the number of reproductive cycles per lifetime. Total monogamy will automatically result if females are inseminated, or males are able to copulate only once (e.g. the male Honey Bee).

(b) How exclusive are matings with a given partner? This is influenced by the individual's reproductive lifetime, by population density, environmental polygamy potential and operational sex ratio (Emlen & Oring, 1977). Exclusivity in a single mating act definitely is enhanced through internal fertilisation, but even here may be overcome by males injecting sperm into rival males and letting them carry their own and alien sperm to a female, as is suggested for cimicid bugs (Carayon, 1964; Lloyd, 1979). Exclusivity often is sex-specific, males usually tending towards polygamy. Extramarital courtings and copulations in typically monogamous species (e.g. in Bullfinch, Zebrafinch, Treesparrow, Gulls, Cattle Egret; see Nicolai, 1956; Immelmann, 1962; Deckert, 1962; MacRoberts, 1973; Fujioka & Yamagishi, 1981, respectively) are often treated as an occasional exception from monogamy, as is bigamy (Roell, 1979), which in fact is polygamy. Kleimann's 'facultative monogamy' (1977) – when e.g. a male can only find or afford one female – might better be classified as 'one-female-harem'.

(c) What percentage of the individuals of either sex out of a given population behave monogamously? A species norm is often deduced from a majority and a divergent minority is excused (as faulty) rather than explained, although different mating systems may be appropriate to different circumstances within the same species, including mixed evolutionarily stable strategies (ESS; Maynard Smith, 1980). For humans, cultural norms, rather than the individual's (or even the majority's) behaviour, are taken to describe a population as monogamous.

In any case, too rigid a classification will depict the classifier's mind and typological thinking rather than the natural situation and is likely to lead to misleading conclusions.

Concluding suggestions and suggestive conclusions

(1) One should distinguish between monogamy as a sociographic unit, indicating the togetherness of two heterosexual individuals (with or without further details about their behavioural interactions), and monogamy as the individual's mating strategy, indicating an exclusivity in reproduction. If the two concepts are mixed, generalising statements that 'more than 90 per cent of all bird species are monogamous' (Lack, 1968), but 'less than 3 per cent of mammalian species have been reported as monogamous' (Kleimann, 1977) are (at least) difficult to interpret.

(2) Monogamy is one out of several possible types of reproductive symbioses between individuals. Each partner's costs and benefits have therefore to be judged separately; monogamy as a mating strategy refers to the individual.

(3) A monogamous social structure may result if:

  (a) monogamy is the preferable mating tactic for both partners (mutual monogamy); or

  (b) monogamy is the preferable mating tactic for one partner only and if this one is able to overcome the other's divergent tendencies (one-sided monogamy); or

  (c) secondary ecological constraints (carrying capacity, predator avoidance) call for a minimum number of adults to be present.

(4) Mutual monogamy may be based on:

  (a) Each partner's tendency to avoid a rival of its own sex. This is mutual mate monopolisation; (e.g. he monopolises her reproductive capacity, she monopolises his food-bringing capacity). In this case one will observe aggression mainly between rivals of the same sex. A harem will result if only one sex avoids rivals.

  (b) Each partner's tendency to avoid another individual of its mate's sex. This seems plausible only with respect to ecological or time- and energy-constraints (e.g. female avoiding unnecessary time investment in additional males). Fights will be expected against heterosexual strangers. Again a harem will result, if only one sex follows this tendency.

(5) Partner-restricted behaviour, if it is non-sexual, and especially parental roles, should not be used to identify mating systems (understood as procreation strategies), since living together, even of heterosexual

individuals, may have various selective consequences. Permanent monogamy in the simultaneous hermaphroditic fish *Serranus tigrinus* is an
adaptation to effective foraging in a jointly-defended territory (Pressley,
1981); two are better than one, sex being irrelevant here. With different
sex roles involved, the same may apply to monogamy in chaetodont fish.

(6) Partner fidelity comprises two different and independent aspects:

(a) the *duration* of a relationship, neglecting the number of individuals
involved (fidelity may matter even in a harem); and

(b) the *exclusivity* of a relationship, that is the number of partners,
neglecting the duration.

(7) Studying widely different species is the only way to sort out the
essential factors underlying monogamy (or any other mating system) and
to assess their relative importance in a given case. Basic principles become
evident from convergencies rather than from homologies. For instance, in
species with pre-copulatory male investment and a male potential to
increase offspring survival by paternal brood care, concealed ovulation in
the female will increase the male's tendency to stay with that female to
ensure his paternity. This has been discussed to explain human monogamy
and the human female's concealed ovulation, that is unique among
primates (Linton, 1936; Benshoof & Thornhill, 1979). But it is not unique
to humans (as Alexander suggests, 1979); the same factor combination,
including concealed ovulation, occurs again in the monogamous family
system of the Desert Wood Louse *Hemilepistus* (Linsenmair, 1979).
Comparisons wih other Isopoda in the case of the Wood Louse, and among
different human populations in case of Man, strongly suggest that a key
factor in both systems seems to be the necessary division of labour by sex
in food getting activities (see Wickler & Seibt, 1981).

Summary

The term 'monogamy' is used in different ways. First, sociologists
use it to describe the togetherness and co-operation of two heterosexual
adults as a social unit. Secondly, evolutionary biologists and sociobiologists
used it to describe a mating tactic of the individual (which reproduces
sexually with only one partner of the opposite sex). Finally, population
geneticists use it to describe the male/female gametic contribution ratio to
the zygotes produced in any mating season. These different monogamy
concepts are outlined and their conceptual consequences analysed. The
different concepts sometimes lead to contradictory statements and to
erroneous generalisations about *the* biological basis for monogamy.

Since the rate of evolutionary change is positively correlated with the amount of genetic variation, and the amount of hereditary variation in a population is directly proportional to the changes in allelic frequencies, and because allelic frequencies correlate with mating systems, we feel that an evolutionarily oriented monogamy concept is of particular importance and should have priority over other concepts.

We discuss the researcher's problems in ascertaining monogamy in a given species, as well as several basic factors which sometimes only collectively lead to monogamy, and also a reasonable biological origin for ongoing fidelity beyond the partner's death. We point out that biparental brood care is not a general phylogenetic prerequisite, but rather a later consequence of monogamy.

We finally offer some technical as well as conceptual suggestions for those who look for monogamy in a particular species or for important properties of monogamy in general.

References

Alexander, R. D. (1979). *Darwinism and Human Affairs*. University of Washington Press: Seattle and London.

Apfelbach, R. (1966). Maulbrüten und Paarbindung bei *Tilapia galilaea* L. *Naturwissenschaften*, **53**, 22.

Barash, D. P. (1981). Mate guarding and gallivanting by male hoary marmots (*Marmota caligata*). *Behavioral Ecology & Sociobiology*, **9**, 187–93.

Beecher, M. D. & Beecher, I. M. (1979). Sociobiology of bank swallows reproductive strategy of the male. *Science*, **205**, 1282–5.

Benshoof, L. & Thornhill, R. (1979). The evolution of monogamy and concealed ovulation in humans. *Journal of Social Biology and Structure*, **2**, 95–106.

Bischof, N. (1980). Biologie als Schicksal? In *Geschlechtsunterschiede – Entstehung und Entwicklung*, ed. N. Bischof & H. Preuschoft, pp. 25–42. C. H. Beck: München.

Brown, J. L. (1975). *The Evolution of Behaviour*. W. W. Norton & Co.: New York.

Burchard, J. E. (1965). Family structure in the Dwarf Cichlid *Apistogramma trifasciatum* Eigenmann and Kennedy. *Zeitschrift für Tierpsychologie*, **22**, 150–62.

Carayon, J. (1964). Les aberrations sexuelles 'normalisées' de certains Hémiptères Cimicoidea. In *Psychiatrie Animale*, ed. A. Brion & H. Ey, pp. 283–94. Desclée de Brouwer: Paris.

Colin, P. L. (1972). Daily activity patterns and effects of environmental conditions on the behavior of the yellowhead jawfish, *Opistognathus aurifrons*, with notes on its ecology. *Zoologica*, **57**, 137–69.

Coulson, J. C. (1980). A study of the factors influencing the duration of the pair-bond in the kittiwake gull *Rissa tridactyla*. *Acta XVII. International Congress of Ornithologists*, 823–33: Berlin.

Crook, J. H., ed. (1970). *Social Behaviour in Birds and Mammals*. Academic Press: London and New York.

Deckert, G. (1962). Zur Ethologie des Feldsperlings (*Passer m. montanus* L.). *Journal für Ornithologie*, **103**, 428–86.

Deegener, P. (1918). *Die Formen der Vergesellschaftung im Tierreiche*. Veit & Co.: Leipzig.

Dowsett-Lemaire, F. (1979). The sexual bond in the Marsh Warbler, *Acrocephalus palustris*. *Le Gerfaut*, **69**, 3–12.

Emlen, S. T. & Oring, L. W. (1977). Ecology, sexual selection, and the evolution of mating systems. *Science*, **197**, 215–23.

Fernald, R. D. (1973). A group of barbets. II. Quantitative measures. *Zeitschrift für Tierpsychologie*, **33**, 341–51.

Fisher, H. I. (1967). Body weights in Laysan albatrosses *Diomedea immutabilis*. *Ibis*, **109**, 373–82.

Foltz, D. W. (1981). Genetic evidence for long-term monogamy in a small rodent, *Peromyscus polionotus*. *American Naturalist*, **117**, 665–75.

Fricke, H. W. (1973). Behaviour as part of ecological adaptation. *Helgoländer wissenschaftliche Meeresuntersuchungen*, **24**, 120–44.

Fricke, H. W. (1975). Evolution of social systems through site attachment in fish. *Zeitschrift für Tierpsychologie*, **39**, 206–10.

Fujioka, M. & Yamagishi, S. (1981). Extramarital and pair copulations in the cattle egret. *The Auk*, **98**, 134–44.

Gosling, L. M. (1969). Parturition and related behaviour in Coke's hartebeest. *Journal of Reproduction and Fertility*, Supplement **6**, 265–86.

Gowaty, P. A. (1981). An extension of the Orians-Verner-Willson model to account for mating systems besides polygyny. *American Naturalist*, **118**, 851–9.

Harrington, R. W. jr. (1961). Oviparous hermaphroditic fish with internal self-fertilization. *Science*, **134**, 1749–50.

Hastings, P. A. & Bortone, S. A. (1980). Observations on the life history of the belted sandfish, *Serranus subligarius* (Serranidae). *Environmental Biology of Fishes*, **5**, 365–74.

Heinroth, O. (1911). Beiträge zur Biologie, namentlich Ethologie und Psychologie der Anatiden. *Report of the Vth International Ornithological Congress*, pp. 582–702. Berlin.

Immelmann, K. (1962). Beiträge zu einer vergleichenden Biologie australischer Prachtfinken (Spermestidae). *Zoologische Jahrbücher* (Systematik), **90**, 1–196.

Kleimann, D. G. (1977). Monogamy in mammals. *Quarterly Review of Biology*, **52**, 39–69.

Klingel, H. (1967). Soziale Organisation und Verhalten freilebender Steppenzebras. *Zeitschrift für Tierpsychologie*, **24**, 580–624.

Lack, D. (1968). *Ecological Adaptations for Breeding in Birds*. Methuen: London.

Lamprecht, J. (1973). Mechanismen des Paarzusammenhaltes beim Cichliden *Tilapia mariae* Boulenger 1899 (Cichlidae, Teleostei). *Zeitschrift für Tierpsychologie*, **32**, 10–61.

Linsenmair, K. E. (1979). Untersuchungen zur Soziobiologie der Wüstenassel *Hemilepistus reaumuri* und verwandter Isopodenarten (Isopoda, Oniscoidea): Paarbindung und Evolution der Monogamie. *Verhandlungen der Deutschen zoologischen Gesellschaft*, 60–72.

Linsenmair, K. E. & Linsenmair, C. (1971). Paarbildung und Paarzusammenhalt bei der monogamen Wüstenassel *Hemilepistus reaumuri* (Crustacea, Isopoda, Oniscoidea). *Zeitschrift für Tierpsychogie*, **29**, 134–55.

Linton, C. R. (1936). *The Study of Man*. Appleton-Century Crofts: New York.

Lloyd, J. E. (1979). Mating behavior and natural selection. *The Florida Entomologist*, **62**, 17–34.

Lorenz, K. (1963). *On Aggression*. Harcourt, Brace & World Inc.: New York.

MacRoberts, M. H. (1973). Extramarital courting in lesser black-backed and herring gulls. *Zeitschrift für Tierpsychologie*, **32**, 62–74.

Mason, L. G. (1980). Sexual selection and the evolution of pair-bonding in soldier beetles. *Evolution*, **34**, 174–80.

Maynard Smith, J. (1978). *The Evolution of Sex*. Cambridge University Press: Cambridge.

Maynard Smith, J. (1980). Power and limits of optimization. In *Evolution of Social*

Behavior: Hypotheses and Empirical tests, ed. H. Markl, pp. 27–34, Dahlem Konferenzen. Verlag Chemie: Weinheim.

Morris, R. L. & Erickson, C. J. (1971). Pair bond maintenance in the ring dove (*Streptopelia risoria*). *Animal Behaviour*, **19**, 398–406.

Nelson, J. B. (1969). The breeding ecology of the red-footed booby in the Galapagos. *Journal of Animal Ecology*, **38**, 181–98.

Nicolai, J. (1956). Zur Biologie und Ethologie des Gimpels. *Zeitschrift für Tierpsychologie*, **13**, 93–132.

Nicolai, J. (1968). Die isolierte Frühmauser der Farbmerkmale des Kopfgefieders bei *Uraeginthus granatinus* (L.) und *U. ianthinogaster* Reichw. *Zeitschrift für Tierpsychologie*, **25**, 854–61.

Orians, G. H. (1969). On the evolution of mating systems in birds and mammals. *American Naturalist*, **103**, 589–603.

Parker, G. A. (1974). Courtship persistence and female-guarding as male time investment strategies. *Behaviour*, **48**, 157–84.

Pianca, E. R. (1978). *Evolutionary Ecology*. Harper & Row: New York.

Pleszczynska, W. K. (1978). Microgeographic prediction of polygyny in the lark bunting. *Science*, **201**, 935–7.

Pressley, P. H. (1981). Pair formation and joint territoriality in a simultaneous hermaphrodite: the coral reef fish *Serranus tigrinus*. *Zeitschrift für Tierpsychologie*, **56**, 33–46.

Rechten, C. (1980). Brood relief behaviour of the cichlid fish *Etroplus maculatus*. *Zeitschrift für Tierpsychologie*, **52**, 77–102.

Roell, A. (1979). Bigamy in jackdaws. *Ardea*, **67**, 123–9.

Rothe, H. (1975). Some aspects of sexuality and reproduction in groups of captive marmosets (*Callithrix jacchus*). *Zeitschrift für Tierpsychologie*, **37**, 255–73.

Scott, D. K. (1980). Functional aspects of the pair bond in winter in Bewick's Swans (*Cygnus columbianus bewickii*). *Behavioral Ecology & Sociobiology*, **7**, 323–7.

Scott, J. P. (1950). Foreword. *Annals of the New York Academy of Sciences*, **51**, 1003–5.

Seibt, U. (1980). Soziometrische Analyse von Gruppen der Garnele *Hymenocera picta* Dana. *Zeitschrift für Tierpsychologie*, **52**, 321–30.

Selander, R. K. (1972). Sexual selection and dimorphisms in birds. In *Sexual Selection and the Descent of Man*, ed. B. Campbell, pp. 180–230. Heinemann: London.

Tinbergen, N. (1973). *The Animal in Its World*, vol. 2. Allen & Unwin: London.

Trillmich, F. (1976). Spatial proximity and mate-specific behaviour in a flock of budgerigars (*Melopsittacus undulatus*; Aves, Psittacidae). *Zeitschrift für Tierpsychologie*, **41**, 307–31.

Trillmich, F. (1976a). The influence of separation on the pair bond in budgerigars (*Melopsittacus undulatus*). *Zeitschrift für Tierpsychologie*, **41**, 396–408.

Trivers, R. L. (1972). Parental investment and sexual selection. In *Sexual Selection and the Descent of Man*, ed. B. Campbell, pp. 136–79. Heinemann: London.

Tutin, C. E. G. (1979). Mating patterns and reproductive strategies in a community of wild chimpanzees (*Pan troglodytes schweinfurthii*). *Behavioral Ecology & Sociobiology*, **6**, 29–38.

Verner, J. & Willson, M. L. (1966). The influence of habitats on mating systems of North American passerine birds. *Ecology*, **47**, 143–7.

Weatherhead, P. J. (1979). Ecological correlates of monogamy in tundra-breeding savannah sparrows. *Auk*, **96**, 391–401.

Wickler, W. (1970). Social behaviour as an adaptive feature. *Verhandlungen der Deutschen Zoologischen Gesellschaft*, **64**, 291–304.

Wickler, W. (1973). Ethological analysis of convergent adaptation. *Annals of the New York Academy of Sciences*, **223**, 65–9.

Wickler, W. (1976). The ethological analysis of attachment. *Zeitschrift für Tierpsychologie*, **42**, 12–28.

Wickler, W. & Seibt, U. (1972). Über den Zusammenhang des Paarsitzens mit anderen Verhaltensweisen bei *Hymenocera picta*. *Zeitschrift für Tierpsychologie*, **31**, 163–70.

Wickler, W. & Seibt, U. (1981). Monogamy in crustacea and Man. *Zeitschrift für Tierpsychologie*, **57**, 215–34.

Wiley, R. H. (1974). The evolution of social organization and life-history patterns among grouse. *Quarterly Review of Biology*, **49**, 201–27.

Wilson, E. O. (1975). *Sociobiology*. Harvard University Press: Cambridge, Mass. and London.

Wittenberger, J. F. (1979). The evolution of mating systems in birds and mammals. In *Social Behavior and Communication. Handbook of Behavioral Neurobiology*, vol. **3**, ed. P. Marler & J. G. Vendenbergh, pp. 271–349. New York: Plenum Press.

II: CHARACTERISTICS OF SEXUAL SELECTION

3

Sexual selection by female choice

PETER O'DONALD

Female choice and female preference

Darwin thought that males would compete for females and females would choose between males. By these two mechanisms of sexual selection Darwin explained the evolution of male weapons for fighting and male adornments to attract the females. It has always been accepted that sexual selection occurs when rival males fight for possession of the females. This selection will 'add to the size, strength and courage of the males, or to improve their weapons' (Darwin, 1871). Males compete for females in more subtle ways than simply by fighting for them. They may compete by holding larger or better territories or by courting the females more vigorously or persistently. The females may also prefer to mate with particular males. Male adornments may more readily elicit the mating responses of some females who will thus mate preferentially in favour of the adorned males. Female choice may thus operate in two different ways. Imagine a woman buying a hairdryer. How does she choose between the different makes and models? She may have no prior preference in favour of a particular model. Her choice may depend solely on the pressure of the salesmanship she has been subjected to: she chooses between the salesmen. Or she may already have decided what model she wants. Sales pressure may have no effect on her choice. Or both prior preference and salesmanship may influence her choice. In a similar manner, a male bird may succeed in mating by his greater ability to court the females. Or females may prefer males with particular characteristics, choosing the males they prefer regardless of how well they sell themselves. Either way, the females make the choices. But if they have prior preferences, females will differ between themselves as well as males: some females prefer one kind of male; others prefer another kind, or have no preference at all.

These two mechanisms of choice can be distinguished only by carefully controlled experiments. For example, female sticklebacks prefer to lay their eggs in the nests of red-throated males: given a choice, females are much more likely to lay their eggs in a red male's nest (Semler, 1971). Are the females turned on by the red throat, or are the red-throated males more active and assiduous in courting the females? In birds, plumage characters for sexual display are developed in the presence of the male sex hormone, testosterone, which also determines males' other sexual activities and aggressive behaviour. The more attractive and highly adorned males may also be the sexually more active and aggressive males. If red-throated male sticklebacks are more active in courting the females, they will increase their chances with all females, both those who may have a prior preference for red throats and those with no preferences. Semler (1971) used genetically red and non-red males in experiments to distinguish between the two mechanisms of female choice. He set up aquaria in which two males had built their nests on either side of a central glass partition. One of the males was red-throated, the other was not. After removing the partition, a female was placed in the aquarium. Semler noted whether she laid her eggs in the nest of the red or non-red male. The females usually chose the red male's nest. Semler then carried out a similar experiment using two non-red males in the same aquarium. But one of the males had a red throat painted on with lipstick or nail varnish. The females still chose the red male. The following table shows the numbers of females choosing red and non-red males:

	Naturally coloured males	Artificially coloured males	All males
Red males	20	18	38
Non-red males	8	7	15

Suppose a proportion α of the females express a preference for red males, while the remaining females, the proportion $1-\alpha$, mate at random. Since half of the random mating females will mate with red males together with all α of the preferring females, the red males mate at a total frequency

$$\alpha+\tfrac{1}{2}(1-\alpha) = \tfrac{1}{2}+\tfrac{1}{2}\alpha$$

The observed proportion of these matings is 38/53, showing that

$$\hat{\alpha} = 0.434$$

This is the maximum likelihood estimate of α. Semler's data are thus consistent with a model in which about 43% of females express a preference for red males (O'Donald, 1973). These females must have had a prior preference for red males, since, genetically, the artificial red males were identical to the non-red males. They differed only in the red throat. This character alone must have determined the females' preference for them.

The immediate effect of female choice is the same regardless of whether females have prior preferences or not: in polygynous species, the sexually favoured males mate more often than the others; in monogamous species, they are chosen before the others, gaining an advantage, as Darwin suggested, from the increased reproductive success of pairs that breed early in the breeding season (O'Donald, 1980a, b). But the two mechanisms of female choice may differ in their long-term effects. When females have prior preferences, the preferred males gain an advantage that must necessarily depend on their relative frequency in the population. When the preferred males are rare, they take part in a larger number of preferential matings than when they are common. Suppose, for example, that one per cent of males have the preferred phenotype, and 10% of females prefer them. The preferred males mate preferentially with a frequency of 0.1 and randomly with a frequency of 0.9×0.01, or a total frequency of 0.109. On average, therefore, each preferred male will mate with $0.109/0.01 = 10.9$, or about 11 females. When they have reached a frequency of 90% they still mate preferentially with a frequency of 0.1, but they now mate randomly with a frequency of 0.9×0.9; the total frequency of their matings is 0.91. On average, each preferred male will mate with only $0.91/0.9 = 1.01$ females. From a very great selective advantage when rare, their selective advantage has become small when common. This frequency-dependence in the selective advantage gained by preferred males has been called the 'rare male effect'. It is an inevitable consequence of preferential mating. If two different male phenotypes are preferred by different groups of females, each will gain an advantage over the other while rare. The rare phenotype will thus increase in frequency at the expense of the common phenotype. A genetic polymorphism will be maintained, for neither can be eliminated from the population. If females prefer only one of the male phenotypes, the preferred males obviously gain an advantage over the others at all frequencies, but their advantage is much greater when they are rare. Rare male effects have often been observed in experiments on mating choice (for a general review, see Ehrman, 1972; for discussion of rare male effects in *Drosophila*, see Spiess & Ehrman, 1978, and O'Donald, 1978; for fitting models of preferential mating to data of rare male effects, see O'Donald, 1980a).

When females have no prior preference and exercise their choice by responding more readily to the more active and persistent of the males competing for their attention, differences in male behaviour alone determine the operation of sexual selection. There is no inevitable frequency-dependence in the advantage the males gain. In specific models of male competition, the males' advantage may increase slightly as they increase in frequency (Charlesworth & Charlesworth, 1975). This is the reverse of the strong negative frequency-dependence found in models of preferential mating. To give rise to a rare male effect, the male competition itself would have to be a function of frequency. The advantageous males would have to compete less strongly as they became more common. As a general mechanism this is implausible.

Ehrman & Spiess (1969) suggested that females may prefer males simply because they are rare: the unusual male excites the females' attention and they respond more readily to him. This can be considered as a special model of preferential mating in which preferences are expressed in proportion to the rarity of the preferred males (O'Donald, 1980a). As in other models of preferential mating, some females mate preferentially while others mate at random. In all models of preferential mating, females differ between each other in their behavioural responses to the different males: some respond more readily to one phenotype of male; others respond more readily to another phenotype, or show no preference by responding equally to all males.

Evolution of preferences

Fisher (1930) produced an argument to show that female preferences would evolve as a result of the sexual selection they gave rise to. The sexual selection would thus reinforce itself. Fisher stated his argument concisely enough to be quoted in full:

> If instead of regarding the existence of sexual preference as a basic fact to be established only by direct observation, we consider that the tastes of organisms, like their organs and faculties, must be regarded as the products of evolutionary change, governed by the relative advantage which such tastes may confer, it appears, as has been shown in a previous section, that occasions may be not infrequent when a sexual preference of a particular kind may confer a selective advantage, and therefore become established in the species. Whenever appreciable differences exist in a species, which are in fact correlated with selective advantage, there will be a tendency to select also those individuals of the opposite sex which most clearly discriminate the difference to be observed, and which most decidedly prefer the more advantageous type. Sexual preference originating in this way may or may not confer any

direct advantage upon the individuals selected, and so hasten the effect of the Natural Selection in progress. It may therefore be far more widespread than the occurrence of striking secondary sexual characters.

Certain remarkable consequences do, however, follow if some sexual preferences of this kind, determined, for example, by a plumage character, are developed in a species in which the preferences of one sex, in particular the female, have a great influence on the number of offspring left by individual males. In such cases the modification of the plumage character in the cock proceeds under two selective influences (i) an initial advantage not due to sexual preference, which advantage may be quite inconsiderable in magnitude, and (ii) an additional advantage conferred by female preference, which will be proportional to the intensity of this preference. The intensity of preference will itself be increased by selection so long as the sons of hens exercising the preference most decidedly have any advantage over the sons of other hens, whether this be due to the first or to the second cause. The importance of this situation lies in the fact that the further development of the plumage character will still proceed, by reason of the advantage gained in sexual selection, even after it has passed the point in development at which its advantage in Natural Selection has ceased. The selective agencies other than sexual preference may be opposed to further development, and yet the further development will proceed, so long as the disadvantage is more than counterbalanced by the advantage in sexual selection. Moreover, as long as there is a net advantage in favour of further plumage development, there will also be a net advantage in favour of giving to it a more decided preference.

The two characteristics affected by such a process, namely plumage development in the male, and sexual preference for such developments in the female, must thus advance together, and so long as the process is unchecked by severe counterselection, will advance with ever-increasing speed. In the total absence of such checks, it is easy to see that the speed of development will be proportional to the development already attained, which will therefore increase with time exponentially, or in geometric progression. There is thus in any bionomic situation, in which sexual selection is capable of conferring a great reproductive advantage, the potentiality of a runaway process, which, however small the beginnings from which it arose, must, unless checked, produce great effects, and in the later stages with great rapidity.

Such a process must soon run against some check. Two such are obvious. If carried far enough, it is evident that sufficiently severe counterselection in favour of less ornamented males will be encountered to balance the advantage of sexual preference; at this point both plumage elaboration and the increase in female preference will be brought to a standstill, and a condition of relative stability will be attained. It will be more effective still if the disadvantage to the males of their sexual ornaments so diminishes their numbers surviving to the breeding season, relative to the females, as to cut at the root of the process, by diminishing the reproductive advantage to be conferred by female preference. It is important to notice that the condition of relative stability brought about by these or other means, will be of far longer duration than the process in which the ornaments are evolved. In most existing species the runaway process must have been already checked, and we should expect that the more extraordinary developments of sexual plumage were not due like most characters to a long and even course of evolutionary progress, but to sudden spurts of change. The theory does not enable us to predict the outcome of such an episode, but points to a great advantage being conferred by sexual preference as its underlying condition.

For many years, I thought that Fisher's theory removed the main difficulty that had been raised against Darwin's original theory of the evolution of male adornment by female preference. Critics had asked: why should females express preferences for the more colourful and adorned males? If they do, why should they be consistent in their preferences: why should they consistently prefer one type of male adornment to another? If they were not consistent, the males might be selected this way and that, first in one direction and then in another, no continuous line of development being followed. Fisher's theory resolves only part of this difficulty. His argument contains what I now see as a glaring non-sequitur. He has certainly shown (in the second paragraph quoted) that the intensity of sexual selection must increase, since the selection of the preferred sons of preferred fathers selects the preference as well. Fisher then immediately assumes that this will produce further development of the plumage character that is the object of the preference. But why should this follow? According to Fisher's theory, females are selected who can discriminate the fitter males by some associated or pleiotropic character and who then mate with them. The proportion of the females with the preference must increase, as Fisher has shown, thus producing more intense sexual selection. This inference does not imply that the females, having been selected originally to prefer males with the character by which they could be discriminated, would then automatically prefer males with more extreme developments of the character. The increase in frequency of females with preferences in no way entails a change of preference to favour more highly developed males. But Fisher's argument does show that a preference can evolve and will persist in a population: it does not show that a runaway process will produce more and more extreme developments of the character – developments such as the peacock's tail or the plumes of birds of paradise.

Relative expression of preference

To complete Fisher's argument, it is necessary to show that preferences will evolve that are expressed relative to the development attained by the preferred character. The third paragraph I quoted shows that Fisher believed he had demonstrated this. But he has jumped straight from his demonstration that the selection increases in intensity to an assumption that more extreme characters will be selected. This would follow only if females always preferred males with a more than average development of the character: they would always prefer the more extreme males. This relative expression of preference will occur if the male character acts as a 'supernormal stimulus' to the females (O'Donald, 1977, 1980a). Greater responsiveness to more extreme stimuli has been observed in animal training experiments. If animals are rewarded when they respond to one stimulus and punished if they respond to another, their peak response after training is usually displaced beyond the point at which they received a reward and in a direction away from the negative stimulus (Hanson, 1959). Staddon (1975) suggested that in the evolution of behaviour favourable selection would correspond to a reward and unfavourable selection to a punishment. The 'peak shift' of response towards supernormal stimuli might be produced by asymmetrical selection pressures. If not to respond to the favourable stimulus produces an extra cost in terms of a reduction in the chances of survival or the numbers of offspring, while to respond to a more extreme stimulus has little or no extra cost, then this asymmetry in the fitness function of response to varying levels of the stimulus will select for extra responsiveness to supernormal stimuli. This might be a general effect, or only applicable to particular stimuli. Staddon's theory can be applied to the evolution of female response to the stimuli of male sexual display. If female preferences evolve by the selective advantage of being more responsive to males whose phenotype indicates higher fitness, a peak shift in their responses will select the more extreme phenotypes as Fisher postulated, eventually producing a character so extreme that its mating advantage is balanced by its deleterious effects on survival. When this point is reached, the selection of the females' responses will no longer be asymmetrical in relation to fitness: stabilising selection will maintain a constant phenotype. According to this argument, the females' preferences are expressed relative to the point in the development of the character at which they have their peak response. Suppose a preference evolves for a mutant phenotype with a value x_0 of the preferred character, while the females' peak response occurs at the greater value α. The same preference that evolved for the original mutant will also select later mutants with values $x_1, x_2, \ldots, x_i$, provided that $x_i < \alpha$; for the preference expressed will be some function of the difference $\alpha - x_i$. Fisher's runaway process of sexual selection can continue until $x_i = \alpha$. Response to a supernormal stimulus provides a mechanism for the relative expression of preference and thus completes the chain of inference that constitutes the theory of sexual selection by female preference.

Genetical models of the evolution of preferences

Genetics has not yet entered our discussion of the evolution of preferences. Fisher explained his theory in non-genetical terms which Darwin himself might have used. Yet the possibility of the evolution of preference depends on the genetics of preference: a gene that gives rise to the expression of female mating preference must increase in frequency as a result of selection for the preferred males. Fisher simply assumed that the preference is passed to the preferred sons born of the preferential matings. Females prefer them and they increase in frequency. Fisher concluded that the preference they carry would increase proportionately with the level of preference and hence exponentially. But non-preferential matings will also produce preferred males by genetic segregation; preferential matings will produce non-preferred males. By recombination, the preference will pass to non-preferred males as well as to preferred males. Selection raises the frequency of the preference gene in the preferred males, but lowers it in the non-preferred males. Its overall frequency increases only if preferred males are more likely to carry the preference gene than non-preferred males. To select for preference, therefore, the preference gene and the gene for the preferred character must segregate together when gametes are formed. When the preferred character is selected, then so too is the preference. In population genetics, this is known as hitch-hiking. A gene with no advantage by itself increases in frequency because it occurs in combination with an advantageous gene. Unless genes are closely linked, however, genetic recombination rapidly breaks up particular combinations of genes. The hitch-hiking gene is soon dropped unless selection continually regenerates its association with the advantageous gene. To some extent, this is what sexual selection does. Preferential mating combines the genes for the preferred character with the preference genes. Fisher's runaway process can thus occur. How far it goes depends on the genetics of the character and the preference. The appropriate combination of genes is maintained at a higher level in some genetical models than in others.

Associations between genes are measured by the linkage disequilibrium between them. This is the difference between the actual frequency of a particular combination and the frequency it would have if the genes were combined at random. Suppose that at two loci A and B, two alternative alleles can be found to segregate – A_1 and A_2, B_1 and B_2. Let these alleles occur at the relative frequencies p_1 and p_2 for A_1 and A_2 and q_1 and q_2 for B_1 and B_2. If the alleles combine at random, the four possible combinations will be found at the following frequencies:

Combination	Frequency
$A_1 B_1$	$p_1 q_1$
$A_1 B_2$	$p_1 q_2$
$A_2 B_1$	$p_2 q_1$
$A_2 B_2$	$p_2 q_2$

If the combination $A_1 B_1$ actually occurs at frequency P_{11}, then the difference

$$D = P_{11} - p_1 q_1$$

is the linkage disequilibrium. Under random mating with no selection, this difference is reduced in the course of successive generations until

$$D = 0$$

Suppose that A_1 determines the preferred character and B_1 the females' preference. Provided that

$$D > 0$$

selection for A_1 gives B_1 a hitch-hike: the preference is selected. Fisher's argument, although stated in non-genetical terms, does suggest that linkage disequilibrium of the genes for the preferred character and preference will be generated: the offspring of the preferential matings must have a chance of at least 50% of receiving the gene for the preferred character from the male parent and the gene for the preference from the female parent.

By extensive computer simulations, I showed that preferential mating always produces some linkage disequilibrium of the genes, at least in the early stage of sexual selection (O'Donald, 1967, 1980*a*). How far the preference gene can hitch-hike depends on the genetics of the character and the preference, the frequencies of the genes at the start of selection and the behavioural model of how the preference is expressed. If females who carry a preference gene always express their preference and thus mate preferentially, the sexual selection is then most intense and the preference shows the greatest possible increase in frequency. Generally a recessive male character is selected more rapidly than a dominant, for a preference gene is maintained in greater linkage disequilibrium with a recessive. When a recessive preferred character is selected and spreads through a population to reach complete fixation, the preference shows a three- to five-fold increase in frequency. During the selection of a preferred dominant, the preference shows a two- to four-fold increase. Assuming that the preference is expressed relative to the development of the character, new mutants that increase the value of the character will also be selected, thus producing further increases in the preference. But as the preference gene becomes more common, it shows smaller and smaller increases in frequency. It never reaches fixation. The population never consists solely of females with preferences. Only at the start of selection, when both character and preference genes are rare, does the rate of selection become exponential and only then for a brief initial period. In some models of selection for a dominant, the preference hardly increases at all. Yet Fisher's argument appears to show that the preference must always increase exponentially. This completely erroneous conclusion results from Fisher's non-genetical analysis of his theory. The evolution of preference depends on a complex genetic interaction: the preference gene is selected through its selective effect on the gene for the preferred character. The frequency-dependence of sexual selection by preferential mating also increases the complexity of the evolutionary process. Apart from the increase in frequency that a preference gene may be expected to show during the selection of a gene for the preferred character, no general inferences can be made about the rates of selection or the establishment of polymorphisms. The results of selection often depend on the specific model of mating behaviour or the initial frequencies of the genes. I have described the detailed results of my computer simulations in chapter 8 of my book *Genetic Models of Sexual Selection* (O'Donald, 1980*a*).

My analysis of the theory of preferential mating can be summarised as follows. Female preference will certainly be selected to some extent by the mechanism Fisher postulated, though never as rapidly as he thought and sometimes hardly at all. The evolution of preference can never proceed so far that all females eventually share the same preference. Selection for preference usually stops long before the preference gene becomes fixed in the population. A polymorphic equilibrium is reached at which the preference genes and their non-preference alleles remain at stable frequencies: some females have the preference, others are without it. Any expression of the preference must give rise to frequency-dependent mating. The preferred males gain a relatively greater advantage when they are rare than when they are common. Therefore, when females mate preferentially, the theory of preferential mating predicts that they will be polymorphic in preference and the males will gain a frequency-dependent advantage giving rise to a 'rare male' effect. But when females show no preference and choose males by responding to variations in male courtship, no rare male effect should be observed. On the contrary, if any frequency-dependent mating does occur, it may be expected to favour the common, not the rare, males.

Lande (1981) simulated the evolution of preference for a quantitative character. Arnold, in his contribution to this volume, discusses Lande's results, which appear to differ in a number of ways from my own. Lande assumes that an indefinite number of loci contribute to the genetic variances of the preferred character and preference. No genetic limit is thus put on the value of the preferred character which can continue to be selected to infinity. Crucial to the analysis of Lande's model is the assumption he makes about the genetic covariance B and the genetic variance in the male character G. As Arnold remarks, the trajectory of the evolving population turns out to be a straight line specified by the regression slope B/G. This regression is assumed to be linear and hence the ratio B/G to be a constant. This assumption guarantees Fisher's result: since there is assumed to be a constant correlation between preference and preferred character, selection of the one must proportionately select the other, giving rise to the geometric rate of increase of the male and female traits. It is precisely this assumption that my own computer simulations show to be false. The covariance B is determined by the linkage disequilibria. For just two loci, the covariance equals the linkage disequilibrium. Linkage disequilibrium can only be calculated for a specific genetic model using the recursion equations of the frequencies of each genotype. Linkage disequilibria cannot be calculated for polygenic models of quantitative characters. This is the major difficulty of all polygenic models. Unfortunately, it is the essential point of models of the evolution of female preferences. The linkage disequilibrium changes in the course of evolution. It depends on the genetic system, the mating system and the initial gene frequencies. I see no reason to suppose that the ratio B/G is even approximately constant. Fisher's geometric rate of increase is built into Lande's models as a premise. I think it is probably false.

Thoday's experiment on female choice

As we have shown, a rare male effect in experiments on female choice corroborates the theory of preferential mating analysed in previous sections of this chapter. Semler's experiment with sticklebacks showed that females would choose in favour of males with either artificial or natural red throats. Their choice could not have been determined by differences in the males' courtship. This strongly corroborates the theory that the females had prior preferences for red-throated males. If so, then according to the computer models of the evolution of preference, the females should so be genetically polymorphic: some should prefer red males; others should have no preference. To test this prediction, it would be necessary to show that the preference could be increased by selective breeding. A selection line could be set up by breeding only from the offspring of the matings with red-throated males, for these matings would include the preferential matings. The preference in the selection line could then be tested by letting the females choose between red and non-red males from an unselected population kept as a control line. This selection experiment has not been carried out. But in an experiment with *Drosophila*, Tebb & Thoday (1956) found that expression of preference was associated with a genetic marker. This observation corroborates the theory of preferential mating by showing that the females were polymorphic as theory predicts they will be: they differed genetically in their preferences.

Tebb & Thoday used stocks of *Drosophila* marked with the sex-linked mutants *white eye* (w) or *apricot eye* (w^a). Females, genotypically w/w, w/w^a or w^a/w^a, were given a choice of mating with either w or w^a males. The experiments took place at one of two different temperatures. A detailed analysis of the data (O'Donald, 1980*a*) shows that only the following two factors are statistically significant: the preference of heterozygous females for *white* males and the preference of homozygous females for *apricot* males. I estimated that 36% of the heterozygous females had expressed a preference for the *white* males and 26% of the homozygous females had expressed a preference for the *apricot* males. These estimates were obtained by the method of maximum likelihood and are very significant. The males showed no difference in their overall chances of mating. The genotypes of the females who exercised the choice were the only factors that determined the variation in the males' chances of mating. Sexual selection took place because the females differed in their preferences.

Thoday's experiment shows that differences of preference can be associated with differences of genotype. We should not expect that the genetic markers themselves determined the preferences. The genomes of the stocks carrying the markers might differ genetically at a number of loci, the association of the preferences with the markers reflecting the differences between the genomes. But the precise genetic determination of the preferences is unimportant. It is sufficient to show that differences of preference can have a genetic component. They can then be selected. This is the fundamental premise of the models of the evolution of female preferences.

Summary

Female choice may take place by two mechanisms: some males may court the females more actively or persistently than others; some females may prefer to mate with particular male phenotypes. These mechanisms can be distinguished only by carefully designed experiments.

The evolution of female preference is not as inevitable as Fisher suggested in his theory of the runaway process. Selection does not proceed at the exponential rate that Fisher had deduced from his non-genetical model: it is much slower; in some genetical models, the preference hardly evolves at all. Fisher's argument also contains the non-sequitur that the increasing intensity of selection entails selection for more extreme male characters.

If female preference has evolved, the preferred males gain a frequency-dependent advantage that can be observed as a 'rare male' effect. It may also be possible to show, as Thoday did, that females differ genetically in their preferences. Alternatively, experiments can be designed to test whether the preference responds to selection. If it does, it must be inherited. Unfortunately, experiments on mate choice have never been carried out in conjunction with long-term selection experiments. Such experiments are essential in order to give the theory of preferential mating an empirical base.

References

Charlesworth, D. & Charlesworth, B. (1975). Sexual selection and polymorphism. *American Naturalist*, **109**, 465–70.

Darwin, C. R. (1871). *The Descent of Man, and Selection in Relation to Sex*. John Murray: London.

Ehrman, L. (1972). Genetics and sexual selection. In *Sexual Selection and the Descent of Man 1871–1971*, ed. B. Campbell, pp. 105–35. Heinemann: London.

Ehrman, L. & Spiess, E. B. (1969). Rare type mating advantage in *Drosophila*. *American Naturalist*, **103**, 675–80.

Fisher, R. A. (1930). *The Genetical Theory of Natural Selection*. Clarendon Press: Oxford.

Hanson, H. M. (1959). Effects of discrimination training on stimulus generalization. *Journal of Experimental Psychology*, **58**, 321–34.

Lande, R. (1981). Models of speciation by sexual selection of polygenic traits. *Proceedings of the National Academy of Sciences of the U.S.A.*, **78**, 3721–5.

O'Donald, P. (1967). A general model of sexual and natural selection. *Heredity*, **22**, 499–518.

O'Donald, P. (1973). Models of sexual and natural selection in polygynous species. *Heredity*, **31**, 145–56.

O'Donald, P. (1977). Theoretical aspects of sexual selection. *Theoretical Population Biology*, **12**, 298–334.

O'Donald, P. (1978). Rare male mating advantage. *Nature*, **272**, 189.

O'Donald, P. (1980a). *Genetic Models of Sexual Selection*. Cambridge University Press: Cambridge.

O'Donald, P. (1980b). Sexual selection by female choice in a monogamous bird: Darwin's theory corroborated. *Heredity*, **45**, 201–17.

Semler, D. E. (1971). Some aspects of adaptation in a polymorphism for breeding colours in the Threespine Stickleback (*Gasterosteus aculeatus*). *Journal of Zoology, London*, **165**, 291–302.

Speiss, E. B. & Ehrman, L. (1978). Rare male mating advantage, *Nature*, **272**, 188–9.

Staddon, J. E. R. (1975). A note on the evolutionary significance of 'supernormal stimuli'. *American Naturalist*, **109**, 541–5.

Tebb, G. & Thoday, J. M. (1956). Reversal of mating preference by crossing strains of *Drosophila melanogaster*. *Nature*, **177**, 707.

4

Sexual selection: the interface of theory and empiricism

STEVAN J. ARNOLD

The aim of this paper is to point out some interesting directions for research that are inspired by recent developments in sexual selection theory. I touch here on only a few new results that seem important and do not attempt a survey comparable to the excellent reviews of Trivers (1972), Halliday (1978), Borgia (1979), and Thornhill (1979).

Much recent theoretical progress has come about by attaching concise mathematical definitions to familiar, but often ill-defined, concepts such as 'sexual selection', 'intensity of selection', and 'good genes'. In striving for conceptual clarity, the goal is not merely to make such terms mathematical, but to find their explicit relationship to expressions for evolutionary change (dynamic equations). A mathematical conception is important because sexual selection can often be so complex that intuition, unaided by equations, can be an untrustworthy guide.

In the following sections, I am concerned with techniques for measuring the impact of sexual selection and with models for evolution by sexual selection. Field workers are increasingly successful at measuring the key variables needed to characterise the impact of sexual selection (e.g. Downhower & Brown, 1980; Kluge, 1981; Lennington, 1980). Such data can be analysed so that they have a direct relationship to formal evolutionary theory (Wade & Arnold, 1980; Arnold & Wade, MS; Lande & Arnold, MS). This is an improvement over *ad hoc* analysis that lacks theoretical motivation, but it is not a panacea. The aim is merely to characterise sexual selection by its statistical effects on phenotypic characters within a generation. This, of course, tells us nothing about how selection actually worked in the past, nor does it enable us to extrapolate into the future. The goal is simply to understand the process of sexual selection by direct measurement of its contemporary impact.

67

This is a timely approach to the subject. Much confusion has recently been generated by anthropomorphic discussions that rely on charming, but misleading metaphors (e.g. females 'shopping for good genes') rather than on a direct analysis of evolutionary process. Although the approach adopted here is, at first, more difficult to handle than one based solely in metaphor, I believe that in the long run it will yield more penetrating insights.

With regard to evolutionary models of sexual selection, I focus primarily on a model by Lande (1981) that describes evolutionary change in continuous characters (like tail size or bill length) in which variation is produced both by genes at many different loci and by the environment. Most of the characters that interest students of sexual selection are of this kind. The significance of Lande's sexual selection model is two-fold: (1) it probably gives a more realistic portrayal of evolution than one-and-two locus models, and (2) the terms used in equations for evolutionary change can be directly estimated, even in natural populations.

Sexual versus natural selection

It is unfortunate that many modern authors do not use the term 'sexual selection' as it was employed by its originator, Charles Darwin (1859, 1871). The most prevalent mishandlings are to treat sexual selection either as a subcategory of natural selection or as referring to any type of selection dealing with reproduction. Bateman (1948), Ghiselin (1974), O'Donald (1980), Wade & Arnold (1980) already have reviewed various misrepresentations of Darwinian sexual selection but their arguments seem to be unappreciated by most workers in this field. Rather than attempt another review of the sad history of abuse, I shortly present an annotated passage from Darwin (1871) that contains all the essential points.

A central problem for Darwin was to explain the origin of sexually dimorphic characters that probably hindered survival. His solution was a process of sexual selection that would promote characters that were deleterious under ordinary or natural selection. In the following passage, Darwin (1871: 256–7) defines sexual selection by contrasting it with natural selection.

> We are, however, here concerned only with that kind of selection, which I have called sexual selection. This depends on the advantage which certain individuals have over other individuals of the same sex and species, in exclusive relation to reproduction.

In order to illustrate the distinction between sexual and natural selection, Darwin next gives four examples of traits elaborated by natural selection rather than sexual selection. They were obviously carefully chosen to make important, but subtle points. The first example concerns sexually dimorphic traits, like the bills of a Hawaiian bird (*Neomorpha acutirostris*), that are perfected by natural selection.

> When the two sexes differ in structure in relation to different habits of life, as in the cases above mentioned, they have no doubt been modified through natural selection, accompanied by inheritance limited to one and the same sex.

In the second example, Darwin points out that primary sexual characteristics (e.g. genitalia and reproductive tracts), as well as mammary glands and other organs for feeding offspring, evolve by natural selection. This key passage shows that natural selection is not simply selection for survivorship and that sexual selection does not act on all aspects of reproduction.

> So again the primary sexual organs, and those for nourishing or protecting the young, come under this same head; for those individuals which generated or nourished their offspring best, would leave, *caeteris paribus*, the greatest number to inherit their superiority; whilst those which generated or nourished their offspring badly, would leave but few to inherit their weaker powers.

In the third example, he notes that some characters may be favoured by both natural and sexual selection.

> As the male has to search for the female, he requires for this purpose organs of sense and locomotion, but if these organs are necessary for other purposes of life, as is generally the case, they will have been developed through natural selection.

Darwin notes in his fourth example that some secondary sexual characteristics will evolve by natural selection, as will primary sexual characters, even though they are used exclusively in mating.

> When the male has found the female he sometimes absolutely requires prehensile organs to hold her; thus Dr. Wallace informs me that the males of certain moths cannot unite with the females if their tarsi or feet are broken. The males of many oceanic crustaceans have their legs and antennae modified in an extraordinary manner for the prehension of the female; hence we may suspect that owing to these animals being washed about by the waves of the open sea, they absolutely require these organs in order to propagate their kind, and if so their development will have been the result of ordinary or natural selection.

The juxtaposition of this example with the last one suggests that Darwin was swayed by the similarity between prehensile organs needed by males to resist wave action during copulation and primary organs, like testes; both are, as he says, absolutely required for reproduction and hence are perfected by natural selection.

The unifying theme of these four examples is that in each of them evolution is by natural selection, not by sexual selection, even though the characters are sexually dimorphic and reproductive in nature. These are the exceptions that help differentiate the two selection processes. In the next paragraph, Darwin opens by putting aside such troublesome exceptions and focuses on unambiguous instances of sexual selection.

> When the two sexes follow exactly the same habits of life, and the male has more highly developed sense or locomotive organs than the female, it may be that these in their perfected state are indispensible to the male for finding the female; but in the vast majority of cases, they serve only to give one male an advantage over another, for the less well-endowed males, if time were allowed them, would succeed in pairing with the females; and they would in all other respects, judging from the structure of the female, be equally well adapted for their ordinary habits of life. In such cases sexual selection must have come into action, for the males have acquired their present structure, not from being better fitted to survive in the struggle for existance, but from having gained an advantage over other males, and from having transmitted this advantage to their male offspring alone. It was the importance of this distinction which led me to designate this form of selection as sexual selection.

In other words, the chief defining feature of sexual selection is that sexually mature males differ in ability to inseminate females. The main reason for calling this sexual selection, distinct from natural selection, is that structures that confer mating success may hinder the male in the struggle for survival: sexual selection and natural can be opposing processes. In the next passage Darwin indicates that female mate choice need not depend on any aesthetic sense and that rival males may constitute an immediate agent of sexual selection.

> 'So again, if the chief service rendered to the male by his prehensile organs is to prevent the escape of the female before the arrival of males, or when assaulted by them, these organs will have been perfected through sexual selection, that is by the advantage acquired by certain males over their rivals.'

He ends with the disclaimer that, although the action of sexual selection may sometimes be clearly revealed, its effects will often be confounded with those of natural selection.

> But in most cases it is scarcely possible to distinguish between the effects of natural and sexual selection.

It is clear from these paragraphs and other passages that Darwin did not view sexual selection as a subcategory of natural selection. Sexual selection was proposed to explain extraordinary sexually dimorphic characters troublesome to his concept of natural selection. It is also clear that Darwin did not design the concept of sexual selection to cover all aspects of reproduction; differences in offspring survivorship induced by differences in parental care, for example, constitute natural selection.

The key to seeing Darwin's distinction between sexual and natural selection is to focus not on the variety of sexually selected characters but instead to consider the effects of such characters on fitness. Characters that evolve by sexual selection are those that cause differences, or variance, in male mating success. An effect on this component of total fitness is the common denominator of the major categories of sexually selected characters listed by Darwin (1871: 257–8): weapons of offence and defence used in male combat; courage and pugnacity in fighting; male ornaments, sound-producing structures and odours that serve only to attract the female or elicit her sexual response. In this context, male mating success is taken as the number of mates that bear the male's progeny: it is not merely the male's copulatory success, but his success in actually siring progeny with a number of mates. Moreover, mating success is conditional on survival to sexual maturity. If we view sexual selection as arising from variance in mating success and natural selection as arising from variance in all other components of total fitness (e.g. survivorship, fertility per mate, offspring survivorship), we come very close to Darwin's concepts, perhaps as close as we can come in exact, statistical terms (Wade & Arnold, 1980; Arnold & Wade, in preparation). This statistical view has the further advantages that: (a) one need not actually identify the agent of sexual selection (e.g. rival males versus discriminating females) in order to measure its impact, and (b) that sexual selection can be measured with conventional statistics.

Dynamic models of evolution by sexual selection

It is important to approach theoretical models with the proper expectations. The goal of a model is to determine what *can* happen: only empirical work can determine what actually *does* happen in the real world. Models are always designed to solve a particular theoretical issue under specified assumptions. In other words, the goal of a model is to explore the consequences of assumptions about the real world rather than to show how the world actually operates. Models should be viewed as guides for field and laboratory work: only empirical work can produce generalisations about the natural world.

Modelling strategies

Dynamic models have many advantages over other formal approaches to evolution by sexual selection. Such models specify how the composition of the population changes through time, from generation to generation. It is worth reviewing the virtues of dynamic models, since they often require more involved mathematics than short cut methods, such as optimisation and evolutionarily stable strategy (ESS) approaches, that merely describe the population at equilibrium. The two sets of approaches have been recently compared by Lewontin (1979), Maynard Smith (1978*b*, 1980) and Lande (1982*a*). The principal advantages of the dynamic approach are: (a) it permits genetic constraints to affect the evolutionary outcome; (b) it does not rely on an optimisation principle; and (c) it specifies the rate and direction of evolution as well as the location and stability of the outcome or equilibrium.

In contrast, short-cut methods suffer from severe limitation. For example, the principle that selection will maximise fitness or optimise behaviours that contribute to fitness (e.g. mate choice) does not apply in the case of sexual selection. Because the fitness of males varies according to the frequencies of female phenotypes exercising mate choice and rival male phenotypes, sexual selection is a form of frequency-dependent selection. In general, neither mean population fitness nor average inclusive fitness is maximised when selection is frequency-dependent (Wright, 1969: 121–2). Thus optimisation arguments about the fate of populations evolving by sexual selection can be very misleading.

ESS models of sexual selection suffer from a milder problem. Since such models implicitly assume asexual reproduction, genetic phenomena (e.g. meiosis and pleiotropy) can play no role in evolution. This too can be misleading since dynamic models of sexual selection indicate that inheritance as well as selection determines how fast the population evolves and where it goes (O'Donald, 1980; Lande, 1980, 1981, 1982*b*; Kirkpatrick, 1982).

Fisher's runaway sexual selection model

R. A. Fisher seems to have been the first person to examine the genetic consequences of sexual selection and to propose a specific, dynamic process. Fisher (1915) sketched the outlines of a model in which mate choice by females led to a self-reinforcing process of evolution. Fisher (1930, 1958) later presented a more explicit version and reached the surprising conclusion that a male character and female preferences could evolve together at ever increasing speed. He reached this conclusion by noting that females choosing the most sexually favoured males would produce sexually favoured sons as well as daughters with strong preferences.

Fisher never presented a mathematical development of his runaway sexual selection model. O'Donald (1967, 1977, 1980) modelled the essential features of sexual selection with genetic models in which one or two loci specified the male character and another locus specified female mating preference. These models did reveal that the assortative mating aspect of sexual selection can create a genetic coupling between male attribute and female mate preference and demonstrated the possibility of polymorphism at equilibrium, but O'Donald was unable to confirm the runaway aspect of Fisher's model (O'Donald, 1980). The runaway feature has recently been confirmed in polygenic models for sexual selection developed by Lande (1981, 1982b). These models, as well as those by O'Donald (1980) and Kirkpatrick (1982), have also yielded results not predicted by Fisher. In particular, there may be a great variety of outcomes at genetic equilibrium.

Polygenic models for evolution by sexual selection

The following account of a model by Lande (1981) gives only the flavour of the main ingredients and results. The original article and related papers (Lande, 1980, 1982b) should be consulted for a full mathematical development and justification of assumptions.

Lande's (1981) model gives the expected evolution of a sex-limited* male character and the female mate preference based on that character. In the following discussion of this model, it is helpful to conceive of a specific male character, such as tail length in a bird population, that is expressed only in males and female mate choice based on that character. The basic assumptions of the model are as follows. Suppose that male tail length, z, is normally distributed with mean of $\bar{z}$ and a standard deviation of σ. In an actual example, a size-related character, like tail length, first might be transformed by taking the logarithm of tail length (Fig. 4.1).

---

* Sex-limited characters are characters that are expressed only in one sex; they need not be sex-linked in inheritance. A contribution to sex-dimorphism is often made by autosomal genes with different expression in males and females.

Natural selection on male character. Tail length might be subject to selective forces other than mate choice. Suppose that these forces of natural selection are stabilising in nature. For example, an intermediate tail size might be optimal under natural selection because a very small tail produces poor flight performance while an extremely long tail makes the male very vulnerable to predators. This situation can be represented by a concave curve shaped like a normal distribution and known as a Gaussian selection function. The top of this curve denotes optimal tail size, θ, or the adaptive peak under natural selection (Fig. 4.2). The width of this natural selection function, ω, describes the intensity of natural selection on tail size. When the function is broad (large ω), male tail size experiences weak stabilising selection; strong stabilising selection is represented by a narrow width (small ω). This width variable is analogous to the standard deviation of a normal distribution, but here we are dealing with a function rather than with a frequency or probability distribution.

Fig. 4.1. In Lande's (1981) model for evolution by natural and sexual selection, a hypothetical sex-limited character, such as male tail size, is normally distributed with a mean of $\bar{z}$ and a standard deviation of σ.

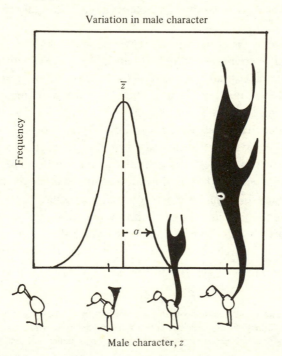

Male character, z

Female mate choice. Consider next the mating preferences of females based on the male character, z. Focusing on a particular female, we imagine that her tendency to mate with a particular encountered male is given by a Gaussian curve like the one shown in Fig. 4.3. Mate preference is assumed to be unaffected by the male composition of the population and in this sense the female's preferences are absolute. Lande (1981) also considers the case in which the characteristic mate preference of the female is relative to the mean of the male population, $\bar{z}$, and the case in which the female's mating preference is an open-ended, increasing (exponential) function of male character. Remarkably, the progress of evolution is qualitatively similar under these disparate models of female choice, so only the absolute preference case is illustrated here.

In order for the mate preferences of females to evolve, there must be

Fig. 4.2. The male's fitness under natural selection is a Gaussian function, shaped like a normal curve, with an optimum at the tail size specified by θ and a characteristic width of ω.

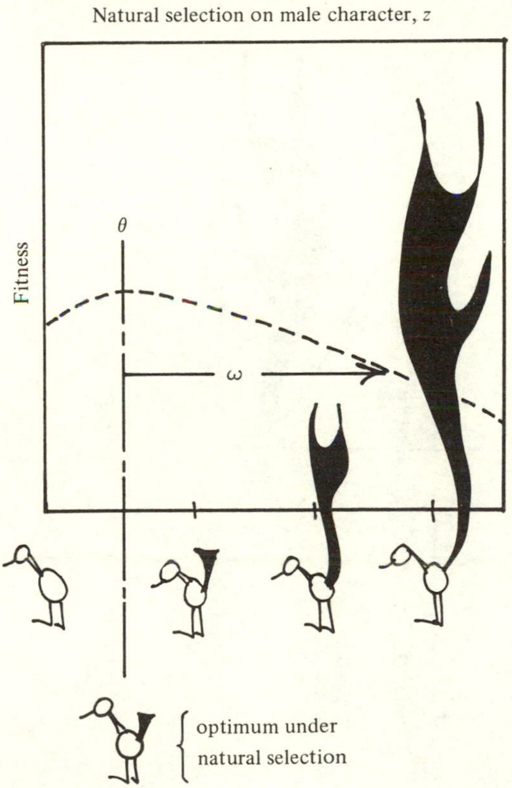

Natural selection on male character, z

optimum under
natural selection

variation among females in mate preference: females must not all prefer the same mate. Let the most preferred mate of a female, y_i, be designated by the male character value corresponding to the maximum of her Gaussian preference function (Fig. 4.3). The females differ in most preferred mate and these are normally distributed with mean $\bar{y}$ (Fig. 4.4).

No selection on female preferences. Assume that males do not protect or provision their mates or offspring, as in many lek-breeding species. Consequently, females have the same number of offspring irrespective of mate choice. There is no immediate benefit to mate choice and in this sense

Fig. 4.3. Suppose that a particular female most prefers mating partners with a tail size of y_i. Her tendency of mating as a function of male tail size falls off on either side of this tail size so that her mating preference function is shaped like a Gaussian curve with characteristic width ν.

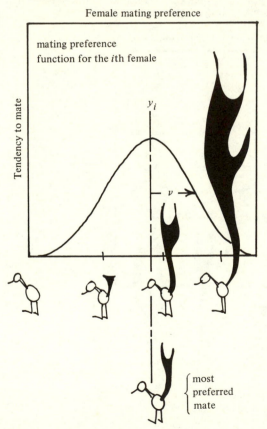

Female mating preference

there is no direct selection of female mating preference. Nevertheless, female mating preferences can evolve, as we shall see, as a correlated response to selection on males.

Polygenic inheritance of male character and female preference. Assume that each character is affected by many genes, each having a small effect, so that inheritance is polygenic. Fisher (1918) showed that the inheritance of such a character can be summarised by a genetic parameter of the population known as the *genic* or *additive genetic variance*. This parameter enables us to predict the phenotypes of offspring from the phenotypes of their parents. One way of estimating the additive genetic variance of the

Fig. 4.4. Females differ in the tail size of their most preferred mate, y_i, but the preference functions of all female (dotted curves) have the same characteristic width, v. The most preferred mates of the females are normally distributed (solid curve) with a mean of $\bar{y}$.

Variation in female mating preference

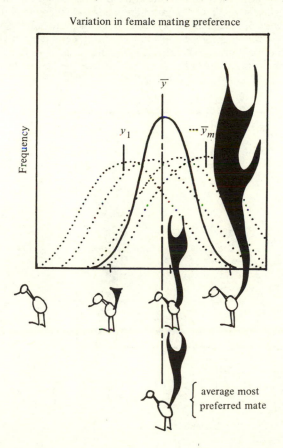

male character z is to calculate the least squares regression of son's character on father's character (Fig. 4.5). This regression slope estimates one half the ratio of genic to phenotypic variance; this ratio of variances is commonly known as the *heritability* of the trait (Falconer, 1960). Likewise, the regression of daughter's most preferred mate on the most preferred mate of her mother would estimate one half the heritability of female mate preference.

We assume now that the genic variances of the male and female characters remain constant during evolution because loss of variance due to selection is balanced by input from polygenic mutation and recombination. The empirical and theoretical justification for this assumption is discussed by Lande (1976).

Fig. 4.5. Each point in the plot represents the average tail size of the sons of a particular male. The data are hypothetical. If there are no non-genetic causes of resemblance between father and sons, the slope of the least squares regression of son's tail size on father's tail size (solid line) will estimate one half the ratio of genic variance in tail size, G, to phenotypic variance in tail size, σ^2, or one half the heritability of male tail size, h^2. Means are indicated with dashed lines.

Inheritance of male character

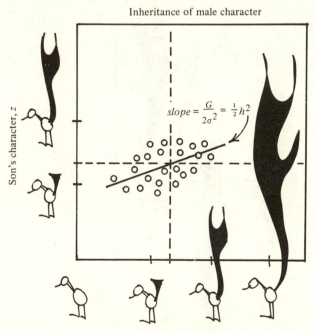

$$slope = \frac{G}{2\sigma^2} = \tfrac{1}{2}h^2$$

Son's character, z

Father's character, z

Genic covariance between the sexes. One of the most important consequences of the model is that a genetic coupling arises between male and female characters. This coupling, or *genic covariance*, is a consequence of assortative mating and heritable variation in the two characters. Genic covariance is not an assumption of Lande's (1981) model but rather one of its results or consequences.

Production of this coupling or genic covariance can be visualised in the following way. In each generation, females with the most extreme preference will tend to mate only with males displaying the most highly developed tails; this aspect of assortative mating yields the points in the upper right-hand corner of Fig. 4.6. Likewise, females preferring males with small tails will tend to mate primarily with such males; this aspect of assortative mating yields the points in the lower left-hand corner of Fig. 4.6. In both cases, mating produces sons that resemble their fathers and daughters that resemble their mothers. Thus the overall effect of assortative mating is to produce a correlation or covariance between sons and daughters. This correlation is known as an additive genetic or genic covariance. It arises from assortative mating and reflects linkage disequilibrium, which is the non-random association or linkage of alleles at different loci in gametes. Thus, in this example, alleles promoting large tails in males tend to become associated with alleles that promote female mating preference for large-tailed males. The regression of daughter's most preferred mate on son's character in Fig. 4.6 estimates the ratio of genic covariance between the sexes to genic variance in male character, B/G. Later this ratio will play a critical role in predicting the joint evolution of female preference and male character.

*Forces of natural and sexual selection.** Natural selection exerts one force, tending to drive the male population towards the optimal tail size, θ. Female mate preferences exert another force that, in general, tends to drive male tail size away from the natural selection optimum. This is the force of sexual selection. It is present whenever the average tail size of sexually successful males differs from the average tail size assessed for the entire

---

* Bradbury & Gibson (this volume) argue that the models of Lande (1981) and Wade and Arnold (1980) are misleading because they do not incorporate natural selection during or after the episode of sexual selection. This is not a troublesome issue. Lande's (1980, 1981) models incorporate natural selection on male attributes that acts prior to sexual selection. These models were extended to cover multiple episodes of selection, including natural selection that follows sexual selection, by Arnold & Wade (MS), but Lande's basic conclusions were unaffected.

population of adult males. The force of sexual selection is proportional to this deviation. Similarly, the force of natural selection is proportional to the deviation of average male tail size for the optimum, θ.

From these considerations we can see that, for any force of natural selection forcing male tails towards their optimum, there might be an

Fig. 4.6. Each point in this hypothetical plot represents the averages of female and male progeny from a particular male parent mated to a large sample of females. These progeny averages are proportional to the males' breeding values for female mate preference and male tail size, respectively. The covariance of breeding values for two such traits is known as the genic covariance, B. The variance in breeding values for the male tail size is the genic variance, G, so the least squares regression of daughters' male preference on sons' tail size is the genetic regression, B/G. Dashed lines show the means for the two characters.

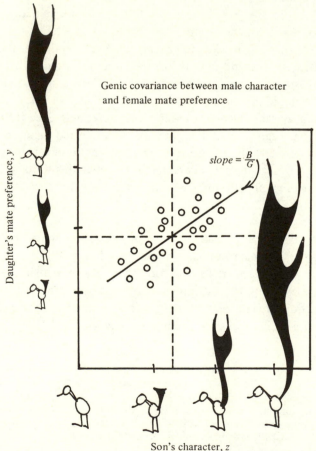

Genic covariance between male character and female mate preference

$slope = \dfrac{B}{G}$

Daughter's mate preference, y

Son's character, z

exactly equivalent force of sexual selection, forcing tail size in the opposite direction. When these two forces are equal, there is no net force of selection on male tail size; thus mean tail size ceases to evolve and the population is said to be in genetic equilibrium. When there is no immediate penalty associated with extreme mate preference, very strong preferences can evolve. Consequently, it is conceivable for there to be a tremendous force of sexual selection exerted by females, a force strong enough to balance the force of natural selection when the average tail is very large and far from the optimum. In this model, female mate choice is selectively neutral and there is no force to oppose directly the development of extreme preferences in the population. Thus, it is not surprising that Lande (1981) finds that there is no unique combination of average male and female traits at genetic equilibrium, rather there is a line of equilibria (Figs. 4.7 and 4.8). In other words, the evolutionary outcome is indeterminate because the balance between natural and sexual selection can be achieved in many different ways. As we shall see, the outcome of evolution depends largely on the starting point of the population.

The proposal that female mate preference might be selectively neutral is counter to intuition and to some popular views of sexual selection. It is commonly argued that females are favoured by selection if they mate with the fittest males. But if only male gametes are transferred to the female, as in lek-breeding birds, the argument is circular, since it is the females themselves that confer the purely sexual advantage on males. The theoretical justification for the view that female mate choice might be selectively neutral is taken up in a later section.

Evolutionary outcomes. Some of the following results will probably not be intuitively obvious unless one is fluent with basic concepts in quantitative genetics. Strained intuition commonly engenders mistrust, but in the present case it should encourage consultation of Falconer's (1960) excellent text and Lande's (1981) own account of his model.

The evolution of the population can be represented by the movement of a point in two-dimensional space in which one axis describes the average of the male character and the other describes average female mating preference. Because natural and sexual selection act directly *only* on the male character, the trajectory of evolving population turns out to be a straight line specified by the genetic regression slope, B/G (Fig. 4.7). A further consequence of selection not acting directly on female mate preference is, as just mentioned, that there is no unique evolutionary equilibrium. Instead, if the line of equilibria is stable, the population

Fig. 4.7. The evolution of the population is described by its change in average female mate preference and average male tail size. The tail size of males most preferred as mates is shown on the vertical axis. In Lande's model the population will evolve along trajectories specified by the genetic regression, B/G. The male tail size that is optimal for survivorship and other non-sexual aspects of life is indicated with the dashed line, θ. Populations stop evolving when they reach the line of equilibria specified by the diagonal heavy line. Thus the composition of the population at equilibrium depends on its starting point. There are many possible combinations of mate preference and tail size at equilibrium.

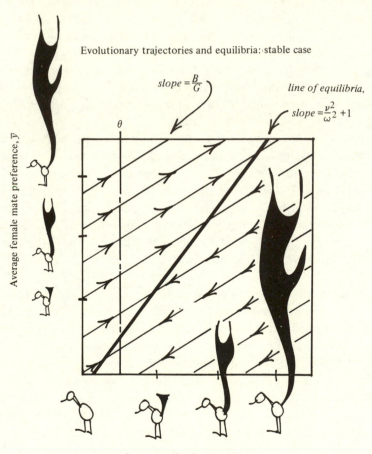

Evolutionary trajectories and equilibria: stable case

$slope = \dfrac{B}{G}$

line of equilibria,

$slope = \dfrac{\nu^2}{\omega^2} + 1$

θ

Average female mate preference, $\bar{y}$

Average male character, $\bar{z}$

gradually decelerates and finally stops evolving when it encounters any point along the line of equilibria (Fig. 4.7). The composition of the population at equilibrium is in large part a consequence of its starting position.

Furthermore, a population starting on the left side of the line of equilibria in Fig. 4.7 will experience a gradual elaboration of male tail size

Fig. 4.8. According to Lande's (1981) model, Fisher's runaway process of sexual selection is triggered when the genetic regression B/G (see Fig. 4.6) exceeds a critical value determined by the stereotypy of female mating preference, ν, and the strength of natural selection on male tail size, ω. When this condition is satisfied, populations will evolve away from the line of unstable equilibria, denoted by the heavy diagonal line, at ever increasing speed. Notice that male tail size might be exaggerated or diminished. Other conventions as in Fig. 4.7.

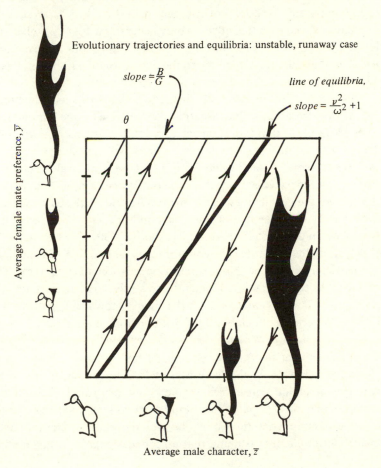

Evolutionary trajectories and equilibria: unstable, runaway case

$slope = \dfrac{B}{G}$

line of equilibria,

$slope = \dfrac{\nu^2}{\omega^2} + 1$

θ

Average female mate preference, $\bar{y}$

Average male character, $\bar{z}$

and female preference, but a population starting on the right side will actually evolve a smaller male tail size by sexual selection.

In general, the male tail size at equilibrium will not be the optimal size, θ, specified by natural selection. Notice in Fig. 4.7 that there is only one point of intersection between the line corresponding to the optimum, θ, and the line of equilibria. If we drew in contour lines on Fig. 4.7, connecting points with equal mean fitness, we would see a ridge along the vertical dashed line, θ, with mean fitness falling off on both the left and the right. Fig. 4.2 shows the ridge in cross-section but its width would be $\sqrt{(\omega^2 + \sigma^2)}$ rather than ω. (In general such adaptive topographies change with time when selection is frequency-dependent but, in the present case, since by assumption all females are inseminated, the effect of sexual selection is merely to distribute fitness among males without affecting mean fitness. Consequently only natural selection contributes to the adaptive topography and it does not change with time.) Whenever evolving populations pass over this ridge, as they generally will, they evolve towards lower average fitness, towards a state of maladaptation. It is even possible for sexual selection to contribute to the extinction of a population (Lande, 1980).

The sexual selection process can lead to stable or unstable equilibria. Fig. 4.7 illustrates the stable case. It is also possible for the line of equilibria to be unstable, so that evolution corresponds to Fisher's runaway process. This will happen when females have such strong, stereotyped mating preferences (small ν^2) and when there is such weak natural selection on the male character (large ω^2) that the slope of the line of equilibria ($[\nu^2/\omega^2] + 1$) is less than the genetic regression, B/G. When this is the case, populations evolve away from the line of unstable equilibria at ever increasing speed (Fig. 4.8). In direct confirmation of Fisher's (1930, 1958) account, Lande (1981) finds that the rates of evolution of male and female traits increase geometrically with time. Notice that a population starting above the line of unstable equilibria will accelerate towards large male tails while a population starting below the line will run away towards smaller tails. Thus Fisher's process could elaborate or diminish male attributes.

Evolutionary predictions. Four promising lines of research are suggested by Lande's (1981) sexual selection models. The models are predicted on variation in female mate choice, yet we know surprisingly little about such variation in natural populations. Many workers seem to have a typological attitude, assuming that there might be preferences of females for particular males, but implicitly assuming that all females concur in this preference, so that there is no variation. A full characterisation of female variation would require testing individual females so that their separate response curves can be specified. If the aim is to relate the results to sexual selection in nature, it is critical to offer females choices of natural, not artificial, variation in male phenotypes (e.g. natural variation in plumage, songs or pheromones). It may be practical to estimate response curves accurately by testing individual females with many simultaneous stimuli using, for example, multiple viewing chambers like those described by P. Bateson, in this volume. It is also important to relate behavioural responses of females in such a choice apparatus to actual mating inclination, since we want a behavioural indicator of actual mate choice. This could be accomplished in a separate experiment, in which females are given actual access to males, so that behavioural responses can be calibrated against mating responses.

The lack of actual data on the form of female mating response curves thwarts further development of sexual selection theory. We do not know whether female responses to particular attributes of males commonly are open-ended or unimodal. Statistical techniques for identifying the characters used by females in mate choice are described in a later section. Such statistical analysis of responses to a random sample of males from a particular natural population might be a useful precursor to detailed experimental work; assessments of this sort can quickly narrow the field of possible characters used in mate choice.

In addition to investigating the nature of variation in female mate choice a second line of research suggested by Lande's models concerns the prediction that a genetic correlation will arise between the sexes during sexual selection. This prediction can be directly tested in natural populations. Both polygenic and two-locus models indicate that the assortative aspect of mating in sexually selected populations should produce and maintain a genetic correlation between male character and female mate choice based on that character (O'Donald, 1980; Lande, 1981; Kirkpatrick, 1982). Thus genetic analysis emerges as an obvious step in studies of sexual selection. Such analysis requires the development of assays for female mate preference. One can then estimate the magnitude of genetic correlation between the two traits by calculating the regression of daughter's mate preference on father's character or from the regression of son's character of mother's mate choice. Alternatively, one can make character measurements in only a single generation; for example, by siring offspring from several females for each of a few dozen males and plotting the means of sons and daughters for each male as in Fig. 4.6. Falconer (1960) and

Bulmer (1980) discuss these and other estimation procedures. A design that permits the estimation of genic covariance beween the traits will usually also yield estimates of genic variances (or heritabilities).

The third prediction based on Lande's models is that the forces of sexual and natural selection will balance at genetic equilibrium. This prediction can be tested by actually measuring the forces of selection on characters. Measurements of this kind are most feasible using organisms with short life spans and non-overlapping generations since the estimation of the forces of selection is more complicated in age-structured populations. Estimation procedures are discussed by Arnold & Wade (MS), Lande & Arnold (MS) and in a later section.

Fourth, Lande's models predict very different evolutionary scenarios depending on whether there is direct selection of female preferences. In the case discussed above, there is no direct selection on female mating preferences. Species of this type (e.g., lek-breeding species and those with no paternal care of mates and offspring) should show extraordinary geographic variation in male attributes for several reasons:

(a) The evolutionary outcome is indeterminate (Figs. 4.7 and 4.8), so that the composition of the population at equilibrium depends on its starting point. Small differences in starting point can be amplified by sexual selection into large differences at equilibrium (Fig. 4.7). Such small differences in starting point could be produced by random drift or by geographic differences in natural selection.

(b) Once populations reach equilibrium, further diversification may occur by an interaction of drift and selection (Lande, 1981). Suppose, for example, that two populations lie close together on the equilibrium line in Fig. 4.7. If one population should drift a short way above the line, while the second drifts a short distance below the line, the male character will be elaborated in the first population and diminished in the second as they are driven by selection back towards the line of equilibria in opposite directions. Furthermore, once a population reaches the line of stable equilibria, there is no force impeding movement along the line. Again, drift can promote diversification by causing movement along the line. Drift due to sampling is not unlikely in sexually selected populations. Intense sexual selection (one or a few males siring most progeny) creates a small effective population size which encourages drift (Wright, 1931; Crow & Kimura, 1970).

(c) When many male characters are subject to female mate choice, a tremendous variety of evolutionary outcomes is possible. In the stable case there can be a hyperplane of possible equilibria, rather than the simple line of equilibria shown in Fig. 4.7 (Lande, 1981). A hyperplane of outcomes can arise either because females choose males using many criteria simultaneously or because one epoch of selection on one male character is later followed by an epoch of selection on other characters.

(d) Speciation as well as geographical variation, is promoted by sexual selection. Lande (1982*b*) has recently confirmed Fisher's (1930, 1958) suggestion that sexual selection arising from mate choice can cause parapatric speciation.

For all these reasons we can expect extraordinary diversity in courtship structures and behaviours in groups where only gametes are transferred to the female. The amazing radiations of birds of paradise and pheasants are probably products of sexual selection.

In contrast to this potential for diversification, Lande's models indicate that there will be much less variation in male attributes if males protect or provision their mates or offspring. In this case natural selection acts directly on female mating choices. The consequence is to change the equilibrium possibilities from a line, plane or hyperplane to a point, a single unique equilibrium (Lande, 1981). There still may be geographic variation in male attributes (e.g. the size of nuptial gift) but this would arise mainly from processes other than sexual selection and the variation would be less extreme. As in the case of pure sexual selection, there can be both stable and unstable cases. Thus, if female preferences are strong and if natural selection on the male character is weak, a Fisherian runaway process can occur even for characters, like size of nest revealed in prenuptial display, that affect the female's fitness directly. It is important to note that in species with male parental investment, Fisher's runaway process could operate (as described above) on male characters that do not influence male parental care.

The origin and cessation of Fisher's runaway process. Fisher (1958) discussed an origin for his runaway process in which a male trait was initially favoured by both natural and sexual selection. Subsequent work indicates that the process can be triggered under a broader class of conditions. Preferences can evolve and the runaway process may be initiated even when there is no directional force of natural selection on the male attribute (Kirkpatrick, 1982; Heisler, MS).

What is the fate of a population experiencing Fisher's runaway process? No limits to the process are specified in Lande's (1981) model. Fisher (1930, 1958) suggested that a stable limit might be achieved once natural selection against extravagant male characters balances the sexual selection that favours them. Lande (1981) has pointed out that the fitness of males must fall off faster than a Gaussian curve, of the type shown in Fig. 4.2, in order to stop the runaway. Such Gaussian curves produce a restraining force of natural selection that is proportional to the deviation of the population mean from the optimum and such linear forces are insufficient to halt the runaway. Another possibility, also suggested by Fisher (1930, 1958), is that the survivorship of males may become so low that some females with extreme mating preferences fail to find a mate, and this selection directly on female mating preferences may stop the runaway process.

Panglossian females, 'Good genes' and genetic variance for fitness

In contrast to the Darwinian and Fisherian views of sexual selection, the Panglossian view imagines that females always employ adaptive criteria in mate choice. The essential features of this position can be seen most clearly in the case where females receive no direct or immediate benefit from mate choice, as in lek-breeding species. According to the Panglossian view, the 'good genes' of the female's mate might indirectly benefit the female by promoting the fitness of her progeny. The female is likened to a shopper in a supermarket, striving to bring home the best genes for her family. There is competition among shoppers for the best genes and eventually the best shopper prevails in the population. According to the metaphor of the Panglossian female, females using arbitrary, non-adaptive criteria for mate choice will be replaced in evolutionary time by females using the most direct, failsafe indicators of male fitness and hence of good genes. Rigorous formulations of the sexual selection process indicate that these conclusions often may be erroneous.

The Panglossian view of sexual selection leads to indefensible conclusions for two major reasons:

First, there is no guarantee that sexual selection will promote adaptation in the population. Because the mating success of male phenotypes varies both with the frequency of other male phenotypes and with the ensemble of females choosing mates, sexual selection is frequency-dependent. In general, fitness is not maximised when selection is frequency-dependent; nor is inclusive fitness maximised (Wright, 1969; Crow & Kimura, 1970; Lewontin, 1974). Consequently there is no theoretical justification for the optimism that females will arrive at the most adaptive criteria for mate choice. Moreover, there is an irony to supposing that females use only adaptive criteria: Darwin originally proposed the concept of sexual selection to explain structures that were maladaptive under natural selection. Especially in species with no male parental care, we expect equilibrium populations to settle below adaptive peaks, rather than on top of them, so that the mate most preferred by females is actually suboptimal or maladaptive (Lande, 1981; Kirkpatrick, 1982).

The vulnerability of populations to maladaptive evolution by sexual selection has recently been illustrated by Kirkpatrick (1982). He shows with genetic models that even when males are maladaptive at equilibrium, due to sexual selection exerted by females, there is no inherent tendency for more adaptive female preferences to evolve. Indeed there seems to be no known mechanism operating within populations that can unfailingly rescue populations from maladaptation promoted by sexual selection (Lande, 1980; Kirkpatrick, 1982). However, if the maladaptation induced by sexual selection is so severe that it enhances the possibility of local extinction then selection among leks or demes may lessen regional maladaptation.

Second, it is misleading to imagine a selective force on female mating preference if the social system involves only transfer of gametes by males. Under these circumstances the most manageable theoretical formulation is to describe the evolution of female mating preferences as a correlated response to selection (Lande, 1981; Kirkpatrick, 1982). Since the number of progeny produced by the female is unaffected by her mate choice, there is no immediate cost or benefit, no direct force of selection on mating preferences. This formulation follows the tradition in population genetics of tallying fitness by simply counting the number of progeny produced by a particular zygote (Crow & Kimura, 1970). The value of this approach is that inheritance can be cleanly separated from fitness (or selection) in equations for evolutionary change. Thus the circumstance that the sons of females exerting mate choice might experience higher than average mating success is best treated as an issue of inheritance (the genic regression that enables us to predict son's phenotype from mother's phenotype). An alternative but less manageable approach (the so called 'sexy-son' approach) is to tally the fitness of females by counting grandchildren or great-grandchildren. This practice appears logical since females exerting mate choice might produce an above average number of grandchildren through their sexually superior sons. Unfortunately this mode of fitness accounting does not permit a precise dynamical formulation since it confounds selection and inheritance. A further logical difficulty with the tallying of distant descendants is that there is no obvious stopping point. Should we tally great-great-great grandchildren?

Thus recent theoretical results yield a new perspective on the question 'What does the female of lek-breeding species get out of mate choice?' Quite possibly she gets nothing. This is an excellent hypothesis for empirical work not only because of its strong theoretical justification but because it can be unambiguously falsified. Bradbury & Gibson (this volume) report that there is currently no evidence for selection on female choice in any lek species. In order to test rigorously for selection on female choice one would need to determine the statistical relationship between the relative fitness of sexually-mature females (number of progeny divided by the population mean) and female mate choice. This would be no small undertaking. Although several investigators have successfully measured fitness in natural populations of birds, for example (e.g. McGregor, Krebs & Perrins, 1981; van Noordwijk, van Balen & Sharloo, 1981; Smith, 1981) female mate choice may be even more difficult to measure. The most informative approach would be to score the mating tendencies of individual females under standardised conditions, as well as in the field, to yield a multivariate characterisation of female mate preference (see later section). Once female mate choice has been characterised and measured the most appropriate measure of selection is the selection gradient or partial regression of female relative fitness on each mate choice variable (Lande & Arnold, MS; Lande, 1979; Arnold & Wade, MS). If female mate choice is selectively neutral then these partial regressions should approach zero within the limits of sampling error.

Partridge's (1980) elegant experiment with *Drosophila* should not be construed as a test for selection on female choice, and she does not attach this interpretation to her results. Partridge found that the progeny of females that had free access to mating partners were superior in larval competition to the progeny of females that were assigned mates at random. Thus Partridge performed artificial selection on female mate choice and detected a correlated response to this selection in larval competitive ability. This clever experiment suggests that there may be heritable variation for one component of fitness (larval competitive ability) and there may be a genetic correlation between this component and some sexually selected attribute (Partridge, 1980). The experiment does not indicate whether there was any natural variation in the mate choice behaviour of females nor does it demonstrate natural selection on female choice.

'*Good genes*'. The concept of 'good genes' has produced much confusion in discussion of sexual selection. The argument is often made that females are selected to prefer males with genes that produce a phenotype that is optimal for survival and male combat. By the use of such reasoning (e.g. Trivers, 1972) one is forced to maintain that all sexually dimorphic characters, no matter how extravagant, are optimal for survival and combat. However, this argument is fallacious because it ignores the fact that mating preferences, once established, constitute a selective force in their own right. 'Good genes' must then be defined with respect to total fitness, which is composed of both survivorship *and* mating success. Female mating preferences also figure in the determination of 'good genes'. Thus suppose that the evolution of mating preferences has produced a population with an extreme male trait that is deleterious for survival but is strongly preferred by females. This condition can be a stable evolutionary equilibrium for the following reason: a rare female genotype that chooses to mate with a male phenotype that is optimal for survival will produce sons that resemble their father in having high survivorship, but they will go unmated (if there is no inbreeding) since most females prefer males with an exaggerated phenotype. Males with the optimal phenotype for survival may be ignored by females. Thus the metaphor of females 'shopping for good genes' must be used very carefully, if it is used at all. If the potentially conflicting forces of mate choice and survivorship are ignored, the metaphor can easily lead to erroneous conclusions.

Genetic variance for fitness. Williams (1975, 1978) and Maynard Smith (1978*a*) have argued that the tendency for genic variance in total fitness to vanish at genetic equilibrium presents a serious difficulty for the maintenance of female mate choice behaviour. The expectation of no heritable fitness variation at equilibrium is a corollary of Fisher's (1930, 1958) fundamental theorem: the rate of evolutionary change in mean fitness equals the genic variance in fitness. Thus when there is no change in mean fitness (fitness equilibrium), there must be no heritable fitness variance. If there is no male contribution to the female besides gametes, as in lek-breeding species, then 'a female who selects as a mate a male of high fitness does not increase the expected fitness of her own offspring' (Maynard Smith, 1978*a*), because there can be no heritability of fitness at equilibrium. This is, however, not a serious difficulty for several reasons: (1) The absence of selection of female preference at equilibrium cannot be construed as a problem because female mate choice can be maintained, and even evolve, in the absence of any direct selection on mate preference (Lande, 1981; Kirkpatrick, 1982). (2) Even equilibrium populations may be vulnerable to episodes of evolution driven by the sexual selection exerted by females (Heisler, MS). (3) Zero genic variance in fitness is a most precarious equilibrium. For example, mate choice can actually produce genic variance in male fitness. Imagine a population in evolutionary equilibrium with the mean of some heritable male attribute at an optimum specified by natural selection. Now if the net preferences of females for males with extreme values of this attribute should shift, for any reason, so that a net force of sexual selection is exerted on the male character, this shift will *create* genic variance in total male fitness. This can happen because fitness itself is a function of mating success and other fitness components. Because fitness is a complex variable, even when there is no heritable variance in total fitness, there may be heritable variance in any or all of its components (Lande, 1982*a*). Consequently a change in the balance among the heritable components of fitness can change the genic variance in total fitness. Thus an increase in genic variance for mating success can create genic variance in total fitness where none existed. We might expect equilibrium populations to vacillate between production and erosion of heritable fitness variance but not to exist long without it. Finally, as Lande (1976) showed, there may be an appreciable input to genic variance in fitness each generation from polygenic mutation and recombination.

The analysis of selection: a special case of the analysis of variance

Many enigmatic aspects of selection can be understood by breaking selection into its component parts. Crow (1958) showed how this can be done. He noted that the expression for the change in mean fitness each generation is mathematically equivalent to the product of fitness heritability and the variance in relative fitness.* He called the variance in relative fitness the intensity of or opportunity for selection, since it limits the rate of evolution. When there are no differences in fitness, there is no selection; when there are great differences in fitness, there is great opportunity for selection. The fact that selection can be formally represented by a variance is important. Armed with Crow's insight that the opportunity for selection is proportional to variance in fitness, we can see that many conceptual problems involving selection can be treated as problems in analysis of variance. The sexual difference in variability of reproductive success is the first of several such problems that are considered in the next few sections.

---

* The variance in relative fitness can be calculated by dividing the absolute fitness of each individual (the number of progeny surviving to the age of the parents) by the average absolute fitness and taking the variance of these relative measures. A simpler method is to divide the variance in absolute fitness by the square of average absolute fitness.

The intensity of selection on males and females

Bateman (1948) showed that the fitness of *Drosophila* males was more variable than female fitness. He found that this sexual difference in fitness variance was largely due to the fact that mating success was more variable in males than in females. He suggested that this basis of sexual difference in fitness variances should hold in many plants and animals.

The explicit relationship between fitness variances of males and females can be readily derived for many social systems. A first step is to note that there always will be a simple relationship between the mean fitness of males and females. This is because in sexual species each offspring has exactly one mother and one father. Consequently the total number of progeny produced by females must equal the total produced by males. When the breeding sex ratio (number of adult males/number of adult females) is unity these totals are each divided by the same number of parents to give the mean number of progeny per sex: in this case, the means are the same. When the sex ratio is R, the progeny totals are still the same but the mean fitness of females will be R times the mean fitness of males (Fisher, 1930). This last relationship is general and holds irrespective of the breeding system. The fact that the frequency distributions of fitness for males and females are tied together by this simple relationship in means suggests that they might also be coupled by a relationship in variances. This turns out to be true, but the form of the relationship changes, often markedly, with the social system.

In many social systems the male variance in reproductive success will be greater than the female variance as a mathematical necessity (Wade & Arnold, 1980). In the present discussion the units for reproductive success (total fitness) are numbers of progeny and the units for mating success are numbers of mates bearing progeny. For example, consider social systems in which there is no correspondence between the mating success of males and the per capita fertility of their mates and in which all the progeny of a female have the same sire. Under these conditions the total variance in the relative reproductive success of males, I_m, is equal to the variance in the relative reproductive success of females, I_f, times the sex ratio, plus the male variance in relative mating success, I_s,

$$I_m = RI_f + I_s$$

The three terms representing variances in relative fitness can also be viewed as opportunities for selection. Thus the opportunity for selection on males will often exceed the opportunity for selection on females because of sexual selection on males, I_s, just as Bateman (1948) argued.

There are two prevalent misunderstandings about the sexual relationship in fitness variances or selection opportunities discussed by Wade (1979) and Wade & Arnold (1980). The first error is to suppose that the results depend on an assumption of normality. This is not the case. The analysis of variance used in the derivation of the results does not depend on normality of distribution. (Analysis of variance is usually not applied to data that depart markedly from normality, but this is because the F ratio used in significance testing is predicated on normally distributed errors; the analysis itself is perfectly valid, irrespective of normality.) Even though fitness and its components commonly show non-normal distributions, variance is still the most useful measure of dispersion because of its key role in equations for evolutionary change.

A second misunderstanding concerns the goal of the analysis. The aim is not to claim that nature always fits the assumptions of a particular model, but rather to find mathematical guides to empirical work. For example, male mating success may be correlated with the average fertility of mates and when this is true we require a formulation more complicated than the one just given. Thus if the correlation is positive (say, because more fertile females are attracted to or monopolised by the most sexually successful males) then the male variance will generally exceed the female reproductive variance because there will be a positive covariance term added on to the right side of the expression above. But if the correlation is negative (say, because of a trade off between males resources expended on mating and on offspring) then male variance might be less than female variance (Wade, 1979). Results such as these can simplify field work by directing attention to crucial issues such as covariances between mating and parental success. As another example, consider polyandrous breeding systems.

It is commonly supposed that sexual selection is more intense among females in polyandrous breeding systems (e.g. seahorses and other syn-gnathid fish, some dendrobatid frogs, phalaropes). If we characterise selection using variance analysis, we can see how to test this proposition. The analysis is particularly straightforward if the breeding success of each and every adult male is monopolised by particular females. A first goal in field studies might be to see if this is so. If it is, and if the mating success of females is uncorrelated with their brood size per mate, then we can use the above formulation and simply reverse the sexual labels. The opportunity for sexual selection on females is then the variance in relative number of males that sire their broods, and one could reasonably argue that there is no sexual selection on males. If both males and females can have multiple mates then one must actually calculate the variances in relative mating success to see which sex experiences the most intense sexual selection.

Comparing the intensities of natural and sexual selection

It is useful to measure the separate forces of natural and sexual selection so that they can be compared. For example, one might want to test the hypothesis that a particular sexually dimorphic character is at equilibrium due to a balance between the opposing forces of natural and sexual selection. Or one might suppose that a particular structure is favoured by both sexual and natural selection and the question is which force predominates. Howard's (1979) exemplary study of mating dynamics in a Bullfrog (*Rana catesbeiana*) population illustrates a problem of the latter kind.

Howard (1979) suggested that large male body size might be favoured for three reasons in a Bullfrog population: (a) larger males tended to mate with more females (sexual selection); (b) larger males sired larger clutches because they tended to mate with larger females which laid larger clutches (a kind of natural selection); and, finally, (c) larger males controlled territories with fewer predators and better temperatures for egg development, so their progeny's hatching success might be higher than average (another kind of natural selection).

The key in analysing this and similar problems is to realise that the total fitness of an individual can be represented as a product of fitness components (Arnold & Wade, MS). In the case of a male Bullfrog, total fitness (not total lifetime fitness, but the fitness that can be measured during a breeding season) is the total number of eggs that hatch (since tadpoles disperse shortly after hatching, it was not practical for Howard to tally later components of fitness). This total number of hatching eggs is the product of three observed fitness components: (a) the number of mates that spawn with the male (mating success); (b) the average number of eggs laid per mate (average mate fertility); and (c) the production of eggs that survive to hatching (offspring survivorship). Since Howard measured the size of each male Bullfrog, it is possible to calculate the force of selection on male size exerted by each of the three fitness components as well as the total force. The results are shown graphically in Fig. 4.9. In the Bullfrog data it turned out that sexual selection was responsible for most of the selection on male size; forces of natural selection acting through differences in mate fertility and offspring survivorship were not statistically significant. The predominant effect of sexual selection is revealed by the large shift in the size distribution of males that can be attributed to differences in mating success (Fig. 4.9, top).

Such shifts in mean are called *selection differentials*; they play a key role in equations that predict evolutionary change. In order to see the

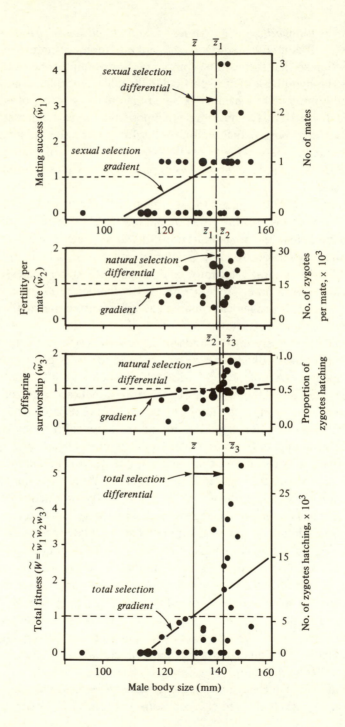

relationship between the selection differential and evolution, it is necessary to review some recent developments in quantitative genetics.

We require information about inheritance in order to predict evolution (the response to selection that occurs across generations), but selection itself is a purely phenotypic event and no knowledge of genetics is required to measure its immediate effects, within generations. When selection acts only on a single character, one that shows neither phenotypic nor genetic correlations with other characters, we can readily predict how much evolution will occur just by knowing the heritability of the character and the selection differential: the expected change in mean from one generation to the next is simply the product of heritability and the selection differential (Falconer, 1960). The measure of selection that figures in the equation is purely phenotypic: the shift in average character value or the difference in means measured before and after selection.

Multivariate selection. Most evolutionists and behaviourists, however, are concerned with selection as it occurs in nature: selection acting simultaneously on many characters that may be intercorrelated. In order to predict evolutionary response to such multivariate selection, we must know more than heritabilities and selection differentials (Falconer, 1960; Robertson, 1968). We must also know the patterns of genetic and phenotypic correlation among characters (Lande, 1979). The complication introduced by phenotypic character correlations is the easiest to visualise. A selection differential, or shift in mean within a generation, may occur either because selection has acted directly on the character (*direct selection*) or because selection has acted on a correlated character and indirectly induced a shift in mean (*indirect selection*) (Pearson, 1903). Thus, in the

Fig. 4.9. An analysis of selection on male body size in a Bullfrog (*Rana catesbeiana*) population studied by Howard (1979) and reanalysed by Arnold & Wade (MS). Each data point represents the mating success (top panel), average mate fertility (second panel from top), offspring survivorship (third panel from top) and total fitness (bottom panel) of a particular male Bullfrog. In each panel relative fitness is shown on the left-hand scale and absolute fitness is shown on the right-hand scale. Mean fitnesses are shown with horizontal dashed lines. The total shift in the mean size of males ($\bar{z}_3 - \bar{z}$) within a breeding season, the total selection differential, can be partitioned into three parts corresponding to the effects of sexual selection (top panel) and natural selection (middle and bottom panels). Likewise, the total, univariate selection gradient (the regression of total relative fitness of male body size) can be partitioned into three additive parts corresponding to sexual selection and two kinds of natural selection.

case of Howard's Bullfrogs, the total selection differential on male body size (illustrated in Fig. 4.9) may represent indirect selection on characters correlated with body size as well as direct selection on body size. For example, female mate choice based on loudness of mating call could have caused the observed shift in average male body size if larger males called louder (indirect selection on size); however, some of the selection differential may have been due to actual size advantages (direct selection on size).

When only a single phenotypic character is measured, it is impossible to tell whether selection has acted on that character or on a phenotypically correlated character. It is only possible to separate the direct and indirect effects of selection by measuring the selection differentials of a set of characters and correctly accounting for their phenotypic intercorrelations. The measure of selection that accomplishes this task is the *selection gradient*, which is equal to the partial regression of relative fitness on the character, holding all other characters constant (Lande, 1979; Lande & Arnold MS). The selection gradient measures only the direct force of selection on the character, whereas the selection differential measures both the direct and indirect forces of selection. The selection gradient on each character can be readily calculated from the table or matrix of phenotypic correlations (or from covariances) and selection differentials. This is because Robertson (1966) showed that selection differentials are mathematically equivalent to covariances between relative fitness and the character, irrespective of the form of selection.

Selection is not evolution. In order to predict how a character will evolve we must know the magnitude of genetic coupling with other characters as well as the selection gradients on each character. Genetic coupling, properly known as *additive genetic or genic covariance*, can arise from pleiotropy (particular genetic loci affect two or more characters) or from linkage. The genic covariance between two characters can be estimated by regressing the values of one character in the offspring on the values of another character in their parents (e.g. Fig. 4.5; Falconer, 1960). The consequence is that, when selection acts on one character, it can cause evolution in other characters that are genetically correlated with it. Thus the expected evolution of a character will be due both to direct selection on that character (acting on its additive genetic variance) and to direct selection on other characters (acting through additive genetic covariances). This can be expressed mathematically by defining three terms: (1) let β_{wz_i} represent the selection gradient, or direct force of selection, on character z_i; (2) let G_{11} represent the genic or additive genetic variance for character

z_1, and (3) let G_{1i} represent the genic covariance between x_1 and character z_i. Lande (1979) shows that the expected change (across one generation) in the mean value of the character, z_1, is

$$\Delta \bar{z}_1 = G_{11}\beta_{wz_1.} + G_{12}\beta_{wz_2.} + G_{13}\beta_{wz_3.} + \ldots + G_{1k}\beta_{wz_k.}.$$

The term $G_{11}\beta_{wz_1.}$ represents the contribution of selection on the character to its own evolution, while the other terms represent the contributions through genetically correlated characters. These latter contributions are known as *correlated responses to selection* on other characters (Falconer, 1960). Notice that the genic covariances could be negative and that the selection gradients on the characters may differ in sign. Because of this, it is possible for a character to evolve in the opposite direction from the direct force of selection acting on it. This can happen if the correlated responses to selection swamp the direct response to selection.

These points can be made more tangible with the Bullfrog example. We wish to predict the evolution of male body size from the observed selection differential on size (a differential which summarises the observation that large males leave more progeny during a breeding season). The first problem, already discussed, is that we need to account for the phenotypic correlations among characters. Let us suppose that we have solved this problem by measuring a variety of characters on each male, as well as reproductive success, so that we can calculate the selection gradients, $\beta_{wz_i.}$. Let $\beta_{wz_1.}$ represent the selection gradient on male body size* and let G_{11} be the additive genetic variance of body size. We cannot predict the amount of evolution in body size merely by taking the product of genic variance for body size and the selection gradient, $G_{11}\beta_{wz_1.}$. Suppose, for example, that call loudness, z_2, also has a direct positive effect on mating success, so that $\beta_{wz_2.}$ is positive. If there is a positive genic covariance between male body size and call loudness (e.g. because some loci affect variation in both male characters), then male body size will also evolve because of a correlated response to direct selection on call loudness, $G_{12}\beta_{wz_2.}$. Now, suppose that pulse rate of the male's call, z_3, also has a direct effect on mating success (thus accounting for the selection gradient, $\beta_{wz_3.}$), but

---

* If the axes in Fig. 4.9 actually were the residual values of relative fitness and body size holding all other characters besides male body size constant, then the illustrated repressions would actually be the desired, multivariate selection gradients. Although the linear regressions of relative mating success and of total fitness on male body size in Fig. 4.9 appear to give poor fits to these data, the slopes of these lines are nevertheless the desired selection gradients. Curvilinear regressions would give better fits to these data but the linear terms in such equations would be identical to the ones graphed in Fig. 4.9 (Lande & Arnold, MS).

that this character has negative genic covariance, G_{13}, with body size: the sons of larger males tend to have slower pulse rates, for example because loci with positive effects on body size tend to have negative effects on pulse rate. It is even possible that the correlated response to selection on pulse rate, $G_{13}\beta_{wz_3}$, is so large that it swamps out both the direct response to selection on size and the correlated response to selection on call loudness and other characters. Thus the population might evolve towards a smaller male body size even though selection actually favours larger males each generation!

This example, of course, was contrived to illustrate the worst evolutionary prediction that can be made with purely phenotypic data. The basic point is that 'natural selection is not evolution' (Fisher, 1958: vii): evolution cannot be predicted from measures of selection only. Nevertheless, there are many valid questions that can be answered with data on selection. Is male body size under sexual selection? Is large size also favoured by natural selection? Another series of questions deals with the analysis of variance in fitness itself. Here again we encounter the issue of correlation in the form of *co-intensities or covariances between fitness components*.

The analysis of fitness variance. The total opportunity for selection, or the total variance in relative fitness, can be broken down into segments corresponding to different episodes of selection. This analysis breaks down the total opportunity for selection but does not address the issue of how much selection acts on any particular character. However, one advantage of the analysis is that it does not depend on character measurements. Unlike the estimates of selection gradients, it is insensitive to the particular sample of phenotypic characters that were measured. The essential points are easier to grasp with an example, such as Howard's (1979) study of selection in Bullfrogs, reanalysed by Arnold & Wade (MS).

We can partition the total selection opportunity, or fitness variance, in Howard's Bullfrog population into three parts corresponding to sexual selection (mating success) and two types of natural selection (variances in fertility of mates and in offspring survivorship). In general these three selection opportunities will not add up to the total because of covariances between them. For example, in Howard's (1979) data there was a positive covariance between the total number of eggs laid in a male's territory ($w_1 w_2$) and the average fertility of his mates (w_2). This positive association may have been caused by a tendency for larger, more fecund females to be attracted to territories where eggs had already been laid. But whatever the causes of this covariance, $COI_{12,2}$, it accounted for 13% of the total opportunity for selection on males (Table 4.1) and was more important than either natural selection exerted through mate fertility, I_2, or through offspring survivorship, I_3. The three other co-intensities in Table 4.1 were of minor importance but they each have biological interpretations. For example, $COI_{1,2}$ measures the tendency of sexually successful males to mate with the most fecund females. If this covariance were negative, it would have indicated a trade off between mating success and mate fertility. The other two co-intensities, $COI_{12,3}$ and $COI_{123,3}$, measure respectively the statistical trends between the male's total count of eggs or tadpoles and his offspring survivorship rate. There is certainly no indication that hatching rate is depressed in large egg masses, say due to crowding; it may have been slightly enhanced.

Triver's (1972) concept of parental investment is an important example of a selection co-intensity. In Trivers' argument there is a trade off between current parental effort per offspring and future fertility. This often may

Table 4.1. *Partitioning of the total opportunity for selection on a reproductive population of male Bullfrogs* (Rana catesbeiana) *studied by Howard (1979), and reanalysed by Arnold & Wade (MS)*

Source of variance in fitness	Contribution to total opportunity for selection		
	Symbol	Value	Percentage
Sexual selection (number of mates, w_1)	I_1	1.382	59
Natural selection (number of eggs per mate, w_2)	I_2	0.212	9
Natural selection (offspring survivorship, w_3)	I_3	0.160	7
Covariance between number of mates (w_1) and number of eggs per mate (w_2)	$COI_{1,2}$	0.081	3
Covariance between total number of eggs ($w_1 w_2$) and number of eggs per mate (w_2)	$COI_{12,2}$	0.312	13
Covariance between total number of eggs ($w_1 w_2$) and offspring survivorship (w_3)	$COI_{12,3}$	0.032	1
Covariance between total number of eggs that hatch (= number of tadpoles, $w_1 w_2 w_3$) and offspring survivorship (w_3)	$COI_{123,2}$	0.150	6
Total selection (number of tadpoles, $w_1 w_2 w_3$)	I_T	2.238	100

be present since most parents have limited resources to expend on reproduction and survival. In the analysis of fitness variance, parental investment (along with other covariances between fitness components), is represented by a co-intensity (Arnold & Wade, MS). This is certainly not a cause of sexual selection and Trivers' (1972) definition of parental investment as the 'single variable controlling sexual selection' is misleading. Parental investment is but one of many co-intensities that contribute to overall selection. Furthermore, the intensity of sexual selection can vary independently of parental investment (Wade, 1979), and the evolutionary effect of parental investment will be exerted through the additive genetic version of the covariance and not by the more readily observed phenotypic covariance (Lande, 1982a).

Partitioning sexual selection

Many puzzling aspects of sexual selection can be resolved by focusing on its separate aspects (Arnold & Wade, MS; Arnold & Houck, 1982). We can, for example, break down mating success (number of mates bearing progeny) into parts due to separate phases: winning combat with other males, encounter with females, insemination success and paternity. Mating success, w_m, can be represented as a product of fitness components corresponding to these four phases (e.g. $w_m = w_c w_e w_s w_p$). A trait may affect one or more of these components of mating success. For example, Waage (1979) has described a genital device in male Damselflies that is used to extract the spermatophores of rival males from the female's tract as a prelude to mating. Presumably the elaboration of this device affected the conditional probability of paternity, but probably no other aspect of mating success.

Sexual selection through male combat and female mate choice. Darwin (1859, 1871) and Fisher (1930, 1958) emphasised the common features of sexual selection exerted by male combat and female choice. Most modern authors stress the distinction between them and complain about the difficulty in separating their effects. In general, it will be difficult to ascribe a particular structure of behaviour to evolution by sexual selection exerted through mates or rivals. The separation may be possible, however, in some experimental situations and sometimes in the field.

We can distinguish the effects of female choice from those of male combat if we carefully arrange a sequence of encounters and measurements. Whether this distorts the social biology of the population will depend on the peculiarities of the species and the inventiveness of the investigator.

It is possible to separate statistically the effects of the two kinds of selection if they are separated in time. This is accomplished in two experimental phases: a combat phase followed by a mate choice phase. Before the first phase, a series of behavioural and morphological characters are measured in each sex. These characters are chosen so as to include the most likely candidates for effects on combat or mating success. During the combat phase, the aim is to assign to each male a value, achieved from combat with as many males as possible, that predicts as accurately as possible his relative success in winning combat, w_c. Success in male combat (or, more properly, male-male encounter since bluffing may be the form of interaction) could be tallied from a design that rotates males among opponents in a random order, perhaps with replication of the opponent list or sequence. The difficult problem of ranking or scaling males by combat outcome is discussed by Boyd & Silk (MS). With this accomplished we begin the mate choice phase.

We desire a randomised sequence of encounters between mates that gives good estimates of male and female mating successes as well as interaction terms describing the complementarity of mating partners. If the females can mate with many males (as in some fish and salamanders) then both sexes can be assigned a sequence of mates using Latin Square or other designs. Our principal concern is with the relative insemination success of the males, w_s, holding constant by design the probability of mate encounter. From this, and from the combat success, we can calculate the forces of selection exerted by combat and mate choice. The contribution of each feature in males (e.g. antler size, running speed, body size) to combat success is measured as the partial regression of relative combat success on the character, holding all other characters constant: this is the *combat selection gradient* that measures the direct force of selection, accounting for character intercorrelation, $\beta_{w_c z_i.}$. Likewise we can calculate the partial regression of relative insemination success on the character: this is the *mate selection gradient*, measuring the independent contribution of each character, z_i, to success in mate choice, $\beta_{w_s z_i.}$. These can be calculated so that they sum to the total force of sexual selection on the character (Arnold & Wade, MS).

A standard multiple regression equation sets expected relative insemination success equal to a sum of contributions from separate characters,

$$\overline{w}_s = \beta_{w_s z_1.}\bar{z}_1 + \beta_{w_s z_2.}\bar{z}_2 + \ldots + \beta_{w_s z_k.}\bar{z}_k$$

where $\bar{z}_i$ is the population mean of a particular character and $\beta_{w_s z_i.}$ is the corresponding mate selection gradient or partial regression. Each mate selection gradient represents the amount that insemination success is enhanced by a unit increase in a particular character. If mating success given encounter with the female is wholly controlled by the female, rather than by physical overpowering by the male, then the mate selection gradients can be construed as the weights attached to each male character by the average female during the mate choice process (the terms, $\beta_{w_s z_i} . \bar{z}_i$, give the average contributions of the characters to insemination success). Thus, in a hypothetical lek-breeding bird, $\beta_{w_s z_1} . = 0$ indicates that the first character, say eyebrow size, has no effect on mating success, whereas a positive value of $\beta_{w_s z_2} .$ indicates that a second hypothetical character, z_2, or tail size has a positive effect on mate choice. These effects, $\beta_{w_s z_i} .$, can be added to the combat selection gradients to give the total force of sexual selection on each character (Arnold & Wade, MS).

The interaction between the combat and mate choice phases of sexual selection could be evaluated with an analysis of fitness variance. We can calculate the separate intensities of combat and mate selection. The total opportunity for selection includes also two co-intensities representing the correlation between combat and mating success (Arnold & Wade, MS). When these co-intensities are zero, or nearly zero, either there is no overlap in the sets of characters effective in combat or mate choice, or their effects cancel. When the co-intensities are positive and large, some characters are effective in both combat and mate choice. Negative co-intensities would describe the enigmatic result that losers in male combat are the most successful in mate choice. Thus the co-intensities provide a convenient way to test for correspondence between combat and mate choice phases of sexual selection.

Summary

1 Darwin's distinction between natural and sexual selection can be formulated in statistical terms that permit measurement of the two processes. Sexual selection arises from variance in mating success whereas natural selection arises from variance in other components of fitness (e.g. survivorship, fertility of mates).

2 Dynamic models of sexual selection with polygenic inheritance confirm the possibility of Fisher's runaway process: male characters and female mating preferences based on those characters can advance together at ever increasing speed. Alternatively, there may be many possible evolutionary outcomes, but no runaway process. The nature of the process depends on genetic parameters, the form of and variation in female mating preferences and the restraining force of natural selection.

3 Because sexual selection is frequency-dependent, there is no theoretical justification for the opinion that females will always employ adaptive criteria in mate choice.

4 The mathematical relationship between male and female variances in reproductive success can be specified for particular breeding systems. Such analyses confirm Bateman's supposition that sexual selection will often be the cause of greater reproductive variance in males.

5 It is possible to break down the total force of selection on particular characters into parts due to natural and to sexual selection.

6 In some situations it may be possible to identify the male attributes used by females in mate choice and to distinguish advantage conferred in mate choice and in male combat.

I am grateful to C. Boake, P. Harvey, L. Heisler, L. Houck, M. Kirkpatrick, R. Lande and M. Wade for their comments on the manuscript. This work was supported by NSF Grants BNS 80-14151 and by PHS Grant 1 KO4 HD00392-01.

References

Arnold, S. J. & Houck, L. (1982). Courtship pheromones: evolution by natural and sexual selection. In *Biochemical Aspects of Evolutionary Biology*, ed. M. Nitecki, pp. 173–211. University of Chicago Press: Chicago.

Arnold, S. J. & Wade, M. J. (MS). On the measurement of natural and sexual selection. *Evolution* (in revision).

Bateman, A. J. (1948). Intra-sexual selection in *Drosophila. Heredity*, **2**, 349–68.

Borgia, G. (1979). Sexual selection and the evolution of mating systems. In *Sexual Selection and Reproductive Competition in Insects*, ed. M. S. Blum & N. A. Blum, pp. 19–80. Academic Press: New York.

Boyd, R. & Silk, J. (MS). A method for assigning cardinal dominance rank.

Bulmer, M. (1980). *The Mathematical Theory of Quantitative Genetics*. Oxford University Press: Oxford.

Crow, J. F. (1958). Some possibilities for measuring selection intensities in man. *Human Biology*, **30**, 1–13.

Crow, J. & Kimura, M. (1970). *Introduction to Population Genetics Theory*. Harper and Row: New York.

Darwin, C. (1859). *The Origin of Species by Means of Natural Selection or the Preservation of Favoured Races in the Struggle for Life*. John Murray: London.

Darwin, C. (1871). *The Descent of Man and Selection in Relation to Sex*. John Murray: London.

Downhower, J. F. & Brown, L. (1980). Mate preferences of female mottled sculpins, *Cottus bairdi. Animal Behaviour*, **28**, 778–34.

Falconer, D. S. (1960). *Introduction to Quantitative Genetics*. Ronald Press: New York.

Fisher, R. A. (1915). The evolution of sexual preference. *Eugenics Review*, **7**, 184–92.

Fisher, R. A. (1918). The correlation between relatives on the supposition of Mendelian inheritance. *Transactions of the Royal Society of Edinburgh*, **52**, 399–433.

Fisher, R. A. (1930). *The Genetical Theory of Natural Selection*. Oxford University Press: Oxford.

Fisher, R. A. (1958). *The Genetical Theory of Natural Selection*. Dover: New York.

Ghiselin, M. T. (1974). *The Economy of Nature and the Evolution of Sex*. University of California Press: Berkeley.

Halliday, T. (1978). Sexual selection and mate choice. In *Behavioural Ecology, an Evolutionary Approach*, ed. J. R. Krebs & N. B. Davies, pp. 180–213. Sinauer Associates: Sunderland, Mass.

Heisler, I. L. (MS). A quantitative genetic model for the origin of mating preferences. *Evolution* (submitted).

Howard, R. D. (1979). Estimating reproductive success in natural populations. *American Naturalist*, **114**, 221–31.

Kirkpatrick, M. (1982). Sexual selection and the evolution of female choice. *Evolution*, **36**, 1–12.

Kluge, A. G. (1981). The life history, social organization, and parental behavior of *Hyla rosenbergi* Boulenger, a nest-building gladiator frog. *Miscellaneous Publications of the Museum of Zoology, University of Michigan*, **160**, 1–170.

Lande, R. (1976). The maintenance of genetic variability by mutation in a polygenic character with linked loci. *Genetical Research*, **26**, 221–35.

Lande, R. (1979). Quantitative genetic analysis of multivariate evolution, applied to brain:body size allometry. *Evolution*, **33**, 402–16.

Lande, R. (1980). Sexual dimorphism, sexual selection, and adaptation in polygenic characters. *Evolution*, **34**, 292–305.

Lande, R. (1981). Models of speciation by sexual selection of polygenic traits. *Proceedings of the National Academy of Sciences of the USA*, **78**, 3721–5.

Lande, R. (1982*a*). A quantitative genetic theory of life history evolution. *Ecology* **63**, 607–15.

Lande, R. (1982*b*). Rapid origin of sexual isolation and character divergence in a cline. *Evolution*, **36**, 213–33.

Lande, R. & Arnold, S. J. (MS). Measuring selection on correlated characters.

Lennington, S. (1980). Female choice and polygyny in redwinged blackbirds. *Animal Behaviour*, **28**, 347–61.

Lewontin, R. C. (1974). *The Genetic Basis of Evolutionary Change*. Columbia University Press: New York.

Lewontin, R. C. (1979). Fitness, survival, and optimality. In *Analysis of Ecological Systems*, ed. D. J. Horn, G. R. Stairs & R. D. Mitchell, pp. 3–21. Ohio State University Press: Columbus.

Maynard Smith, J. (1978*a*). *The Evolution of Sex*. Cambridge University Press: Cambridge.

Maynard Smith, J. (1978*b*). Optimization theory of evolution. *Annual Review of Ecology & Systematics*, **9**, 31–56.

Maynard Smith, J. (1980). Power and limits of optimization. In *Evolution of Social Behavior: Hypotheses and Empirical Tests*, ed. H. Markl, pp. 27–34, Dahlem Konferenzen. Verlag Chemie: Weinheim.

McGregor, P. K., Krebs, J. P. & Perrins, C. M. (1981). Song repertoires and lifetime reproductive success in the great tit (*Parus major*). *American Naturalist*, **118**, 149–59.

Noordwijk, A. J. van, Balen, J. H. van & Sharloo, W. (1980). Heritability of ecologically important traits in the great tit, *Parus major*. *Ardea*, **68**, 193–203.

O'Donald, P. (1967). A general model of sexual and natural selection. *Heredity*, **22**, 499–518.

O'Donald, P. (1977). Theoretical aspects of sexual selection. *Theoretical Population Biology*, **12**, 298–334.

O'Donald, P. (1980). *Genetic Models of Sexual Selection*. Cambridge University Press: Cambridge.

Partridge, L. (1980). Mate choice increases a component of offspring fitness in fruit flies. *Nature*, **283**, 290–1.

Pearson, K. (1903). Mathematical contributions to the theory of evolution. XI. On the influence of natural selection of the variability and correlation of organs. *Philosophical Transactions of the Royal Society of London Series A*, **200**, 1–66.

Robertson, A. (1966). A mathematical model of the culling process in dairy cattle. *Animal Production*, **8**, 93–108.

Robertson, A. (1968). The spectrum of genetic variation. In *Population Biology and Evolution*, ed. R. C. Lewontin, pp. 5–16. Syracuse University Press: Syracuse.

Smith, J. M. (1981). Does high fecundity reduce survival in song sparrows? *Evolution*, **35**, 1142–8.

Thornhill, R. (1979). Male and female sexual selection and the evolution of mating strategies in insects. In *Sexual Selection and Reproductive Competition in Insects*, ed. M. S. Blum & N. A. Blum, pp. 81–121. Academic Press: New York.

Trivers, R. L. (1972). Parental investment and sexual selection. In *Sexual Selection and the Descent of Man, 1871–1971*, ed. B. Campbell, pp. 136–79. Chicago University Press: Chicago.

Waage, R. L. (1979). Dual function of the damselfly penis: sperm removal and transfer. *Science*, **203**, 916–18.

Wade, M. J. (1979). Sexual selection and variance in reproductive success. *American Naturalist*, **114**, 742–7.

Wade, M. J. & Arnold, S. J. (1980). The intensity of sexual selection in relation to male sexual behaviour, female choice, and sperm precedence. *Animal Behaviour*, **28**, 446–61.

Williams, G. C. (1975). *Sex and Evolution*. Princeton University Press: Princeton.

Williams, G. C. (1978). Mysteries of sex and recombination. *Quarterly Review of Biology*, **53**, 287–9.

Wright, S. (1931). Evolution in Mendelian populations. *Genetics*, **16**, 97–159.

Wright, S. (1968). *Evolution and the Genetics of Population, vol. 1. Biometric and Genetic Foundations*. University of Chicago Press: Chicago.

Wright, S. (1969). *Evolution and the Genetics of Populations, vol. 2. The Theory of Gene Frequencies*. University of Chicago Press: Chicago.

5

Leks and mate choice

JACK W. BRADBURY AND ROBERT M. GIBSON

Leks are assemblies of adult males which females visit solely for the purpose of copulation. Males of lek species provide neither resources nor parental care for females, and females of most species appear free to pick the male of their choice for mating. Usually there is fair unanimity in female choice such that only a few males account for most of the matings at a given site. Although uncommon when compared to other mating systems, leks recur in a wide variety of taxa and in an equally diverse set of environmental contexts (cf. reviews by Davies, 1978a; Wittenberger, 1981; Bradbury, 1981; Oring, in press).

At first glance, leks seem ideal for testing many of the current theories of sexual selection and mate choice. Since females are usually free of male herding or restraint, leks would seem the proper system in which to demonstrate and measure the often-debated process of Female Choice (Huxley, 1938; Thornhill, 1980; Borgia, 1979; O'Donald, 1980; Lande, 1981). This seems particularly apropos because in principle, lek females may exercise choice at two levels; (a) choice between leks, and (b) choice between males on a given lek. Choice between leks is of considerable interest because it both affects, and is affected by, the spatial dispersion of displaying males. The actual patterns of male dispersion can thus tell us something about the relative leverages of each sex in determining the mating system. Female choice within a lek is of interest because it provides one of the few systems in which one can hope to analyse the process of female choice without the usual confounding of 'material' and 'genetic' benefits (*sensu* Borgia, 1979): in lek species, the only benefit a female can hope to gain by mate choice is genetic. Finally, leks ought to be prime systems in which one can identify and measure the specific benefits and costs of sexual selection. The benefits to males are direct functions of the

109

numbers of matings obtained, and the costs to these males are matings lost due to reduced survivorship or mating success at later ages. This is in contrast to many other mating systems in which male benefits and costs are confounded by second-order effects such as male-induced mortality of young (Le Boeuf & Briggs, 1977; Hrdy, 1977), unequally distributed paternal effort (Martin, 1974), and discrepancies between male and female assessments of resource value (Wittenberger, 1979). The costs and benefits of mate choice for females are still an issue of considerable theoretical dispute (see below), but one expects that the simpler transactions generated by deleting material benefits in lek species might actually facilitate a clarification of these issues. As a bonus, the ecological and taxonomic diversity of lek species would seem more than sufficient for a comparative separation of general rules of mate choice from taxon-specific variations in these rules.

As so often happens with naive first glances, leks have turned out to be much more complicated than was originally anticipated. For one thing, the extreme variance in male mating success on leks has fostered the simultaneous or subsequent evolution of alternative and parasitic male strategies. In addition, different males on the arena can adopt different strategies (*e.g.* Ruffs), or the same male might adopt a mixture of strategies (personal observations on Sage Grouse). Untangling these options, determining their relative frequencies, and measuring their relative successes has slowed down the testing of general models considerably. For example, the discovery that in some, but not all, lek species, males interrupt each other's mating attempts sufficiently often to curtail free female choice, has led some authors to question whether female choice occurs at all on leks (Diamond, 1981). The complexity of male options may in turn have aggravated the already complicated co-evolutionary interplay between the sexes, thereby making the kinds of cues used by females subtle and difficult to identify. Finally, strong sexual selection such as occurs on leks ought to reduce the heritable variation in male characters to low (but given the recent work of Lande (1977), non-zero) levels. Measuring any genetic benefits in the midst of the large environmental 'noise' is clearly very challenging.

Despite these problems, we believe leks will in the long run shed considerable light on the processes of sexual selection. One simply must accept the facts that high mating skew may lead to complex assortments of strategies, that these alternatives and other complex feedbacks must be controlled for in data collection, and that all measures of costs and benefits will have to be extracted from high levels of noise. With this cautious optimism in mind, we shall review the questions posed above from the point of view of leks, discuss some of the problems with prior studies, and suggest some areas which we think deserve the most urgent attention in future work.

Male dispersion and female choice between leks

One of the characteristics of lek species is that males are clumped in space. The degree of clumping varies from classical leks in which males are densely packed within a lek but leks tend to be far apart, to a number of 'exploded lek' species in which males within an aggregation have fairly large display territories and leks may be closer together (cf. Bradbury, 1981; Oring, in press). These patterns of male dispersion are related to mate choice in two ways. On the one hand, if males themselves determine how they will be dispersed, the females' options for finding leks and comparing males within a lek will be consequently constrained. The dispersion thus may limit female choice. If, on the other hand, it is the females who initiate male clumping by preferring clumped males, then the male dispersion will reflect both this preference and the degree to which females have leverage in exerting it. In this case, female choice might regulate dispersion. Insofar as male- and female-initiation of clumping lead to different spatial patterns of males, we can examine the actual dispersions to infer which sex initiates clumping and the degree to which the other sex has leverage over the final outcome.

There are a number of hypotheses which have been advanced to explain male dispersion in lek species. For the reasons given above, these can be divided into those in which males initiate display aggregations for their own benefit, and those in which females favour males which aggregate and thus force males to aggregate if they want to mate. Male-initiated reasons for clumping include:

(1) Males clump to reduce predation on themselves while displaying (Koivisto, 1965; Hjorth, 1970; Wiley, 1974).
(2) Males clump to increase signal range or amount of time signals are being emitted (Lack, 1939; Snow, 1963; Hjorth, 1970; Otte, 1974).
(3) Males require specific display habitats which are limiting and patchily distributed (Boag & Sumanik, 1969; B. Snow, 1974; Gullion, 1976).
(4) Males clump near 'hotspots' through which the largest numbers of females are likely to pass (Lill, 1976; Emlen & Oring, 1977; Payne & Payne, 1977; J. P. Kruijt, personal communication).

Female-initiated reasons for clumping include:

(5) Females prefer clumped males because this reduces predation on the females (Wittenberger, 1978).

(6) Females prefer males which clump in less-desirable habitats thus reducing competition between the sexes for resources (Wrangham, 1981).

(7) Females prefer larger clumps of males because this facilitates mate choice (Alexander, 1975; Bradbury, 1981).

Several of these hypotheses can be dismissed as general reasons for male clumping. The two predation models (1 and 5) may well play an important role for grouse and frogs, but it is very unlikely they play any role in male spacing for manakins, Hammer-headed Bats, or cotingids (Wiley, 1973; Hartzler, 1974; Tuttle & Ryan, 1981; Bradbury, 1977; Lill, 1974, 1975; B. Snow, 1961, 1973). The competition reduction model of Wrangham (6) really does not appear to fit the data even in the species he has suggested: in Hammer-headed Bats, for example, the two sexes tend to concentrate on different fruit species for food but these species are so mingled as to ensure sexual overlap in space. In addition, those fruit species used in common by the two sexes *are* shared spatially with both sexes frequently feeding at the same trees (J. Bradbury, personal observations). The signal efficacy model (2) has been criticised as being unlikely by several authors (Bradbury, 1981; Oring, 1982) because it requires that the numbers of females must increase on a *per male* basis to justify the aggregation and this seems improbable on physical grounds. Cade (1981) has recently shown that broadcasting cricket songs from increasing numbers of speakers does attract more females, but not on a per speaker basis. Similar conclusions were reached by Lill (1976) on Golden-headed Manakin leks and Koivisto (1965) on Blackcock leks. The only data suggesting that larger leks do attract more females per male are those of Hamerstrom & Hamerstrom (1960) on Prairie Chickens. Unfortunately, these results did not correct for different local densities of females, a necessary correction in such a contrast. Finally, although it is clear that males are selective in their choice of display sites (Model 3), it has never been demonstrated to our knowledge that such sites are limiting. Studies of a number of lek species have reported changes in lek location over time under conditions in which it is unlikely that the distribution of available sites had also changed (Rippin & Boag, 1974; Stiles & Wolf, 1979; Oring, 1982; Kruijt, de Vos & Bossema, 1972). Although the appropriate statistical analyses have not been done, it does appear that for many lek species the spacing of known leks is too even, and/or the characteristics of used locations too diverse for suitable sites to be limiting (cf. Patterson, 1952; Dalke *et al.*, 1963; Hoffman, 1963). Habitat selection by males thus seems an unlikely contender as a general determinant of male dispersion in lek species.

This leaves two general models: a male-initiated model (4: hotspots) and a female-initiated model (7: larger leks/easier mate choice). The hotspot model has usually been proposed with an environmental determination component. That is, certain locations such as foraging or nesting or roosting sites occur in an uneven pattern spatially and hence females will tend to aggregate in such sites. The model thus requires both a clumping of resources and a consequent clumping of females. Following a suggestion by Oring (in press) that males ought to display at 'the point having the lowest cumulative distance to the activity centres of all females in the population', we have been modelling some simple hotspot models which do not require an underlying clumping of resources (Bradbury & Gibson, submitted MS). As stated, Oring's suggestion would lead to only one lek per population, or alternatively, an *a posteriori* definition of a population as that served by one lek. Clearly, there is nearly always more than one lek per population in the general sense of the latter term.

Our basic models all begin with a random dispersion of female home range centres. If female home ranges are at least contiguous, or more likely in lek species, overlapping, the points of overlap or contiguity with the most females will be by definition the 'hotspots'. We allow males to settle successively at any point in the sample habitat. The first male of course settles in the hottest spot. The next male must be more circumspect: if he settles within one female home range of the first male, there will be some females which encounter both males and therefore must be shared. Should one of these hotspots be sufficiently 'rich', this sharing might be better than settling elsewhere. In most cases, locations within one female home range diameter from the first male are not sufficiently rich, and hence the second male does better to settle outside this diameter where he has exclusive use of all females encountered (at least until other males settle). This means that hotspots within one female home range diameter of a settled male are 'devalued' relative to hotspots not near a settled male. The usual result is that the first males settle further apart from each other than would be expected if there were no sharing of females. Once all the best hotspots are occupied, subsequent males must choose between sharing females at settled locations or looking for secondary spots between the settled locations. The outcome of all of our models is that males will clump even when females are randomly distributed. It even seems reasonable that males will clump when females are uniformly distributed, if female home ranges are at least contiguous, and especially so if they are overlapping. Our simulations generate similar outcomes when we let males settle despotically (*sensu* Fretwell, 1972) instead of in an ideal free manner. The despotism in our lek models is exhibited not as larger territories than in equitable settlement, but as larger than equitable fractions of matings per location. Our despotic models, using skew values similar to those of real lek species, tend to be 25% less clumped than the free models, but in all other respects, the outcomes are identical.

Because the clumping of males arises from local devaluation of hotspots within one female home range diameter of settled males, one might expect female home range size to affect the degree of male clumping. In all of our models, female home range size accounts for about 25–30% of the variance in male clumping: the larger the home ranges of females, the more males per assembly and the greater the distance between sites. The hotspot model thus leads to a positive correlation between female home range size and the distances between male assemblies. In addition, nearly all parameter configurations of the hotspot models allow leks to be less than one female home range apart. Not only are large leks closer than this limit, but one also obtains binary leks with small separations and 'satellite leks' (small leks a short distance from a large one). It is thus relatively easy in a hotspot model for a female to be able to visit any of several leks and still remain within her current home range. The importance of these outcomes will become obvious below.

The second remaining model for male dispersion is a female-initiated one: females are better able to choose between males when the latter are clumped and thus clumping arises in males in response to this female preference. (This of course presumes that females already have evolved some reason to choose between males.) Once females prefer males which are clumped, it is reasonable to suppose that a female encountering clumps of different sizes would at least discriminate against the smallest clumps and at most would select the largest clump within her home range. If female home ranges are sufficiently overlapping, and if female choice between leks is sufficiently unanimous, matings would be concentrated at a few widely separated leks and interstitial leks would receive no matings at all. Males on the ignored assemblies would most likely disband and either join the successful leks or adopt alternative mating strategies. The process would end when leks were far enough apart that individual females could no longer exert a preference without enlarging their usual home ranges: that is, when leks were approximately one female home range diameter apart. At this point, most females would include only a single lek within their usual home range, and would be likely to visit only this lek before mating. A few females, situated by chance equidistant between two or three leks might visit all of these and exert a choice. While this latter choice would constitute a force for wider spacing, it would be exactly balanced by an opposite tendency for itinerant or low-ranking males to move into the home ranges of females who would have no lek within their ranges at wider spacings. This model thus provides both a force for increasing the clumping of males and a quantitative limit on how clumped females can force males to be.

The original formulation of the female preference model by Bradbury (1981) was a verbal model which relied on several strong assumptions. The most vulnerable assumption was that females were 100% unanimous in their choice of the largest lek in their home range. It seems possible that if females were not able or inclined to exert this degree of discrimination, the diminution of interstitial leks might halt before these leks went totally extinct. We have examined this assumption quantitatively with the following results. Unanimity of female choice between leks rests on two parameters: (a) the strength of a female's preference for one of two leks of size N and size M, and (b) her ability to make the right discrimination given such a size difference. The product of these two probabilities is the joint probability of exercising a correct choice. One minus this value is the probability of her not exercising the choice or of making the wrong choice. These joint probabilities are critical to a male's decision either to remain on an interstitial lek or to resettle on a larger one. In addition, note that in all lek species studied, the distribution of matings within a lek is highly skewed (cf. Bradbury, 1981). In short, a male occupying an interstitial lek must compare the product of the probability a female will select his lek and the fraction of matings he can expect to obtain there, with the equivalent product for a larger lek. Whereas a larger lek might obtain a greater fraction of the total matings, a low-ranking male on a small lek obtains a larger fraction of those which do occur than would a low-ranking male on a larger lek.

Using a power function approximation to the skew curve on a typical vertebrate lek ($i = 1.5$, Bradbury, 1981), it only takes a 55–60% probability of a female preferring the larger lek to force males away from the smaller of two leks which differ slightly in size. As more males relocate and the size difference between the two leks increases, it requires an increasingly stronger and/or more accurate female preference to continue the process: for a lek of five males and a lek of 50 males, the preference must be 96.9% in favour of the larger lek to justify the next male's transfer. Once all the males have joined the large lek, it requires a continued 99.9% preference for the larger lek to keep the lowest-ranking males on a lek of 50 from re-settling in an interstitial position. If the females fail to exert these minimal levels of preference for larger leks, then the process will stop before interstitial leks are completely eliminated.

Are these levels of preference restrictive? In fact, we think they are not. As the difference between lek sizes increases, the acuity component of the preference ought to move quickly to nearly 100% accuracy. Should females exert this level of discrimination? It seems likely that if it paid for a female to exert a preference for larger clumps when leks were similarly sized, it should be even more worth her while to favour leks of 50 males over leks of one or even five males. In other words, while the minimal preference required increases as interstitial leks die off, it seems likely that both the acuity of discrimination and the rewards of exerting a preference ought to keep step. We conclude that it takes a very mild preference and discrimination ability on the part of females to get such a process going, and that there ought to be little problem on the part of females in keeping the process active up to the final limit suggested by the verbal model.

We thus have two alternative models which make rather different predictions. The hotspot model (a male-initiated process), predicts that the spacing between leks will be positively correlated with the size of female home ranges, but that leks can and will be less than one female home range diameter apart. As a corollary, females will typically be able to visit several leks before mating without increasing their usual home ranges. The female preference model (a female-initiated process) also predicts a positive correlation between female home range size and inter-lek spacing, but it does not predict leks closer than one female home range diameter and it suggests that most females should visit only a single lek before mating. Note that both processes may co-occur but the outcome will be more similar to the female preference model: that is, leks may be initially spaced according to a hotspot process, but a subsequent evolution of female choice between leks would lead to typical inter-lek spacing of about one female home range by eliminating interstitial leks. Turning the argument around, the existence of typical lek spacings at distances less than a female home range would argue that females do not choose between leks, or that their acuity or benefit in so choosing is limited by other factors.

What are the data? Bradbury (1981) presented data for two species of Epomorphorine bats with leks which appear to fit the females preference model. The mean distances between leks are very close to the average diameter of one female home range. However, the variations in the inter-lek distances for both species are about 50% of the mean. Whereas the longer than expected distances could easily be due to the presence of unsuitable intervening habitat, the shorter distances could be explained by the female preference model only if female home ranges were smaller in some areas or female preferences were fixed at some level less than 100%.

More damaging to female preference models are data on Ruffs and Sage Grouse. Ruff leks are often quite close together, even to the point of being in sight of each other (Hogan-Warburg, 1966; van Rhijn, 1973). Our own work on Sage Grouse (unpublished), which was prompted by the female preference models, has convinced us that binary leks, satellite leks, and the like are quite common in Eastern California populations of these birds. Although female home ranges have not yet been adequately measured, some of these binary and satellite patterns are clearly more closely spaced than the distances females are observed to fly in approaching the leks. Finally, a number of workers have noted that females of lek species may visit several leks (Kruijt *et al.*, Lill, 1976; Oring, in press; van Rhijn, personal communication). These observations alone do not disprove a female preference model. It is instead necessary to show that *most* females visit more than one lek. However, the evidence does seem to be accumulating against female preference models and in favour of a male-initiated model such as hotspots.

What does this suggest for future work? It is clear that there are too few data for any lek species to be sure that female preferences for male clumping, and thus choice between leks, are not major factors in lek evolution. The importance of obtaining such data ought to be clear. It is also important to devise means to falsify the general hotspot model in the way that the female preference models have been made falsifiable. While it is true that this model allows for leks to be closer than one female home range, it does not follow that there is not a parameter set which would also allow the leks to be just that distance apart. One problem with the generalised hotspot model is that it is essentially a null model. It makes minimal assumptions and simply allows males to settle on random patterns of female accessibility in the same way as most animals are expected to settle on any resource (Fretwell, 1972). Such simple models often have sufficient flexibility that they are difficult to disprove. However, the hotspot model would be falsified were we to map out home ranges of females and find that male display sites were totally unrelated to areas of maximal female home range overlap. Direct mapping of female ranges is clearly required for both hypotheses, and thus this test can be applied to the same data used to test the female preference model. It should also be pointed out that combinations of hotspots and some of the lek-spacing mechanisms which were discounted as insufficiently universal might provide the best explanations for spatial pattern. Males might not display exactly at a given point of maximal home range overlap but nearby where cover or terrain allowed for better and/or safer display. Because hotspots or female preference models may interact with habitat suitability, predator defence, etc., or because there may be no universal determinant of male spacing, it is clearly wise to continue to consider *all* of the hypotheses listed earlier when studying spacing of lek males.

Do females choose between males on leks?

There seem to be two issues relevant to this question. First, do interactions between males either prior to or during female visits pre-empt the control of mate choice away from females in lek species? Secondly, what is the evidence that females are really exercising their option to make choices among males on a lek?

Interactions by males prior to female visits have been implicated in mate choice for a small subset of the exploded lek species. All of these forms exhibit co-operative displays by two to five males at a common site. Although the data are scanty, it appears that a single male obtains most of the matings within such a group (B. Snow, 1961; D. Snow & D. Goodwin, 1974; Schodde & Mason, 1974; Foster, 1977; LeCroy, Kulupi & Peckover, 1980). Diamond (1981) has suggested that dominance interactions between males in such a group eliminate any opportunity for a female to make a choice of mate. While this might be true for choice within a group, it need not be true if the home range of a female encompasses several such groups. For example, we were able to radiotrack a female of one of these species (*Chiroxiphia linearis*) in Costa Rica, and found that its foraging range included the display grounds of three pairs of co-operatively displaying males. Thus, while strong dominance in small 'leks' may reduce female options within an assembly, it is necessary to know female home range sizes and dispositions before arguing that female choice has been completely pre-empted.

It seems very unlikely that the type of strong dominance outlined above can be enforced and maintained on any but the smallest and most stable of leks. For example, in a lek of 50–100 Sage Grouse or Hammer-headed Bats, it would be very difficult for a central and dominant male to prevent a female from mating with a low-ranking male on the lek periphery, and the evidence is that they do not (Bradbury, 1977; Hartzler, 1972). It is more likely, however, that neighbouring males might interfere with each other's copulation attempts and thus modify female choice. Interference between males occurs in a variety of, but not all, lek species. The best studied examples are Ruffs (Hogan-Warburg, 1966), Buff-breasted Sandpipers (Myers, 1979), Black Grouse (Kruijt & Hogan, 1967), Prairie Chickens (Hamerstrom & Hamerstrom, 1960), Sage Grouse (Hartzler, 1972; Wiley, 1973), and White-bearded and Golden-headed Manakins (Lill, 1974, 1976). In all of these species, males enter the territories of their neighbours to disrupt copulation attempts. That such interference can halt a copulation sequence successfully has been shown in manakins (Lill, 1976) and grouse (Wiley, 1973; Robel & Ballard, 1974). Is it likely that female choice is sufficiently curtailed by male interference to alter the presumed processes of sexual selection on leks?

The extent to which male interference curtails female choice should depend upon (a) the proportion of copulation attempts which are disrupted, (b) the distribution of disrupted copulations among the various males on the lek, and (c) whether interference alters the subsequent mate choices of the disrupted females. Current evidence suggests that male interference plays a minor role in the mate choice process for most lek species. Considering each component in turn:

(a) Even in species where interference is most common, the rates of *effective* copulation disruption are generally low (e.g. 1% in White-bearded Manakins (Lill, 1974); 4% in Black Grouse (Kruijt & Hogan, 1967); 10–18% in Sage Grouse (Hartzler, 1972; Wiley, 1973); 6–18% in Prairie Chickens (Hamerstrom & Hamerstrom, 1960; Robel & Ballard, 1974); and 26% in Golden-headed Manakins (Lill, 1976)). In many other species such as Hammer-headed Bats (Bradbury, 1977), copulation disruption has either not been seen or is very rare.

(b) Although there may be a trend in some cases, there is no statistically significant evidence that interference is differentially distributed within a lek according to status. Males who obtain the most copulations are neither more likely nor less likely to have a copulation attempt disrupted than are less-successful males (Hartzler, 1972; Wiley, 1973; Lill, 1976).

(c) There is no convincing evidence that females significantly change their preferences for a given male as a result of experiencing a disrupted copulation (Lill, 1976; personal observations on Sage Grouse). In fact, we have on several occasions observed a female Sage Grouse return persistently to the same male following a disruption until she was able to mate with him.

This suggests that females of lek species retain considerable latitude in making a choice of mate. Do they exercise this option? A simple demonstration that they do, once male interference has been relegated to minor status, is to point out that mating success among males is significantly non-random for every lek species which has been studied. More elegant evidence, of course, would be to identify all cues used by females and quantify the relative contributions made by each to the overall patterns of male mating success. Unfortunately, elegance requires careful analysis and large sample sizes. Were sufficient data available, one would like to be able to partition the total variance in male mating success into a minimum of four categories: (a) that explained by female choice using specific male cues; (b) that explained by male behaviour unrelated to female choice such as interference; (c) that due to female–female effects, such as possible copying of choices (see below); and (d) a residual which is due to error in female mate choice. There might be statistical interaction terms as well.

We have argued above that the male interaction term is probably a small part of this variance in most species. A female copying component has not been considered in most studies and will be discussed below. Given that both of these *were* known, the remaining variance is that specifically related to independent female choice. What is important is how much of this remaining variance is explained by any one cue or set of cues. The analysis requires that a large list of alternative cues be considered at the outset of the study. If it is not, an important but measured cue could show up in the residual term, and/or a cue may appear important only because it is correlated with another, unmeasured cue, which is. If the copying and male interference terms are not known, then sample sizes will probably have to be large to obtain significant relations with specific cues. Nearly all studies on leks to date fail to meet some requirement above. Either interaction and copying terms were not considered and samples were too small, or lists of alternatives were not exhaustive, or a simple (often non-parametric) correlation was accepted as evidence of an effect without consideration of its size or its possible explanation as a result of correlations with unmeasured variables.

Accepting that the ideal has yet to be accomplished, and keeping the potential problems in mind, we shall review existing data concerning cues females may use for mate choice on leks. Three types of cues have been suggested: (a) proximity to some reference point, such as the lek centre, (b) dominance status, and (c) other male phenotypic traits such as age, size, or vigour.

Position effects

Nearly all lek species that have been studied show a clustering of the more successful males at some point or points within the lek. In small leks, there is usually a single such cluster, whereas in the large leks of 50–100 Sage Grouse or Hammer-headed Bats, there may be several such clusters simultaneously (Hartzler, 1972; Wiley, 1973; Bradbury, 1977). It has been suggested by several authors (e.g. Wiley, 1974; Borgia, 1979) that female choice is based in part on male proximity to some reference point. Two types of reference points seem possible: a relative point such as the centre of gravity of the male assembly, and an absolute point, such as a traditional location or topographical feature. Such a choice cue would generate both the clustering of successful males and the apparent competition among males of some species to occupy territories closer to such a cluster (Ballard & Robel, 1974; Buechner & Roth, 1974; Floody & Arnold, 1975; Lill, 1974; Kruijt *et al.*, 1972).

The evidence for a position effect in female choice on leks is mixed. One problem is that a very reasonable alternative explanation for both the clustering of successful males and the male competition for sites has often been ignored. If females pick males on the basis of cues other than position, we might expect the less-successful males to move to those portions of their territories and/or even move their territories so as to be closer to the successful males and hence the females. Hartzler (1972) and Wiley (1973) have described just such behaviour in Sage Grouse. Both a centripetal movement of males and a clustering of successful males will result from such a process. In addition, one might encounter both processes at once: females might choose males in part because of position *and* less successful males might then move to be closer to the more successful males. In short, discrimination between a true position effect and a male relocation effect requires more than demonstrations of successful male clustering and male competition for positions.

One way to discriminate between these alternatives is to see the degree to which removal of specific males (either naturally or experimentally) shifts the loci of major mating activity. Lill (1974) showed that White-bearded Manakin hens returned for renesting matings to the territory in which they had mated earlier that year even when the male occupants had changed. While this does show a fidelity to a location for remating, it does not argue that the female used location instead of other male traits in making the original choice. In Uganda kob, turnover of successful males is very high. Despite this turnover in occupants, certain central territories continue to be the major sites of matings (Buechner & Roth, 1974). The problem with this result is that the same small subset of males generates the entire turnover by recycling in turn between successful territory and bachelor herd (Buechner *et al.*, MS). Were these particular males distinguishable by features or behaviour, the observed fidelity by females for 'central' territories would be as compatible with a male relocation model as with a position effect. Finally, and in contrast to manakins, Hartzler (1972) found that Sage Grouse hens *lost* interest in the territories of successful males when those males disappeared and were subsequently replaced by others.

A qualitative disproof of some position models is to show that certain types of reference points cannot be related to male success. The only relative point which appears to be reasonable is a centre of gravity one. If female choice is based primarily on proximity to this centre, then we expect the successful male cluster to be close to the geometric centre of the lek. In fact, a careful examination of published studies indicates to us that the observed clusters of successful males are rarely at the geometrical centres of the leks. In Ruffs, the successful males may even be on the lek periphery (Shepard, 1975). Absolute position effects which might involve landmarks or conventional topographic features are equally hard to justify. Sage Grouse mating centres vary from day to day within a season as well as between seasons (Hartzler, 1972). It is possible that the landmarks could be as fleeting as melting snow spots or changing vegetation, but current evidence is too scanty to evaluate this notion (Hartzler, 1972; our own observations). Despite considerable effort, Lill (1974) was unable to identify any kind of landmark or territorial character which correlated with male success in manakins.

Returning to the variance analysis, the final quantitative test of either alternative is to see how much of male mating success can be explained by male position using any reference point. In Hammer-headed Bats, successful males are clustered in the sense that the pooled copulations of the 10–12 males in each 100-m segment of the linearly-shaped lek show large differences between segments (Bradbury, 1977). However, mapping of individuals shows that successful males are often separated from each other by from one to ten unsuccessful males. Whether the geometrical centre of the lek or proximity to the most successful male is used, and regardless of the scaling of proximity, a maximum of 10% of the variance in male success can be explained by male position alone. Hartzler (1972) obtained a similar result for Sage Grouse: the nearest neighbours of successful males often fail to copulate at all. While it is true that neither analysis controlled for male interference or female copying effects, the spatial discontinuities in male success argue against any strong position effects in these species by either mechanism.

It thus appears either that (i) position effects are real but act only in conjunction with other cues for female choice, or (ii) the data supporting position effects reflect a spurious outcome of another process such as male relocation around successful males. Future success in distinguishing between these alternatives will depend on having much larger sample sizes, paying more careful attention to male settlement and resettlement, and either excluding or correcting for the role of other types of cues.

Dominance

A second cue which might be used in female choice is dominance of males. There are two levels at which male dominance status might come into play: global status within the lek as a whole, and local status in comparison with nearest neighbours. To our knowledge, the first level of status has never been statistically partitioned from concomitant benefits of a possible position effect. It is true that males often appear to fight for the more central territories on a lek during the early part of each lek season (see above), and that if central males are removed, peripheral males may take over their territories (Ballard & Robel, 1974). From this one can infer that those males which succeeded in obtaining the central territories are in one respect 'dominant' to those which did not. However, unless males can exhibit dominance in some other manner as well, no additional cue information is being supplied to females than already existed through a position effect, and this we have already argued is insufficient to explain the overall patterns of mate choice.

It seems most likely that after a lek is settled, the ability of a male to enforce dominance on any one of its fellows falls off with the distance between their territories. Therefore, any additional demonstrations of dominance that a female might use as a cue would be local interactions. Alexander (1975) and Borgia (1979) have argued that the ability to display and/or copulate without being interrupted by neighbouring males is a measure of a male's 'prowess' or 'dominance'. By this, they must mean local dominance in the sense above. We have already summarised the relevant data on copulation interference. To date, there is no significant evidence that successful males are interrupted less often than they themselves interrupt other males, that effective interruption is very common, or that females, once interrupted, alter their choice of mate. It is possible that dominance is more subtle. Perhaps dominant males attack those neighbours that display more vigorously than they do and over time reduce the conspicuousness of these other males. Perhaps harassment by dominants is sufficiently costly to their neighbours that the latter must leave the leks to feed earlier. Other mechanisms are possible, but in lieu of any substantiating data, we feel that whether male dominance is a choice cue or not is an open question.

Other cues

A variety of other phenotypic cues have been invoked in mate choice. Age, size, and vigour are all traits which females might use to choose males in conjunction with centre effects. Dominance status might be one indirect measure of these cues if success in winning battles was partially dependent on these traits. For example, Wiley (1973) argued that older males were more likely to win contests for central territories and thus location, age, and status were all correlated. Again, this does not provide an adequate explanation of mate choice unless some additional index of age is available to females. It is perhaps possible that some experience-dependent performance of displays (e.g., Kruijt *et al.*, 1972) could be used by females as an additional measure of age, but to date no one has provided the requisite evidence.

Body size in manakins is not related to mating success, and Stiles & Wolf (1979) could find no relation between body size and proximity of a male's territory to the lek centre in Hermit Hummingbirds. In frogs, large size (and deeply-pitched croaks) seem to be correlated in many species, but only a subset of these (*e.g. Physalaemus pustulosus*) appear to qualify as true leks (cf. Howard, 1979; Davies & Halliday, 1978; Ryan, 1980). In *Physalaemus*, body size of males is significantly correlated with mating success, but it explains only a portion of the overall variance and is a less effective predictor than is time spent calling. Male size and time spent calling are not correlated in this species (Ryan, MS).

Finally, vigour has been measured in a number of ways in various lek species. Lill (1974, 1976) was unable to find any measure of display vigour or frequency which was a significant predictor of mating success. Local trends for higher rates in successful males were always obscured by very high variations within each male. Hartzler (1972) and Wiley (1973), both studying Sage Grouse, came to different conclusions as to whether successful males strutted at higher rates than unsuccessful males. The differences in opinion stem from different ways of correcting for the proximity of females and prior success of males. The strongest evidence in favour of a vigour cue is that of Payne & Payne (1977) in Indigo Birds.

This study examined durations of display in males both early and late in the breeding season and concluded that those males who displayed longest early in the season continued to do so and had the highest reproductive success later in the season.

It should be clear that we are only beginning to understand which cues are used by females to choose mates on leks. Many careful attempts (e.g. Lill, 1974; Wiley, 1973; Kruijt *et al.*, 1972; Payne & Payne, 1977) have failed to come up with unequivocal sets of cues which explain most of the variation in male mating success. We noted earlier that if either male–male interference or female copying make large contributions to the overall variance in male mating success, it will be difficult to extract any actual choice without correcting for these effects in the analyses. Since male interference is limited to a subset of lek species, high levels of female copying (or similar second-order effects) might be the more ubiquitous cause for the failure to identify cues used in female choice. What is the evidence for copying?

Female copying of each other's mate choices has been suggested by a number of authors (e.g. Hogan-Warburg, 1966; Wiley, 1974; Lill, 1974). Although female Hammer-headed Bats do not visit leks in large groups like Prairie Grouse, the loud post-copulatory squeal emitted by females might be used (intended?) as a cue for copying. On the negative side, van Rhijn (1973) was unable to demonstrate copying in Ruffs. Because copying has not yet been measured quantitatively in any lek species, we wondered whether the results of mate choice on leks might be used to infer copying. Specifically, if each female were to have a finite likelihood of correctly assessing the relative cue values for any pair of males, would one expect the degree of unanimity in mate choice which is found if choices were independent? We have run some simple computer simulations of this type of process using choice based on a single cue, and we have examined three kinds of cues: (a) normally distributed cues such as body size in birds and mammals, (b) site-specific cues such as might occur with position effects, and (c) age-specific cues such as body size in frogs or display technique in longer-lived animals. Using typical coefficients of variation for weight and linear dimensions, rates of growth, survival rates of adults, a number of lek sizes, and a variety of female discrimination curves, the models suggest that it is extremely unlikely that the degree of unanimity in female choice for any of the lek species simulated can be explained by females choosing independently with a single cue (Bradbury, submitted MS).

The unanimity in female choice which *is* observed could be explained if (a) females had much better discrimination abilities than expected, (b) females used combinations of cues which were considerably better than single cue discriminations, and/or (c) females copied each other. The first alternative seems unlikely given available data and the range of female discrimination functions used. The second is more likely, especially given the rest of the evidence arguing for multiple cues in mate choice on leks. However, for sets of normally distributed cues, the improvement would have to be near an order of magnitude better. It is not clear to us that this level of improvement is likely, and it seems prudent to accept the possibility that extensive copying may occur and account for a significant amount of the variance in male mating success on leks. If copying is extensive, then it is unwise to use the acute skew on leks as evidence for careful female choice. Female choice may be either accurate or not if copying occurs and still one might get the degree of skew observed.

The force of this section is that the identification of the cues used by females in choosing males on leks is fraught with numerous pitfalls. Effects such as male interference and female copying must be measured and removed from the overall variation in male mating success before attempting to rate or exclude potential female choice cues. This in turn requires both a large data base and sufficiently diverse combinations of male success, female visitation rates, and interruption frequencies to tease apart the separate components. Given that these conditions are met, one must then be careful to collect the kinds of data which will allow one to remove spurious correlations and compare the relative contributions of the large list of potential cues. As seems likely, several cues may be combined to generate the overall patterns of mate choice observed on leks, and this outcome must be allowed for in the field design. It should not be concluded from these comments that the contributions from prior studies of leks should be devalued. To the contrary, it is only because of careful work such as that of Lill (1974, 1976) that we can now ask these questions in a more formal way.

The benefits and costs of mate choice on leks

If one accepts that females do choose males on leks, even if we have not yet identified all the cues used, one must ask what a female is getting for her efforts. There are two quite alternative opinions on this matter. The first position is exemplified in the recent work of Lande (1980, 1981) and Kirkpatrick (1982) who have shown that all of the classical processes of female choice envisioned by Fisher (1958) (e.g., the initiation of sexual selection, 'runaway' phases of change in male trait and female preference, and approach to equilibria) *can* evolve with a female preference for a male trait which is totally arbitrary (see Arnold, this volume, for a review). In other words, all that a female *need* get to justify making a choice is a set of sons who will themselves be preferred by females. The alternative position is that evolution ought to lead preferentially to female preferences for that subset of male traits which not only produce 'preferred sons' but also produce better 'adapted' daughters and/or sons (Williams, 1966; Trivers, 1972; Zahavi, 1975; Eshel, 1978; Borgia, 1979). Put another way, proponents of 'adaptive cues' suggest that judicious instead of arbitrary choice of cues might lead to sufficient benefit above and beyond having preferred sons that they would occur more commonly in actual systems.

It is difficult with the available literature to formulate these two alternatives in sufficiently demographic terms that one could contrast them in a real system such as a lek. One problem is that there are as many versions of the 'adaptive cue' position as there are publications on it. Another is that the discrediting of specific versions, such as Zahavi's (1975) 'handicap principle' (cf. Bell, 1978; Davis & O'Donald, 1976; Maynard Smith, 1976, 1978; O'Donald, 1980), has fostered in some quarters a categorical dismissal of all adaptive cue models. It seems to us that there are at least three different versions of the adaptive cue position, and that each needs to be considered separately. Specifically, nearly all female choice models include the opposition of increased mating success through a female preference for some cue and concomitant decrease in the viability of males possessing or displaying the cue. This is true of both adaptive and arbitrary cue models. Adaptive cue hypotheses all add to this base some additional demographic 'benefit' of making a specific choice in a specific way. Thus, one adaptive cue scenario argues that given a choice, female preferences for cues which lead to higher adult male viability ought to be more likely than those which lead to lower adult male viability. A second version accepts the lowered adult male survivorship, but suggests that the expression of certain male cues in females and/or juvenile males might be sufficiently beneficial that *net* fitness would be higher than with arbitrary cues. It is then assumed that a cue leading to higher absolute fitness will be favoured over one that leads to lower absolute fitness. Finally, a third version would call a cue adaptive if it enhanced either some female or juvenile male demographic component regardless of whether it led to an enhancement of net fitness or not.

This suggests two separate questions. The first is whether there *are* cues which might attract females for mating, decrease adult male viability, and enhance female or juvenile male survival all at once. We shall return to this question later in this section. Assuming such cues exist, the second is whether such cues are any more likely to evolve than cues which only attract females and reduce male viability, or more extreme, than cues which affect those components and *reduce* female fitness or juvenile male survival. Although it may seem intuitively reasonable that the latter question might be answered in the affirmative, the recent analyses of Lande (1981) and Kirkpatrick (1982) show quite the opposite: in their models, no adaptive benefit is needed to initiate sexual selection through female choice, and in addition, it is relatively easy for a female preference for less-'adapted' males to invade and displace an initial preference for better-'adapted' males. Although the major focus of 'adaptedness' in both formulations was male viability, Kirkpatrick explicitly considers a case in which the female expression of the 'invading' cue is also detrimental and still obtains the same result. In both analyses, initial conditions such as relative starting frequencies of alternative female preferences and existing genetic structure of the populations have a greater effect on the outcomes of sexual selection than do absolute fitness of the alternatives. Put bluntly, if one accepts these models (which rest on quite simple assumptions), there is no reason to expect adaptive cues to be favoured in evolution even if they generally lead to higher absolute fitness. Instead, one expects adaptive cues to be present only at a rate commensurate with their abundance in an overall list of all possible cues (both arbitrary and adaptive). Were we to have such a list and find that adaptive cues were unexpectedly common, we would conclude either that (a) the initial conditions of female choice were not randomly encountered, or (b) the simple models of Lande and Kirkpatrick were wrong or too simple.

At the moment, the theory stops here and the issue becomes an empirical one: what we need to do is identify the cues in female choice species and see with what frequency the cues used do have demographic benefits above and beyond increased male mating success and decreased adult male survival. As an example, consider a lek species in which we have identified some quantitative male trait which is used as the cue for female choice. Suppose the population is stable, that survivorship for both sexes can be partitioned into juvenile and adult annual rates, and that male mating success depends only on a male's cue value and not on his age. (These assumptions could always be checked in the field.) Let z be the value of the trait in a given individual, S_m the annual survival rate of adult males, G_m the annual survival rate of juvenile males, T the age at sexual maturity for males, R the annual number of offspring sired by a given male, S_f the annual survival rate of adult females, G_f the annual survival rate of juvenile females, t the age at sexual maturity of females, and B the annual fecundity of females. In the general case, it is possible that all or any of S_m, S_f, G_m, G_f, T, t, R, and B might be affected by the cue value z. Assuming an equal sex ratio at birth, the expected lifetime output of offspring by an individual with cue value z would be

$$W(z) = 1/2(G_m{}^T \sum_{i=1}^{\infty} S_m{}^i \cdot R) + 1/2(G_f{}^t \sum_{i=1}^{\infty} S_f{}^i \cdot B)$$

This can be simplified by letting

$$G_m{}^T = J(z), \quad \sum_{i=1}^{\infty} S_m{}^i = C(z)$$

and

$$(G_f{}^t \sum_{i=1}^{\infty} S_f{}^i \cdot B) = F(z)$$

so that

$$W(z) = 1/2[J(z) \cdot C(z) \cdot R(z)] + 1/2[F(z)].$$

How would one measure the components of this equation? Once the critical cues were identified, obtaining the functions $C(z)$ and $R(z)$ would be relatively straightforward. In fact, establishing the quantitative relation between R and z would be a necessary part of showing that the proper cues had been identified. The only difficulty might be in obtaining sufficient variation in z; in Sage Grouse, Hammer-headed Bats, and Hermit Hummingbirds, coefficients of variation in obvious linear anatomical measures are only 1–3% whereas equivalent volume and weight measures are only 3–5% (personal observation; Stiles & Wolf, 1979). Since we are not even sure the crucial cues are anatomical, this limited variation may or may not be a problem. Determination of $J(z)$ would be more difficult because it would require a juvenile index of an adult male's eventual cue value. Such indicators of adult male traits have been used successfully in red deer (T. Clutton-Brock, personal communication). Once identified, the index would be measured on a large number of young males, the males marked, and survival rates related to the index as the males matured and died off. Clearly, the most difficult term to measure is $F(z)$. The problem is finding out *how* z is expressed in females. If we have some reasonable assurances of paternity, females sired by males with known z values can be measured on a variety of characters including survival rates and fecundity. Each trait or ensemble of traits can then be regressed on fathers' cue values. Presuming some heritability and no assortative mating, significant regressions would then allow for some estimates to be made of $F(z)$. Paternity in a properly-selected lek species is not as difficult to ascertain as it is in many other mating systems since females may mate only once a season and all matings are directly observable. However, the unanimity in mate choice within a given lek would limit the number of males, and thus the variation in sire z values, which one would have for the regressions. Since there is no *a priori* reason to expect the top males at different leks to have the same absolute z value, one way to obviate this problem would be to collect data from a number of different leks.

Suppose that one were able to measure these variables and functions. Showing that the cues used were adaptive in the first of our defined senses would be quite difficult. If we were to stumble on a number of systems currently in a period of rapid sexual selection, we could look to see whether the changes were away from systems with low $C(z)$ effects to those with higher $C(z)$ effects. The problem is that both current theory (Lande, 1981) and existing observations suggest that most sexually selected species are not now in a state of rapid change: on the contrary, it seems most likely that short bouts of rapid change alternate with longer periods of relative stasis and thus the chances of finding one, much less many systems, in a state of change are small. Trying to show that cues leading to higher male viability are favoured by looking at static systems strikes us as futile. If in the extreme case, it could be shown that only cues which guarantee high male viability are selected, this would be of interest. But we already know that male display in many lek species is quite costly. For example, there is clear evidence that in the frog *Physalaemus pustulosus*, males suffer both increased predation (Tuttle & Ryan, 1981) and energetic (Bucher, Ryan & Bartholomew, 1982) costs as a direct result of their display activities. One is then left with a variety of species in which males suffer viability decreases to greater or lesser amounts, and no way to know what the alternatives were early in their evolution.

Contrasts based on the second definition of adaptive cues might be more feasible. There are three cases. First, there is a slight chance that a given system will still be in a state of rapid evolutionary change. If so, we shall find some directional shifts in the distribution of the observed z values over time. Alternatively the system may have a stable distribution of z values, but it may still be under directional selection. In this case, a plot of $W(z)$ vs. z would show a monotonic function with a maximal value of $W(z)$ at either very large or very low z. Such a system could arise if it had entered a state of runaway change (Lande's 'unstable' case), but had been halted by a lack of sufficient new genetic variation in male trait values. Finally, the system may actually be at an equilibrium (in the sense of Lande and Kirkpatrick), in which case the plot of $W(z)$ vs. z would most likely be unimodal over the range of realisable z values.

Whether the system is in rapid change, at an arrested steady state, or at an equilibrium, there will be some value of z, $\bar{z}$, at which $W(z)$ is maximised. Because we also have the $R(z)$ and $C(z)$ functions in hand, we can identify a second z, $\bar{z}'$, at which the product $R(z) \cdot C(z)$ would be maximised. Since $W(\bar{z}')$ is the maximal fitness which would have been realised if this cue only affected the classical components of male mating success and adult male viability, the difference $[W(\bar{z}) - W(\bar{z}')]$ is the additional adaptive benefit (or *cost* if the difference is negative) of the cue. If we were to examine a number of species and find that this difference was both positive and a large fraction of $W(\bar{z})$, we would conclude that for some reason cues with adaptive benefits were occurring commonly. Whether they occur more commonly than expected depends on the size and composition of the list of likely cues. Although the generation of such a list is the weakest part of the exercise, it seems reasonable that any high frequency of large adaptive benefits in female choice systems would be cause for re-examination of current theory. It is worth noting that such an exercise might produce the contrary result: that is, sexual selection by female choice might turn out to produce *decreases* in juvenile male viability and/or female fitness more commonly than expected.

There is also an indirect way in which the second type of adaptive cue might be studied. One difficulty with measuring $W(z)$ directly is obtaining both the $J(z)$ and $F(z)$ functions. If one is willing to make certain assumptions about the state of the system, it is also possible to infer the presence of adaptive benefits or costs simply by looking at the $R(z)$ and $C(z)$ curves and the actual distribution of z. Specifically, if $R(z)$ and $C(z)$ are the primary determinants of the system, one can predict the mean value of z which ought to occur and compare this to that which actually is found. The deviation of the observed mean z from the classical component expectation can indicate whether the adaptive effects are positive or negative and how large they are relative to the classical male mating success and viability components.

Finally, showing that cues used in female choice systems were adaptive in our third sense would be relatively easy once the separate functions were known. That is, if $R(z)$, $J(z)$, and/or $F(z)$ all could be shown to co-vary positively more often than expected given a list of possible cues, this would be of interest. As noted earlier, there is no obvious theoretical reason to expect this result, but were one to find it, it might suggest links in the evolution of demographic components which should have been included in the sexual selection models.

All of the above presume that there *are* cues which are likely to have the multiple effects and/or differential expressions in different sex and age groups suggested. Is this a reasonable presumption? Traits expressed in adult males of lek species which have been argued to have possible adaptive benefits in young or female animals include dominance status (as evidenced by proximity to some reference point or by immunity from interference), age, size, and vigour of display (Williams, 1975; M. Williams, 1978; Wiley, 1974; Trivers, 1972; West-Eberhard, 1979; Thornhill, 1980; Zahavi, 1975). To date, no one has actually demonstrated any positive relationship between female preferences on leks and any measure of juvenile male viability or female fecundity and survival. Instead, the typical nomination of one of these cues as 'adaptive' is justified by invoking some correlation between a possible cue and male mating success (usually ignoring *how much* of the variation is explained by this trait), then postulating some possible link between the cue and one demographic component (usually ignoring the possible counter-consequences on other demographic components), and then making the assumption that if this cue enhances net absolute fitness, it ought to be favoured. It should be clear by now that there are serious risks and pitfalls in all three phases of this logic, and that the best evidence for or against such traits serving as adaptive cues will be empirical. What can be said is that there are adult male traits which could have demographic effects when expressed in other sex and age classes. The ones which have been noted are included in this list, but there are no reasons to presume that the list is currently exhaustive or that these are more likely because they come to mind first.

There are some other logical problems with the current arguments for specific traits serving as adaptive cues. One of the traits most favoured as an adaptive cue is male dominance. Proponents have argued that it effectively summarises the positive benefits of age, size, and vigour in a single variable and it is easier for a female to assess than is direct measurement of any of those three components (Selander, 1972; Borgia, 1979). While dominance is probably easier to measure than relative size or vigour, this ease of assessment is a red herring. Landau (1951*a*, *b*) and Chase (1974) have both shown that if status is determined only by a cue such as size or vigour (or even by a set of such cues), the correlations between the cue values and status must be unreasonably high to explain the degree of structure seen in most dominance orders. Since the actual correlations are always much lower than that required, both workers concluded that some secondary process was involved in the establishment of a dominance hierarchy. This secondary process appears to be a resetting of escalation probabilities on the basis of an animal's most recent experience in contests (e.g. Alexander, 1969; Ewing & Ewing, 1973).

Because none of the cues are uniformly distributed, it follows that there will always be a sizable group of contestants with similar cue values and thus similar *a priori* chances of winning a contest. The only information available to such a contestant on its relative position in this distribution is its recent experience in the past. While prior experience *will* correlate roughly with actual cue values, the settling of status levels between animals with equal cue values can only be a matter of chance. In fact, the use of prior experience as an assessment mechanism can by chance lead to anomalous associations of rank and cue value. In short, the nice linear ordering of males in a dominance hierarchy does not imply an equivalent ordering of cue values; the two will be correlated, but the correlations are always much lower than the apparent order. This means that a female who uses dominance status as an index of sizes, vigour, or age may be able to make an assessment more easily, but she may have gained nothing in terms of the accuracy of her assessment. It is even possible she will do worse than if she made direct assessments herself. It still may be the case that dominance is a better estimator of overall adaptedness of males, but this must be shown by the means suggested above and not by ease of determination by females.

We are thus left with the challenging empirical problem of measuring the demographic consequences of female choice in various lek species. The issues are complex enough and the possible outcomes diverse enough that one cannot at present predict whether adaptive cues are or are not likely to be common in nature. Most of the intuitive arguments advanced by prior authors in support of adaptive cues have now been challenged from one quarter or another. On the other hand, there is no strong theoretical reason which precludes their frequent evolution. The problem will be resolved only by extensive and careful fieldwork, and lek species seem an obvious place to start.

One peripheral benefit of thinking about these issues is a realisation that careful measures of survival rates for adult lek males might provide crucial information on a number of theoretically important issues. For one thing, the existing models of female choice suggest that both male mating success and male viability are closely linked to adult male cue values. This suggests that if we have difficulty identifying the critical cues solely by examining mate success, we might get some additional hints by looking at the major causes of adult male mortality. Whether we use direct or indirect means to estimate the size and direction of adaptive effects of mate choice, adult male survivorship functions are clearly a major component in the analysis. Most of us studying leks have spent considerable energy examining the positive side of the sexual selection ledger: male mating success and its immediate causes. It now seems clear that we must also direct as much attention to the debit side (e.g. decreased male viability) and do so for the same animals for which we are measuring mating success. Survivorship is never an easy thing to measure in the field, but its importance to our understanding of sexual selection clearly warrants the effort.

Summary

Lek mating has recently been the subject of renewed theoretical interest. Females of lek species obtain only 'genes' by selecting a mate, and thus this system is closer to the classical models of sexual selection by female choice than other better-studied systems in which females obtain resources and paternal care as well. A lek female has the potential option of exercising a choice both between existing leks and between males on a given lek. It is clear that the patterns of male dispersion and the degree to which females do exert choices between leks will interact. Since the dispersion of males is very diverse even among related lek species, a careful examination of this interaction can both characterise the between-lek level of female choice and perhaps explain the observed variations in male spatial pattern. Because we are just beginning to obtain data on these issues in a few lek species, any general patterns remain to be described.

At the level of choice within a given lek, the basic issues are (a) what are the cues used by females to choose males, and (b) what do they get out of making a choice with those cues. The widely-accepted notions that females simply choose the central male on a lek or that females always choose the 'dominant' male are not warranted by the available data. In fact, no one has yet identified the critical cues used by females in making choices within a given lek. One reason for the difficulty in identifying cues, even when females are unanimous in their choices, may be that there are second-order exaggerations of both correct and incorrect choices. For example, some females may copy the choice of others without themselves attempting to discriminate between males. Until these second-order effects are identified and controlled for, it will be difficult to identify the actual cues.

Identifying the cues is important not only in its own right, but is a necessary condition for settling existing disputes about the way in which sexual selection operates. Do females who choose a given male only obtain the genes to produce sons who will themselves be chosen, or are there other demographic advantages such as more viable sons and/or more viable and fecund daughters? Current theory suggests that only the former effect is needed to explain sexual selection. However, there are a number of authors who continue to insist that the latter effects may be important. The issues can only be resolved by identifying the cues and looking for possible additional demographic consequences in species, such as those with leks, in which females choose mates and do so without having to consider access to resources or paternal care.

Steve Arnold, Mark Kirkpatrick, and Paul Harvey provided extensive comments on our original manuscript, and Ted Case, Mike Gilpin, Dan Sulzbach, Mark Taper and Sandra Vehrencamp made a number of suggestions and criticisms which helped us to clarify our positions on these issues. This work was supported by NSF Grant BNS 79-23524.

References

Alexander, R. (1969). Social behavior in crickets. *Behaviour*, **17**, 131–219

Alexander, R. D. (1975). Natural selection and specialized chorusing behavior in acoustical insects. In *Insects, Science, and Society*, ed. D. Pimental, pp. 35–77. Academic Press: New York.

Ballard, W. B. & Robel, R. J. (1974). Reproductive importance of dominant male Greater Prairie chickens. *Auk*, **91**, 75–86.

Bell, G. (1978). The handicap principle in sexual selection. *Evolution*, **32**, 872–5.

Boag, D. A. & Sumanik, K. M. (1969). Characteristics of drumming sites selected by ruffed grouse in Alberta. *Journal of Wildlife Management*, **33**, 621–8.

Borgia, G. (1979). Sexual selection and the evolution of mating systems. In *Sexual Selection and Reproductive Competition in Insects*, ed. M. S. Blum & N. A. Blum, pp. 19–80. Academic Press: New York.

Bradbury, J. W. (1977). Lek mating behavior in the hammer-headed bat. *Zeitschrift für Tierpsychologie*, **45**, 225–55.

Bradbury, J. W. (1981). The evolution of leks. In *Natural Selection and Social Behavior: Recent Research and New Theory*, ed. R. D. Alexander & D. W. Tinkle, vol. **9**, 138–69. Chiron Press: New York.

Bradbury, J. W. (Submitted MS). Skew in male mating success and independent female choice on leks.

Bradbury, J. W. & Gibson, R. (Submitted MS). The hot-spot model of lek dispersion.

Bucher, T. L., Ryan, M. J. & Bartholomew, G. A. (1982). Oxygen consumption during resting, calling, and nest building in the frog, *Physalaemus pustulosus*. *Physiological Zoology*, **55**, 10–22.

Buechner, H. K., Leuthold, W. & Roth, H. D. (Unpublished MS). Lek territory occupancy in male Uganda kob antelope.

Buechner, H. K. & Roth, H. D. (1974). The lek system in Uganda kob antelope. *American Zoologist*, **14**, 145–62.

Cade, W. H. (1981). Field cricket spacing and the phonotaxis of crickets and parasitoid flies to clumped and isolated cricket songs. *Zeitschrift für Tierpsychologie*, **55**, 365–75.

Chase, I. D. (1974). Models of hierarchy formation in animal societies. *Behavioral Science*, **19**, 374–82.

Dalke, P. D., Pyrah, D. B., Stanton, D. C., Crawford, J. F. & Schlatterer, E. F. (1963). Ecology, productivity and management of sage grouse in Idaho. *Journal of Wildlife Management*, **27**, 810–41.

Davies, N. B. (1978). Ecological questions about territorial behavior. In *Behavioral Ecology: An Evolutionary Approach*, ed. J. R. Krebs & N. B. Davies, chapter 9, pp. 317–50. Sinauer Associates: Sunderland, Mass.

Davies, N. B. & Halliday, T. R. (1978). Deep croaks and fighting assessment in toads, *Bufo bufo. Nature*, **274**, 683–5.

Davis, J. W. F. & O'Donald, P. (1976). Sexual selection for a handicap: a critical analysis of Zahavi's theory. *Journal of Theoretical Biology*, **57**, 345–54.

Diamond, J. M. (1981). Birds of paradise and the theory of sexual selection. *Nature*, **298**, 257–8.

Emlen, S. T. & Oring, L. W. (1977). Ecology, sexual selection and the evolution of mating systems. *Science*, **197**, 215–23.

Eshel, I. (1978). On the handicap principle – a critical defense. *Journal of Theoretical Biology*, **70**, 245–50.

Ewing, L. S. & Ewing, A. W. (1973). Correlates of subordinate behavior in the cockroach, *Nauphoeta cinerea. Animal Behavior*, **21**, 571–8.

Fisher, R. A. (1958). *The Genetical Theory of Natural Selection*. 2nd edn, 291 pp. Dover Publications: New York.

Floody, O. R. & Arnold, A. P. (1975). Uganda kob (*Adenota kob thomasii*): territoriality and the spatial distributions of sexual and agonistic behaviors at a territorial ground. *Zeitschrift für Tierpsychologie*, **37**, 192–212.

Foster, M. S. (1977). Odd couples in manakins: a study of social organization and cooperative breeding in *Chiroxiphia linearis. American Naturalist*, **111**, 845–53.

Fretwell, S. D. (1972). Populations in a seasonal environment, Monograph 5: *Monographs in Population Biology*, 217 pp. Princeton University Press: Princeton.

Gullion, G. W. (1976). Reevaluation of 'activity clustering' by male grouse. *Auk*, **93**, 192–3.

Hamerstrom, F. & Hamerstrom, F. (1960). Comparability of some social displays of grouse. In *Proceedings of the 12th International Ornithological Congress, 1958*, pp. 274–93.

Hartzler, J. E. (1972). *An Analysis of Sage Grouse Lek Behavior*. Ph.D. Dissertation Thesis, 234 pp. University of Montana, Missoula, Montana.

Hartzler, J. E. (1974). Predation and the daily timing of sage grouse leks. *Auk*, **91**, 532–6.

Heisler, I. L. (1981). Offspring quality and the polygyny threshold: a new model for the 'sexy son' hypothesis. *American Naturalist*, **117**, 316–28.

Hjorth, I. (1970). Reproductive behavior in *Tetraonidae. Vilfrevy*, **7**(4), 183–596.

Hoffman, D. M. (1963). The lesser prairie chicken in Colorado. *Journal of Wildlife Management*, **27**, 726–32.

Hogan-Warburg, A. J. (1966). Social behavior of the ruff, *Philomachus pugnax. Ardea*, **54**, 1–45.

Howard, R. D. (1979). The evolution of mating systems in bullfrogs, *Rana catesbeiana. Evolution*, **32**, 850–71.

Hrdy, S. B. (1977). *The Langurs of Abu*. Harvard University Press: Cambridge, Mass.

Huxley, J. S. (1938). The present standing of the theory of sexual selection. In *Evolution: Essays on Aspects of Evolutionary Biology Presented to Professor E. S. Goodrich on his 70th Birthday*. Clarendon Press: Oxford.

Kirkpatrick, M. (1982). Sexual selection and the evolution of female choice. *Evolution*, **36**, 1–12.

Koivisto, I. (1965). Behavior of the black grouse, *Lyrunus tetrix*, during the Spring display. *Finnish Game Research*, **26**, 1–60.

Kruijt, J. P., de Vos, G. J. & Bossema, I. (1972). The arena system of black grouse. *Proceedings of the XVth International Ornithological Congress*, pp. 399–423. E. J. Brill: Leiden.

Kruijt, J. P. & Hogan, J. A. (1967). Social behavior on the lek in black grouse. *Ardea*, **55**, 203–40.

Lack, D. (1939). The display of the black cock. *British Birds*, **32**, 290–303.

Landau, H. G. (1951a). On dominance relations and the structure of animal societies, I. Effect of inherent characteristics. *Bulletin of Mathematical Biophysics*, **13**, 1–19.

Landau, H. G. (1951b). On dominance relations and the structure of animal societies, II. Some effects of possible social factors. *Bulletin of Mathematical Biophysics*, **13**, 245–62.

Lande, R. (1977). The influence of mating system on the maintenance of genetic variability in polygenic characters. *Genetics*, **86**, 485–98.

Lande, R. (1980). Sexual dimorphism, sexual selection, and adaptation in polygenic characters. *Evolution*, **34**, 292–305.

Lande, R. (1981). Models of speciation by sexual selection on polygenic traits. *Proceedings of the National Academy of Sciences of the USA*, **78**, 3721–5.

Le Boeuf, B. J. & Briggs, K. T. (1977). The cost of living in a seal harem. *Mammalia*, **41**, 167–95.

Le Croy, M., Kulupi, A. & Peckover, W. S. (1980). Goldie's Bird-of-Paradise: display, natural history, and traditional relationships of people to the bird. *Wilson Bulletin*, **92**, 289–301.

Lill, A. (1974). Social organization and space utilization in the lek-forming white-bearded manakin, *M. manacus trinitatis. Zeitschrift für Tierpsychologie*, **36**, 513–30.

Lill, A. (1976). Lek behavior in the golden-headed manakin (*Pipra erythrocephala*) in Trinidad (West Indies). *Forstschrift Verhaltensforschung*, Heft **18**, pp. 1–84. Verlag Paul Parey: Berlin/Hamburg.

Martin, S. G. (1974). Adaptations for polygynous breeding in the bobolink, *Dolichonyx oryzivorus. American Zoologist*, **14**, 109–19.

Maynard Smith, J. (1976). Sexual selection and the handicap principle. *Journal of Theoretical Biology*, **57**, 239–42.

Maynard Smith, J. (1978). The handicap principle – a comment. *Journal of Theoretical Biology*, **70**, 251–2.

Myers, J. P. (1979). Leks, sex and buff-breasted sandpipers. *American Birds*, **33**, 823–5.

O'Donald, P. (1980). *Genetic Models of Sexual Selection*. Cambridge University Press: Cambridge.

Oring, L. W. (1982). Avian mating systems. In *Avian Biology*, vol. **6**, ed. D. Farner, J. King & K. Parkes, 1–92. Academic Press: New York.

Otte, D. (1974). Effects and functions in the evolution of signaling systems. *Annual Review of Ecology and Systematics*, **5**, 385–416.

Partridge, L. (1980). Mate choice increases a component of offspring fitness in fruit flies. *Nature*, **283**, 290–1.

Patterson, R. L. (1952). *The Sage Grouse in Wyoming*. Sage Books: Denver.

Payne, R. & Payne, K. (1977). Social organization and mating success in local song populations of village idigo birds, *Vidua chalybeata. Zeitschrift für Tierpsychologie*, **45**, 113–73.

Rhijn, J. G. van (1973). Behavioral dimorphism in male ruffs, *Philomachus pugnax. Behaviour*, **47**, 153–229.

Rippin, A. B. & Boag, D. A. (1974). Recruitment to populations of male sharp-tailed grouse. *Journal of Wildlife Management*, **38**, 616–21.

Robel, R. J. & Ballard, W. B. (1974). Lek social organization and reproductive success in the Greater Prairie chicken. *American Zoologist*, **14**, 121–8.

Ryan, M. J. (1980). Female mate choice in a neotropical frog. *Science*, **209**, 523–5.

Ryan, M. J. (MS). Sexual selection and communication in a neotropical frog, *Physalaemus pustulosus.*

Schodde, R. & Mason, I. J. (1974). Further observations on *Parotia wahnesi* and *P. lawesii* (Paradisaeidae). *Emu*, **74**, 200–1.

Selander, R. K. (1972). Sexual selection and dimorphism in birds. In *Sexual Selection and the Descent of Man: 1871–1971*. Aldine Press: Chicago.

Shepard, J. M. (1975). Factors influencing female choice in the lek mating system of the ruff. *Living Bird*, **14**, 87–111.

Snow, B. K. (1961). Notes on the behavior of three *Cotingidae*. *Auk*, **78**, 150–61.

Snow, B. K. (1973). Notes on the behavior of the White Bellbird. *Auk*, **90**, 743–51.

Snow, B. K. (1974). Lek behavior and breeding of Guy's hermit hummingbird *Phaethornis guy*. *Ibis*, **116**, 278–97.

Snow, D. W. (1963). The evolution of manakin displays. In *Proceedings of the 13th International Ornithological Congress*, vol. **1**, pp. 553–61.

Snow, D. W. & Goodwin, D. (1974). The black and gold cotinga. *Auk*, **91**, 360–9.

Stiles, F. G. & Wolf, L. L. (1979). Ecology and evolution of lek mating behavior in the long-tailed hermit hummingbird. *Ornithological Monographs*, pp. 27–88. American Ornithologists' Union: Washington, D.C.

Thornhill, R. (1980). Competitive charming males and choosy females: was Darwin correct? *Florida Entomologist*, **63**, 5–30.

Trivers, R. L. (1972). Parental investment and sexual selection. In *Sexual Selection and the Descent of Man: 1871–1971*, ed. B. Campbell, chapter 7. Aldine Press: Chicago.

Tuttle, M. & Ryan, M. J. (1981). Bat predation and the evolution of frog vocalizations in the neotropics. *Science*, **214**, 677–8.

Wade, M. J. & Arnold, S. J. (1980). The intensity of sexual selection in relation to male sexual behavior, female choice, and sperm precedence. *Animal Behavior*, **28**, 446–61.

West-Eberhard, M. J. (1979). Sexual selection, social competition, and evolution. *Proceedings of the American Philosophical Society*, **123**, 222–34.

Wiley, R. H. (1973). Territoriality and non-random mating in sage grouse, *Centrocercus urophasianus*. *Animal Behavior*, **6**, 85–169.

Wiley, R. H. (1974). Evolution of social organization and life history patterns among grouse (Aves: Tetraonidae). *Quarterly Review of Biology*, **49**, 209–27.

Williams, G. C. (1966). *Adaptation & Natural Selection*, 207 pp. Princeton University Press: Princeton, New Jersey.

Williams, G. C. (1975). *Sex and Evolution*, 200 pp. Princeton University Press: Princeton, New Jersey.

Williams, M. (1978). Sexual selection, adaptation, and ornamental traits: the advantage of seeming fitter. *Journal of Theoretical Biology*, **72**, 377–83.

Wittenberger, J. F. (1978). The evolution of mating systems in grouse. *Condor*, **80**, 126–37.

Wittenberger, J. F. (1979). The evolution of mating systems in birds and mammals. In *Handbook of Behavioral Neurobiology*, vol. **3**, ed. P. J. Marler & J. Vanderbergh, pp. 271–349. Plenum Press: New York.

Wittenberger, J. F. (1981). *Animal Social Behaviour*. Duxbery Press: Boston.

Wrangham, R. D. (1980). Female choice of least costly males; a possible factor in the evolution of leks. *Zeitschrift für Tierpsychologie*, **54**, 357–67.

Zahavi, A. (1975). Mate selection – a selection for a handicap. *Journal of Theoretical Biology*, **53**, 205–14.

III: SEX DIFFERENCES IN CHOOSINESS

6

Mate quality and mating decisions

G. A. PARKER

Since the influential papers of Bateman (1948) and Trivers (1972) it has been evident that parental investment (PI) is important in determining which sex competes, and which sex is choosy. It is usual to argue that when male PI is small or negligible, males will compete and females will be choosy. Alternatively, in cases of sex role reversal in PI pattern, females compete and males are choosy.

My aim in this paper is to propose that active mate choice in fact depends on an interaction between relative PI (or more accurately, investment with a given mate) and relative variance in mate quality for the two sexes. Benefits of choice are an increasing function of the variance in mate quality of the opposite sex; costs of choice relate to the time and effort needed to find an alternative mate (they will therefore decrease as the PI of the opposite sex decreases). Although genetic benefits (choice of 'good genes') are likely to be small or negligible, major benefits of active mate choice may arise through environmental variance in PI ability. Thus both variance in mate quality (benefit of choice) *and* time to find an alternative mate (costs of choice) are likely to increase with PI, a feature which greatly complicates the making of general predictions. Certainly, we should not always expect that the sex with lowest investment will be the least choosy, though this may often be the case.

Active mate choice and passive attraction

If we observe differences in reproductive success between male phenotypes in nature, this does not establish that there is *active* female choice. Apart from the obvious possibility that males may contest directly for females, there are more subtle ways in which the success of a male may relate to its phenotype without involving active female choice. Depending

141

on phenotype, different males may have different optimal sexual advertisement levels (Andersson, 1982; Parker, 1982).

Many instances of apparent mate choice may involve no more than the passive attraction of an individual to sexual cues emitted by an individual of opposite sex (Parker, 1982). Thus where, say, the female finds the male by attraction to some male cue, males that emit the greatest stimulus may obtain most meetings. The female need exert no active preference between males, she simply moves towards the most intense source of the conspecific cue. For active mate choice we would require that the female rejects certain conspecific males in favour of others. As A. Arak (present volume) and T. Halliday (present volume) stress, great caution will be needed in field studies to establish whether this apparent preference for certain males is due to active choice or simply to passive attraction. If a female locates a male by passive attraction, she should simply move towards the male that emits the most intense stimulus at the point she is placed. If she shows active choice, she should reject certain males, even when placed close by them.

I shall explore a model of passive choice in some detail because it is important to illustrate precisely how passive attraction to a sexual cue can generate the apparent effect that there is active mate choice. The model is a summary of that given by Parker (1982); rather similar conclusions had been drawn earlier using a slightly different model by Andersson (1982).

Suppose that females find males by attraction to a visual, auditory, or chemical stimulus. Males compete, within the encounter site for the species, by sexual advertisement. The greater the sexual advertisement (stimulus emitted) relative to competitors, the greater the relative number of matings a male achieves. The result is what can be termed the 'sexual advertisement scramble competition' and we seek a level of advertisement which is an ESS ('evolutionarily stable strategy', Maynard Smith, 1974). Suppose that male i achieves benefits (matings) in proportion to his own advertisement expenditure level a_i relative to the current mean level:

$$\text{benefit}_i = \frac{\text{self's expenditure } a_i}{\text{mean expenditure } \bar{a}}$$

(more complex forms of benefit can be devised, see Parker, 1982). The justification for allocating benefits in this way is that a male with, say, a louder call would have a greater 'circle of attraction' around it and hence obtains greater catchment area of females than its competitors (see Fig. 6.1). A female at a given point simply moves towards the greatest source of stimulus.

Assume also that advertisement carries costs; these may be either energetic losses or increased risks of predation due to enhanced detection by predators. Let the probability c of survival be some monotonic decreasing function of advertisement level a (see Fig. 6.2). It is easy to show that the ESS level of advertisement, a_*, for a large population of competing males has

$$-\frac{\mathrm{d}c(a_*)}{\mathrm{d}a} = \frac{c(a_*)}{a_*}$$

This result can best be demonstrated graphically (Fig. 6.2). At the ESS, the gradient of the function $c(a)$ must equal the slope $c(a)$ divided by a. (This slope is drawn with negative gradient in Fig. 6.2 to counter the negative sign in the above equation and the fact that $c(a)$ has a negative gradient.)

This ESS level of advertisement a_* is in fact a Nash equilibrium, or competitive optimum. When the population is at the ESS, a mutant with $a > a_*$ will sustain too great a level of costs to spread, despite its increased benefits, and a mutant with $a < a_*$ will not gain enough matings despite its reduced costs. It was Fisher (1930) who first proposed that sexual selection may proceed to some form of optimum, though his argument related to active rather than passive choice. Perhaps the most interesting feature of this solution, and not discussed by Fisher, is the fact that different phenotypes will have different ESS levels of advertisement. 'Strong' phenotypes, for whom $c(a)$ is less steeply declining, will have a

Fig. 6.1. Sexual advertisement scramble competition. A mutant male with an advertisement level $a_i > \bar{a}$ (the advertisement level of the rest of the population) will have a larger zone of attraction and will attract more females. It will also sustain greater costs of advertisement.

mutant male
with $a_i > a$

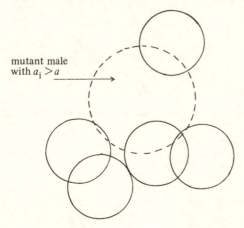

higher ESS level of advertisement than 'weaker' phenotypes for whom $c(a)$ declines more steeply. Thus we should find that 'strong' males attract more females, and vice versa, simply because it will pay them to advertise to a higher level. So by a purely passive process, we should observe that females tend to mate more frequently with certain male phenotypes than others; no active choice whatever by females is required to generate this effect.

This conclusion at first sight bears a startling resemblance to the ingenious 'handicap theory' (Zahavi, 1975; Bell, 1978). Zahavi proposed that females should actively choose mates with the highest level of costly advertisement ('handicap') since this means that they are likely, having survived their handicap, to carry 'good genes' and to be 'strong'. There have been many critical discussions of the handicap theory and the subject is still controversial (see Andersson, 1982). The major problem concerns getting a sex-limited handicap gene to spread. If it is actually to be a handicap, then the handicap gene must be lost when there are no females that prefer it (i.e. all females possess genes coding for random mating). However, if (somehow) enough females in the population possess genes coding for active choice of handicapped males, the handicap characteristic can spread to fixation because of its sexual selection advantage, and in the process the preference gene will also increase in frequency (see later). But if initially choice genes are very rare, selection will act *against* females choosing handicapped males and *in favour* of those choosing non-

Fig. 6.2. Costs of advertisement are assumed to increase with increasing advertisement level. Thus the probability of survival c is a decreasing function of advertisement level a. At the ESS, a_*, $-c'(a_*) = c(a_*)/a_*$. Different phenotypes have different optima, but if $c(a)$ is a negative exponential, all phenotypes have the same level of costs, i.e. $c(a_{*i}) = c(a_{*j})\ldots = c(a_{*n})$; see Parker (1982).

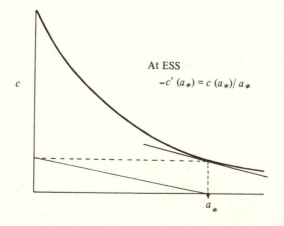

handicapped males, unless the mean fitness of a brood from a handicapped male exceeds the mean brood fitness. This could occur if (i) the mean fitness of daughters is high enough to compensate for the reduced fitness of sons, or (ii) if the mean fitness of sons, despite the handicap, exceeds mean male fitness. However, when both choice genes and handicap genes are rare, handicap genes will be being lost at a fast rate by direct selection, whereas choice genes can at best increase at a slow rate (dependent on meeting of rare individuals).

The sexual advertisement model outlined here is rather different from Zahavi's model. It does not predict that 'strong' males will take on a greater risk of predation than 'weak' males; in fact for some explicit forms of $c(a)$ it can be shown that at the ESS all phenotypes would sustain *equal* costs (Parker, 1982). 'Strong' males, however, always obtain more matings because they will advertise more extensively for the same predation risk.

Do females actively choose males with 'good genes'?

Active female choice concerns the case where the female possesses some mechanism for discriminating between conspecific males. The theoretical arguments in favour of active female choice are well known and need not be stressed (see Trivers, 1972). Suffice it to say that there are two cases:

(1) *Benefits environmental.* The male confers some non-heritable benefit to the female and the offspring. For example, he may have a better territory in which the female may forage, or may have a better prey item on which the female will feed (e.g. Thornhill, 1980*a*). Assuming that variance between males is essentially environmental, the benefits of choice to the female relate entirely to increased resources or reduced risks, etc. This case poses no obvious theoretical difficulties.

(2) *Benefits genetic.* The male confers heritable benefits upon the offspring. Hence the advantage of female choice relies on the assumption that there is genetic variance between males. Stated crudely, females choose males with 'good genes'.

Apart from the fascinating circumstantial evidence (open to various interpretations) that *Drosophila melanogaster* females allowed to choose their mates produce larvae with higher competitive ability than those denied a choice (Partridge, 1980), there is remarkably little empirical data to support the view that females may exert a fine-tuned choice related to 'good genes'. Female choice of central males in lekking species has also been seen as circumstantial evidence for choice of 'good genes', since lekking males typically provide no resources for the female (Maynard Smith, 1978; Borgia, 1979). There are alternative environmental explanations, however (Thornhill, 1980*b*).

The principal difficulty with the 'good genes' argument is whether adequate genetic variance can be maintained amongst males (e.g. Williams, 1975; Maynard Smith, 1978; Thornhill, 1980*b*), especially when mate choice carries costs (Parker, 1982). Costs of mate choice are seldom considered; they have serious theoretical implications for the maintenance of choice strategies where benefits derive from 'good genes'. I shall consider briefly the theoretical implications of these costs separately for the case of major gene effects and polygenic effects.

The major gene model

O'Donald (see 1980 for review) has formulated an extensive series of major gene models based on Fisher's original argument (Fisher, 1930). In the simplest case there are two alternative alleles at a locus active in males, and two alternate alleles at a locus active in females. Thus females can be either indiscriminative or choosy, and males can either possess or not possess the character preferred by choosy females. Fisher envisaged that in order to spread, the preferred male allele (call it M) must initially have a selective advantage unrelated to the choice allele. As M spreads, the choice allele (call it C) also spreads (but at a slower rate) because it gains an advantage due to the advantage of M. As C spreads, the advantage of M increases through sexual selection, which in turn reciprocally increases the advantage of C, and the spread of both alleles accelerates. As M approaches fixation, the selective advantage of C over its alternative allele decreases to zero. It is only back-mutation of M to the allele for the non-preferred characteristic that can allow C to proceed slowly towards fixation.

In the absence of recurrent mutation to the non-preferred allele, C will at best be selectively neutral and will be subject to drift. If there are significant costs associated with the choice allele C, it will crash in favour of the allele for indiscriminateness (a discussion of costs is given later). In this case, M will be held at fixation only by virtue of its original initial selective advantage (see Fig. 6.3). Note that if, in the absence of C, M is selectively neutral or disadvantageous (as in the handicap theory), then M is also unstable and may drift or crash in favour of the non-preferred allele. If allele M is selectively disadvantageous in the absence of C (i.e. M is a handicap), then the frequency of C must somehow rise above a threshold level before M can begin to spread at all.

It is clear from the above arguments that the ESSs to this 2 × 2 strategy game depend critically on the relative costs and benefits of the choice allele C when the preferred allele is at fixation. Benefits will relate entirely to recurrent mutation to the non-preferred allele. Assume first that benefits of choice due to recurrent back-mutation exceed the costs. ESSs are either: (i) preferred males and choosy females, or (ii) non-preferred males and indiscriminate females.

ESS (ii) can occur only if preferred males have a selective disadvantage in the absence of choosy females, i.e. if they are 'handicapped'. Because a very rare gene for preference of handicapped males will be selected against, ESS (i) can arise only after drift to a high enough frequency of allele C.

Assume now that costs of choice exceed the benefits due to recurrent

Fig. 6.3. Possible fate of choice alleles (C, D) and alleles for preferred characters (M, N). Suppose allele M (acting in males) has a natural selection advantage. It begins to spread, and by a Fisherian process a preference allele C (that causes females to choose males with M) will spread and accelerate the spread of M, assuming that the C mutation occurs during the period over which a polymorphism exists at the M locus. C will decline in frequency as M approaches fixation, because costs of choice may be non-negligible, though benefits may diminish towards zero (see text). The process is repeated later with alleles N and D, but because N and D involve quite different loci from M and C, the C allele itself will not sustain any boost from N, and will be lost. This will not be the case for polygenic characters, however (see text).

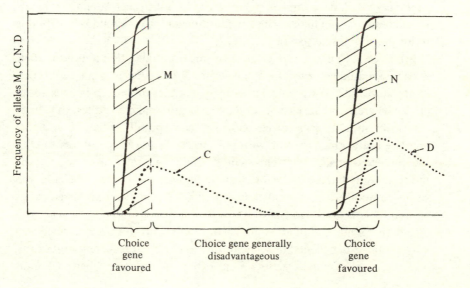

back mutation. ESSs are either: (i) preferred males and indiscriminate females or (ii) non-preferred males and indiscriminate females, and the ESS obtained depends on which allele has greater selective advantage in the absence of choosy females.

In summary, the major gene model will yield choosy females only if recurrent back-mutation can generate enough genetic variance to create significant enough benefits to outweigh the costs of choice. Even then, as Halliday (1978) has noted, female choice appears merely to increase the speed at which a male character would anyhow spread in a population. It seems quite likely, even, that the appropriate choice allele will not be present in the population at the time a favourable male character is spreading, especially if the male characteristic is highly advantageous so that it proceeds quickly to fixation in the absence of female choice.

If costs outweigh benefits, the case for female choice becomes very pessimistic. What are the costs of choice? Costs, like benefits, would appear to diminish to zero when the preferred male character approaches fixation. If virtually all males possess the character, a female with a preference for it finds virtually all males acceptable, and therefore appears to be equivalent to an indiscriminate female. I argue that there are at least two reasons why a choosy female would plausibly sustain greater costs than an indiscriminate female, even when the preferred character approaches fixation:

(i) There may be environmental effects that cause males with the preferred allele to resemble males without it. Alternatively, the preferred gene may not have complete penetrance. In both cases, a choosy female would tend to reject males (a cost without benefit) that would be acceptable to an indiscriminate female.

(ii) Even if (i) never applies, it seems most unlikely that a mutant allele for choice could achieve a perfect discrimination between male genotypes. Quite simply, a choosy female is likely sometimes to make mistakes about choice whereas an indiscriminate female cannot make mistakes. In genetic terms, the mutant gene for choice is (at least initially) likely to code for increased reluctance to mate with both male phenotypes, but less so with the preferred male type. This would again generate costs not felt by indiscriminate females. In short, perfect choice is unlikely to be achieved by an unmodified 'mutant allele'; sometimes it will reject preferred males as well as non-preferred ones.

Whether females should be choosy or not depends on a balance between two second-order effects; the benefits of choice due to recurrent mutations, and the costs of choice arising from errors of the type where a female incorrectly rejects a preferred male. Ultimately, mutations may be rarer than mistakes, and hence costs of choice greater than benefits.

Borgia (1979) has suggested that where heterozygous males have a mating advantage over homozygous males, females will be favoured if they choose heterozygous males. He argues that this strategy would, on average, yield more of the advantageous heterozygous offspring. In fact, it is easy to show that if the population is at polymorphic equilibrium, Borgia's argument is fallacious. Assuming that the female does not 'know' her genetic constitution at the heterotic locus, then mutant strategies for choice of any of the three male genotypes yields exactly the same fitness, and is selectively neutral in a population of randomly mating females (see Partridge, present volume). However, if the female is able to exert a choice that is dependent on her own genotype, then it clearly pays a homozygous female to choose the alternative homozygous male, and a heterozygous female to choose whichever of the two homozygotes that is fitter. Whether fine-grained choice of this type is a plausible possibility seems doubtful.

An alternative mechanism of maintaining genetic variation may relate to spatio-temporal variations in the habitat. Precisely whether this could lead to the maintenance of choice genes through genetic benefits still remains to be analysed. Hamilton & Zuk (in press) have recently shown that gene frequency limit cycles can favour female choice genes.

Polygenic traits

Lande (1980, 1981) has recently analysed polygenic models of mate choice. His fascinating results represent important theoretical developments in sexual selection (see Arnold, present volume). His models, however, do not appear to include costs of choice to females; precisely how this might affect the conclusions is difficult to estimate.

Thornhill (1980*b*) has made the point that if females exert a preference for a quantitative male character – say they prefer males with the highest measure of a given character – they may achieve benefits both by rejecting males with mutations towards low scores and by accepting those with mutations towards high scores. A character such as size may be affected by changes at a vast number of loci, generating a large number of mutants in the population and perhaps a higher potential benefit in choice (Partridge, personal communication). However, if we assume that each locus involved is subject, in its expression, to an equivalent amount of environmental variation, then it is not at all clear that there will be a higher ratio of genetic variation:environmental variation for polygenic characters than for major gene effects. In short, genetic benefits may be higher for choice of polygenic characters, but costs may be correspondingly higher because there will be a vast amount of environmental 'noise' which will obscure the accurate operation of choice. Mutations increasing the character may be relatively common, but the chances that a mutant will achieve, say, the highest score out of the males sampled, is low.

There is one way in which female choice of a quantitative character is easier to maintain than 'major gene' choice. For 'major gene' choice, preference for one male character (due to a particular gene) may require a quite different mechanism (and hence a different choice gene) from the previous mechanism. Hence after their initial boost during the spread of the preferred male character, each choice gene will decline to zero (Fig. 6.3). However, for female choice of a quantitative character, the same choice gene could experience a boost each time a favourable mutation occurs.

Although the case for maintenance of mate choice for reasons of 'good genes' appears rather pessimistic, there are cases where genetic choice seems entirely feasible. These include:

(i) discrimination against non-conspecifics, or different ecotypes.
(ii) avoidance of inbreeding or excessive outbreeding (see Bateson, present volume), and
(iii) avoidance of mating with obviously deleterious mutants,
(iv) gene frequency limit cycles (Hamilton & Zuk, in press).

Mate quality, search costs, and mating decisions

A mating decision is simply an individual's decision whether to mate or not to mate when it meets an individual of opposite sex. In a given encounter between a male and female, there will commonly be sexual conflict over mating decision, i.e. one individual would gain and one individual would lose if mating were to occur. Models of optimal mating decision have recently been constructed for both sexes by Parker (1979), and for females by Janetos (1980).

My earlier approach (Parker, 1979) outlined an 'ideal' degree of mate choice to be exercised by each sex, based on the assumption that an individual could always mate in an encounter if it chose to do so. This approach effectively prescribes the strategy that will spread fastest as a rare mutant in a population that shows random mating. However, it does not offer an ESS to the problem of mate choice unless random mating (indiscriminateness) is the best mating decision for one sex. Where some degree of choice is favourable for both sexes, the ESS for mate choice may be rather different from the best strategy for a rare mutant in a population playing 'indiscriminateness'. As we shall see, an optimal choice may depend on self's mate quality. I attempt below a prospective ESS analysis for mate choice. It includes two important components: the extent of investment in a particular mating, and variance in mate quality. Variance in mate quality in a sex is the variance in fitness experienced by the other sex were it to mate randomly.

Let us make the simplifying assumption that, in order for a mating to occur, both sexes must be willing to mate. Thus if the favourable mating decision for either partner is not to mate, it cannot be forced to mate by the other partner. (This assumption certainly does not hold in all species, and the general problem of resolution of sexual conflict is discussed later.) Secondly, assume that there is a search cost (or search and rejection cost) associated with rejecting a particular mate. Thirdly, assume for simplicity that a given individual has the same mate quality for all individuals of the opposite sex (this is clearly not so for optimal inbreeding and certain other forms of choice; see Bateson, present volume). There will be three types of ESS for mate choice. These are as follows.

(1) *Both sexes indiscriminate* (random mating). This should occur when there is little variance in mate quality in both sexes, and/or when search costs are high (e.g. low encounter rates due to low population densities, low mobility, etc.). Following the optimal diet model of MacArthur & Pianka (1966) this ESS occurs when for both sexes

$$\frac{Q_{min}}{g} > \frac{\bar{Q}}{s+g} \tag{6.1}$$

where

Q_{min} = the value (in fitness units) of a mating with the lowest quality mate

$\bar{Q}$ = the value of a mating with a mate of average quality

g = the reproductive time investment due to mating (time taken to copulate, to replenish the gametes expanded, and to supply PI)

s = the search time (time to find another mate).

(2) *Only one sex discriminate.* If variance in mate quality is similar for each sex, then the discriminate sex will be the sex with lower investment, g. If investment is similar for each sex, then it will be the sex with the least variance in mate quality that will be discriminate. This ESS occurs when equation (6.1) is satisfied for one sex, but not the other. The discriminate sex should reject all mates of quality $Q < Q_{opt}$, where Q_{opt} is defined by:

$$\frac{Q_{opt}}{g} = \frac{\displaystyle\int_{Q_{opt}}^{Q_{max}} p(Q)Q \cdot dQ}{g + \left[\displaystyle\int_{Q_{opt}}^{Q_{max}} p(Q)dQ\right]^{-1} s} \tag{6.2}$$

where
Q_{max} = the value of a mating with the highest quality mate
$p(Q)$ = the distribution of mate quality in the opposite sex.
The right hand side of equation (6.2) is the average value of an acceptable mate (numerator) divided by g+the average search cost to find an acceptable mate (see also the fixed threshold model of Janetos, 1980).

An alternative graphical model can be used to demonstrate the same fixed threshold ESS (Parker, 1979). Fig. 6.4 shows a case where variance in mate quality is the same for each sex, but the investment of a male in a mating is insignificant. We plot $G(bs)$, the fitness G achieved by taking on bs search costs, where b = mean the number of searches sustained for each mating. Thus b is the strategy for mating decision; e.g. if $b = 10$ then 9 out of 10 mates are below the acceptable quality and the fixed threshold is to accept only the top 10% of mates encountered. The ESS for the discriminate sex can be found by the tangent method as outlined in Fig. 6.4 (see Appendix for further explanation).

The value of the graphical model is that it shows directly how important variance in mate quality is in determining the strategy for mate choice. For instance, if females vary in their quality as mates much more than males then $G(bs_m)$ could in fact rise much more steeply than $G(bs_f)$. In reality, this is likely, since male mate quality will hardly vary if males contribute nothing but genes to the mating. Thus it could be males that are discriminate and females that are indiscriminate, despite the fact that male investment in each mating is insignificant compared to female investment.

(3) *Both sexes discriminate.* When (1) cannot be satisfied for either sex, then at the ESS both sexes will exercise some degree of mate choice. This ESS is most likely when there is high variance in mate quality in both sexes and when the search costs to find an alternative mate are relatively low. In these circumstances, the ESS consists *either* of a state in which there will be assortative pairing for mate quality over part of the range of lower mate qualities, and indiscriminate pairing between certain high-quality individuals, *or* of a state in which high-quality individuals mate together randomly and certain lower-quality individuals mate together randomly.

I shall adopt a heuristic approach, since a rigorous analytical solution to this problem becomes tediously complex. I assume that variance in mate quality will be roughly equal in the two sexes; if female quality varies much more than male quality, the labelling of the axes in Figs. 6.5 and 6.6 can be reversed for males and females. In Fig. 6.5, graph (a) shows the lowest quality of male that will be acceptable to a female of quality Q_f; graph

Fig. 6.4. An example of an ESS where one sex should be choosy and one indiscriminate. Curve $G(bs_f)$ shows the increase in female fitness if she takes on a search cost bs_f, in which only the best one in four males is accepted; curve $G(bs_m)$ is the corresponding curve for the male, drawn on the assumption that the variance in mate quality is equal for the two sexes (but see text). The optimal choice b_f is given by the tangent as shown; it is assumed that the female invests time g_f producing and caring for the offspring whereas the male invests nothing. Hence the total search time for the male, if there is a 1:1 adult sex ratio, is $s_m = g + s_f$, where s_f is the search time for the female. In the case shown, it pays females to accept only the best 25% of males encountered ($b_f = 4$), but males should accept all females. After Parker (1979).

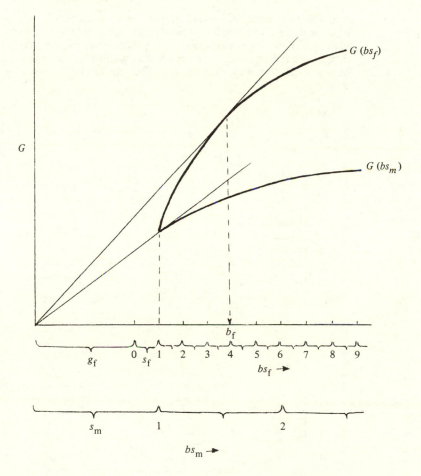

(b) shows the corresponding acceptance threshold for a male of quality Q_m. The case concerns a species in which the male's investment in a mating is significant, but less than the females.

A female (Fig. 6.5a) should accept all males with quality greater than Q_{mt} if her own quality is above Q_{ft}. If her quality is below Q_{ft}, she should be less choosy. Poorer quality females ($Q_f < Q_{ft}$) may show one of two alternative patterns of choice. They may have a single, lower-acceptance threshold than the higher quality females, in which case lower quality males ($Q_m < Q_{mt}$) will be indiscriminate. Alternatively, poorer-quality

Fig. 6.5. An example of an ESS in which both sexes should be choosy to some degree. The graphs are acceptance thresholds for the two sexes: (a) shows the lowest quality male that should be acceptable to a female of quality Q_f; (b) shows the lowest quality female that should be acceptable to a male of quality Q_m. For further explanation see text.

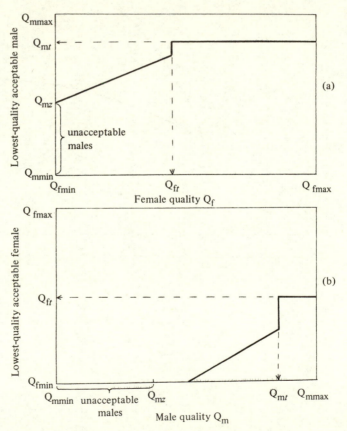

individuals of both sexes will have choice thresholds that correlate positively with their own quality, as shown in Fig. 6.5. Male decisions (Fig. 6.5b) are organised rather similarly. The logic behind these conclusions is explained in the Appendix.

Fig. 6.6 indicates the zones of potential pairings for the case outlined in Fig. 6.5. As discussed, high-quality individuals ($Q_m > Q_{mt}$; $Q_f > Q_{ft}$) should mate with each other randomly. But if choice thresholds correlate with mate quality over some range as in Fig. 6.5, then we should observe some degree of assortative pairing for mate quality for lower-quality individuals (Fig. 6.6). Alternatively, if search costs are so high that males are either choosy or indiscriminate, then potential pairings would occur within two rectangles (indicating two zones of random pairing) – one for high-quality individuals and one for lower-quality individuals. This second rectangle would include all females below Q_{ft}, but only those males between Q_{mt} and the step interval below it. A range of poor quality males is always unacceptable whichever case applies. Again, conclusions about the sexes can be reversed if female mate quality varies more than male mate quality.

It is clear that even when search costs are high so that just two thresholds

Fig. 6.6. The zones (cross-hatching) of mate quality over which mating will occur if acceptance thresholds are arranged as in Fig. 6.5. High quality individuals ($Q_m > Q_{mt}$; $Q_f > Q_{ft}$) will mate randomly. Poorer quality individuals will (in this example) show assortative pairing for mate quality, but some males ($Q_m < Q_{mz}$) will not mate at all. In the zone above and to the left of the cross-hatching, the female will accept but the male will not; in the zone below and to the right of cross-hatching, the male will accept but not the female.

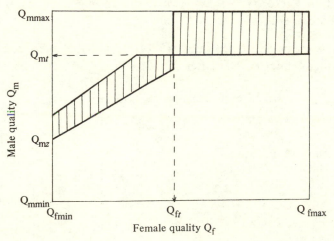

apply for each sex, field data on pairings may well give significant positive correlations for mate quality (assortative pairing). However, it is where search costs are small for both sexes that we would expect the strongest assortative pairing effect. In general, it seems most likely that assortative pairing will be strongest when male investment is high, because although this will increase female search costs (reduce Q_{mf}) it will reduce male search costs (increase Q_{ff}). If male investment is zero, then with a 1:1 sex ratio the minimum possible search cost for a male must be greater than time g_f, the female investment time.

Many varied effects can generate positive assortative pairing (see Ridley, in preparation). For instance, a common cause of positive assortment for size could be that bigger females produce more eggs and hence are more valuable to males than small females; also big males are better at defending their preferred resources than small males. Thus assortative pairing could be due to a mixture of male choice and intermale competition. However, the present model shows that variance in mate quality in each sex should alone be enough to generate assortative pairing for mate quality, provided that variance in mate quality is high enough for both sexes.

Sexual conflict and mating decisions

Fig. 6.7 outlines the three types of outcome that are possible for mating decisions in a sexual encounter (see also Parker, 1979). It is condition (ii) that involves sexual conflict; one individual (usually the male) finds the potential mate acceptable, but the other (usually the female) finds the potential mate to be below the acceptance threshold.

There are several forms of sexual conflict, many of which are discussed at length in Parker (1979). Some of the more interesting cases can be summarised as follows:

(1) *Conflict over incest.* Dawkins (1976) stressed that male and female interests may differ in the matter of inbreeding. Call c the ratio of male

Fig. 6.7. Sexual conflict and mating decisions.

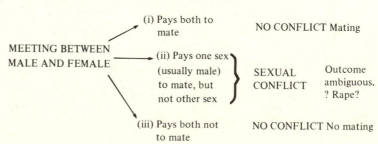

investment in a mating/female investment in a mating. Suppose that offspring from an incestuous mating between two individuals that share half their genes have a fitness of $(1 - D)$ relative to 1 for offspring from outcrossing. It will pay a male to mate with his sister, daughter, or mother, and will pay her not to mate if:

$$3 - 2c - 1 > \frac{D}{3} > 3 - c - 2 \tag{6.3}$$

Where male investment is negligible, c approaches zero and condition (6.3) becomes:

$$\tfrac{2}{3} > D > \tfrac{1}{3} \tag{6.4}$$

(Parker, 1979). Thus if D lies anywhere between $\tfrac{1}{3}$ and $\tfrac{2}{3}$, there will be conflict between male and female mating decisions. Males will be eager to mate, but females do better to avoid mating. The model takes account of kin selection.

(2) *Conflict in rare meetings between different ecotypes or closely related species.* It is often stressed that males have less to lose than females by mating with non-conspecifics. In fact, males may often gain from such matings, and conflict between male and females mating decision may be common. Degrees of hybrid disadvantage over which sexual conflict will occur have been analysed in previous models (Parker, 1979); the male is usually under more intense selection to achieve the mating than is the female to prevent the mating. However, where one species or ecotype has much higher search costs than the other, possibly due to differences in population density, this need not be the case. At least theoretically, a conflict can occur where it pays a female of the low-density population to mate, but pays the male (of the high density population) not to mate.

(3) *Conflict between conspecifics concerning mate quality.* This is the case discussed in the last section. Inspection of Fig. 6.6 indicates the two zones of conflict. In one zone it will pay the female to mate, but not the male; in the other, larger zone, it pays the male to mate but not the female. In this model, there will be no encounters in which it pays *neither* individual to mate because of the assumption that an individual's quality as a mate is equal for all members of the opposite sex. Certain individuals (usually males, see Fig. 6.5; unless variance in female quality much exceeds variance in male quality) will be unacceptable as mates to even the poorest quality individuals of the opposite sex. However it could never pay poorest quality individuals of *both* sexes to avoid mating with each other if this meant that they would never mate at all.

Resolution of sexual conflict over mating decision

What will be the evolutionary outcome of sexual conflict over mating decision? This is a subject of some considerable complexity (see Parker, 1979) and one that is currently developing. I shall attempt only a brief summary.

First, there is the simplistic solution that the individual who does not wish to mate wins, as assumed earlier in the mate choice model. In many cases this is very likely to be the outcome of the conflict. It will occur when one sex can avoid mating at negligible cost, whilst the other sex can persist only at high cost. An obvious candidate here would be the case where, say, a reluctant female can simply remove herself from the vicinity of an unacceptable male, whereas to pursue might be costly for the male in terms of losing his territory, etc. Another obvious candidate may be the unusual case where it pays the female to mate but not the male. It seems generally unlikely that a persistent female could easily 'rape' a male.

However, much of observable behaviour may relate to the typical case where it pays the male to mate but the female not to mate. Males show persistence and females show rejection; the outcome may or may not be successful rape. Two games have been discussed (Parker, 1979, 1983):

(1) *Sexual war of attrition.* In a war of attrition, the winner is simply the individual prepared to continue longer (Maynard Smith, 1974). Sexual conflict over mating decision could resemble a war of attrition in which, say, the male persistently attempts to mate and the female persistently attempts to reject. If the male gives up before the female, there is no mating; if the female gives up first, she is mated. This game will clearly be characterised by the following asymmetries: (i) the male/female asymmetry, (ii) an asymmetry in the value of winning (V_m fitness units for the male; V_f for the female), and (iii) an asymmetry in the rate at which costs will be expended by each opponent (persistence has a fitness cost rate of K_m for the male; rejection has a cost rate of K_f for the female). Set up in this way the game is analogous to the war of attrition with payoff relevant asymmetries (about which information will be imperfect) *and* an arbitrary asymmetry, such as ownership (about which there is perfect information – an individual 'knows' whether it is the prior resident or intruder; or in our case whether it is male or female). The ESS to this game (following the arguments of Parker & Rubenstein, 1981; Hammerstein & Parker, 1982; Parker, 1983) may generally be for the male to retreat without appreciable escalation if $V_m/K_m < V_f/K_f$ or for the female to

retreat without appreciable escalation if the sign is reversed. However over a range where there is no direct information about relative V and K, opponents may simply respect the male:female asymmetry in a way correlated with the above rule. Thus if *on average* $V_m/K_m < V_f/K_f$, the male would retreat, and vice-versa.

(2) *The sexual arms race*. The subject of arms races has been discussed recently in an excellent paper by Dawkins & Krebs (1979). A formal arms race game (the 'opponent-independent costs game') has been discussed by Parker (1979, 1983). It differs from the war of attrition in that costs relate to prior investment in armament (weaponry, body size, etc.). Thus the individual that has invested more heavily in expensive armament than his opponent is the winner. A strategy is now a choice of level of expenditure in armament, not a choice of persistence time. This model is not an alternative to the war of attrition. It is really a consequence of it, since the analyses indicate that asymmetries in fighting ability will be respected in the war of attrition. Conflict over mating decision seems to be an excellent candidate for this arms race game; e.g. by being bigger a male may be able to rape a female without her being able to prevent it. There are various solutions to the independent costs arms race game, depending on assumptions about costs:

(i) if choosing a given investment level specifies *exactly* an armament level (say cost x gives arms level X) there is no ESS (Parker, 1979; Rose, 1978).

(ii) if the opponent with the higher bid does not have to pay *in full* the difference between his bid and his opponents bid, there is a unique ESS (Haigh & Rose, 1980). This solution is unlikely to apply to true morphological arms races, but has applicability to games that are intermediate between wars of attrition and the independent costs game.

(iii) if choosing a given investment level specifies only a probability distribution for the arms level attained (e.g. because of environmental effects), rather than an exact level as in (i), there will be a Nash equilibrium ESS dependent on the forms of the distributions (Parker, 1983). Suppose that for the male, cost x specifies probability density $p(X)$ of achieving arms level X, and for the female cost y specifies $p(Y)$. Then the ESS can consist of a pair of pure strategies x_* for the male and y_* for the female, from which it would pay neither to deviate unilaterally.

For our purposes, solution (iii) appears most plausible. Because of asymmetries between the sexes in the value of winning and in the cost of balancing a unit increase in arms level of the opponent, ESS distributions p(X) and p(Y) may not overlap extensively. This will generate the observable effect that individuals of one sex *usually* win the conflict, but not always.

The effects of parental investment on the two forms of sexual selection

It seems clear that as Darwin (1871), Bateman (1948) and Trivers (1972) envisaged, direct intra-sexual competition will be most intense in the sex that invests least in a given pairing. Usually, therefore, it will be the male that experiences most intense direct competition. The operational sex ratio (reproductive males/reproductive female; Emlen & Oring, 1978) is roughly proportional to female investment/male investment, and it will be mainly this ratio that sets the intensity of sexual competition.

However, operational sex ratio is only a part of the picture for the mate choice component of sexual selection. The effects of a high operational sex ratio in the low-investing sex can be counterbalanced by high variance in mate quality in the high-investing sex. It is the way in which investment interacts with variation in mate quality that generates something of a paradox. The high-investing sex may have much higher variation in mate quality; thus in contrast to intermale competition, selection for mate choice may intensify as male investment increases.

Suppose that male investment with a particular female is zero. The operational sex ratio will be highly male-biased, and consequently the cost to a female of being choosy will be low. But benefits of choice may be negligible, since males may not vary much genetically, and do not contribute resources to the offspring. In contrast, female mate quality may be very variable because of environmental differences in her capacity to produce and provision offspring. Despite this high variance in female quality (high benefit of choice), male choosiness may not be favoured because search costs for alternative females would be great compared to the time taken to copulate and to replenish his sperm content. Thus where there is a very high investment disparity, it is quite likely that both sexes will be indiscriminate. Indeed, if ejaculate costs are high enough it is possibly males that will be choosy rather than females (Dewsbury, 1982).

As male investment in offspring increases, the male quality will increase because of environmental variance in his capacity to contribute to offspring fitness. Hence although the operational sex ratio will reduce – increasing the cost to a female of turning down a particular male – variance in male mate quality will increase. Similarly, for the male, although variance in female mate quality will reduce (because the male now contributes to offspring fitness), so does the cost of searching for an alternative female. Hence over some range of investment, choosiness may be favoured to some degree in both sexes.

This sort of consideration may help to explain why males sometimes appear more choosy than females. For instance in the crustaceans *Asellus* and *Gammarus*, the male guards the female often for several days before mating, and then leaves her. Thus he contributes nothing to the offspring and although male investment is high, male quality as mates may not vary much. Hence females should not be choosy. But female quality varies considerably (because bigger females lay more eggs); males *should* therefore be choosy and there is evidence that they are (Thompson & Manning, 1982; Ward, in preparation).

In summary, we may obtain the paradox that although the intensity of direct intra-male competition increases as male parental investment reduces, the *reverse* may be true for the female choice component of sexual selection. As male parental investment increases, so does the variance in male mate quality, and hence selection may intensify on female choice provided that the simultaneous increase in search costs is not too severe. Precise predictions are not possible until a rigorous model is formulated; much will depend on the rate at which variance in mate quality increases with increased investment versus the rate at which search costs increase with increased investment.

Summary

Apparent mate choice may be observed in the field even when there is no active choice (in the sense that there is discrimination between different potential mates). If females are passively attracted to a male advertisement cue, a mate's reproductive success will be an increasing function of the relative intensity of his cue. An ESS will consist of a state in which observed reproductive success depends on male phenotype because different phenotypes will have different optimal advertisement levels.

There may be difficulty in maintaining active mate choice if benefits of choice relate entirely to 'good genes' because of the costs of choice. Whereas benefits (proportional to genetic variance) diminish towards zero with selection (depending on the extent of recurrent mutation), costs are unlikely ever to become negligible. Mate choice is therefore most likely to occur when benefits relate to environmentally-induced variation.

A mate choice model is proposed in which the two important variables are (i) the degree of variance in mate quality for each sex, and (ii) the costs of choice for each sex; equivalent to the costs of finding an alternative mate. There are three ESSs: both sexes indiscriminate; one sex indiscriminate, one choosy; both sexes choosy to some degree. A prospective analysis suggests that if the ESS is for both sexes to show choice, one solution is that there will be assortative pairing for mate quality over a range of lower-quality individuals. Another solution is that one sex has choosy (high quality) individuals and less choosy (low quality) individuals, and the other sex has choosy (high quality) and indiscriminate (low quality) individuals.

There will commonly be conflict between the sexes over mating decisions (mate or not mate) in a given encounter. When males can achieve a mating by out-persisting a female (the sexual war of attrition), this conflict is likely to be resolved by difference in relative costs sustained during persistence. When males can more readily enforce matings on females (and females more readily resist) by increased investment in armament (the sexual arms race) the result is likely to be an equilibrium development of armament in each sex. In both models, one sex will usually win the conflict, depending on the characteristic asymmetries.

The greater the variance in mate quality of the opposite sex, the greater the relative benefits of mate choice. Because genetic variance may be small, the main contribution to variance in mate quality is likely to be environmental variance in ability to supply parental investment (PI). But as one sex increases its PI, it becomes more costly for individuals of the other sex to be choosy. Both costs and benefits of choice therefore increase with increasing PI of the opposite sex; this makes general predictions difficult. The intensity of selection for female choice may increase as male parental investment increases, in contrast to intermale competition. Assortative pairing for mate quality is perhaps most likely in a species with equal PI and low search costs. When males guard single females but contribute no PI, it may pay the male to be more choosy than the female.

I am indebted to Pat Bateson and Linda Partridge for many helpful suggestions, and to Miss A. Callaghan and Miss S. Scott for typing.

References

Andersson, M. (1982). Sexual selection, natural selection and quality advertisement. *Biological Journal of the Linnean Society*, **17**, 375–93.
Bateman, A. J. (1948). Intra-sexual selection in *Drosophila*. *Heredity*, **2**, 349–68.
Bell, G. (1978). The handicap principle in sexual selection. *Evolution*, **32**, 872–85.
Borgia, G. (1979). Sexual selection and the evolution of mating systems. In *Sexual*

Selection and Reproductive Competition in Insects, ed. M. S. Blum & N. A. Blum, pp. 19–80. Academic Press: New York.

Darwin, C. (1871). *The Descent of Man and Selection in Relation to Sex*. John Murray: London.

Dawkins, R. (1976). *The Selfish Gene*. Oxford University Press: Oxford.

Dawkins, R. & Krebs, J. R. (1979). Arms races between and within species. *Proceedings of the Royal Society of London*, B **205**, 489–511.

Dewsbury, D. A. (1982). Ejaculate cost and male choice. *American Naturalist*, **119**, 601–10.

Emlen, S. T. & Oring, L. W. (1977). Ecology, sexual selection, and the evolution of mating systems. *Science*, **197**, 215–23.

Fisher, R. A. (1930). *The Genetical Theory of Natural Selection*. Clarendon Press: Oxford.

Haigh, J. & Rose, M. R. (1980). Evolutionary game auctions. *Journal of Theoretical Biology*, **85**, 381–97.

Halliday, T. R. (1978). Sexual selection and mate choice. In *Behavioural Ecology: an Evolutionary Approach*, ed. J. R. Krebs & N. B. Davies, pp. 180–213. Blackwells: Oxford.

Hammerstein, P. & Parker, G. A. (1982). The asymmetric war of attrition. *Journal of Theoretical Biology*, **96**, 647–82.

Janetos, A. C. (1980). Strategies of female choice: a theoretical analysis. *Behavioral Ecology and Sociobiology*, **7**, 107–12.

Lande, R. (1980). Sexual dimorphism, sexual selection and adaptation in polygenic characters. *Evolution*, **34**, 292–305.

Lande, R. (1981). Models of speciation by sexual selection on polygenic traits. *Proceedings of the National Academy of Sciences of the USA*, **78**, 3731–5.

MacArthur, R. H. & Pianka, E. R. (1966). On optimal use of a patchy environment. *American Naturalist*, **100**, 603–9.

Maynard Smith, J. (1974). The theory of games and the evolution of animal conflicts. *Journal of Theoretical Biology*, **47**, 209–21.

Maynard Smith, J. (1978). *The Evolution of Sex*. Cambridge University Press: Cambridge.

O'Donald, P. (1980). *Genetic Models of Sexual Selection*. Cambridge University Press: Cambridge.

Parker, G. A. (1979). Sexual selection and sexual conflict. In *Sexual Selection and Reproductive Competition in Insects*, ed. M. S. Blum & N. A. Blum, pp. 123–66. Academic Press: New York.

Parker, G. A. (1982). Phenotype limited evolutionarily stable strategies. In *Current Problems in Sociobiology*, ed. B. R. Bertram, T. H. Clutton-Brock, R. I. M. Dunbar, D. I. Rubenstein & R. Wrangham, pp. 173–201. Cambridge University Press: Cambridge.

Parker, G. A. (1983). Arms races in evolution: an ESS to the opponent-independent costs game. *Journal of Theoretical Biology* (in press).

Parker, G. A. & Rubenstein, D. I. (1981). Role assessment, reserve strategy, and acquisition of information in asymmetric animal conflicts. *Animal Behaviour*, **29**, 221–40.

Partridge, L. (1980). Mate choice increases a component of offspring fitness in fruit flies. *Nature*, **283**, 290–1.

Ridley, M. (in preparation). On being the right-sized mates.

Rose, M. R. (1978). Cheating in evolutionary games. *Journal of Theoretical Biology*, **75**, 21–34.

Thompson, D. J. & Manning, J. T. (1982). Mate selection by *Asellus* (Crustacea: Isopoda). *Behaviour* (in press).

Thornhill, R. (1980a). Mate choice in *Hylobittacus apicalis* (Insecta: Mecoptera) and its relation to some models of female choice. *Evolution*, **34**, 519–38.

Thornhill, R. (1980*b*). Competitive, charming males and choosy females: was Darwin correct? *Florida Entomologist*, **63**, 5–30.

Trivers, R. L. (1972). Parental investment and sexual selection. In *Sexual Selection and the Descent of Man, 1871–1971*, ed. B. Campbell, pp. 136–79. Aldine: Chicago.

Ward, P. (in preparation). The effects of size on the mating decisions of *Gammarus pulex* (Crustacea, Amphipoda).

Williams, G. C. (1975). *Sex and Evolution*. Princeton University Press: Princeton.

Zahavi, A. (1975). Mate selection – a selection for a handicap. *Journal of Theoretical Biology*, **53**, 205–14.

Appendix

A. Mating decisions with only one sex discriminate

The logic behind curves $G(bs_f)$ and $G(bs_m)$ in Fig. 6.4 is as follows. It takes time g_f for a female to produce her eggs, and time s_f for her to find a male to invest in them. The male investment is zero, so if there is a 1:1 sex ratio, on average it takes a male time $g_f + s_f$ to find a female. Since we assume that the distribution of mate quality is equal for each sex, then curve $G(bs_f)$ – the fitness achieved by the female in relation to accepting 1 male in every b encountered – has the same initial value at $b = 1$ as curve $G(bs_m)$ for the male. However, $G(bs_f)$ will rise at $(g + s_f)/s_m$ the rate of curve $G(bs_m)$; hence in the case drawn the ESS for the female is to select the best 25% (1 in $b = 4$) of males, and for males to be indiscriminate.

B. Mating decisions where both sexes are discriminate

Consider first the female's choices (Fig. 6.5a). She should have an optimal fixed threshold, accept all males of quality greater than Q_{mt}, if her own quality is greater than Q_{ft}. This arises from the fact that all males should be willing to mate with any females from this group, because even for the highest-quality males the search costs are too great to turn down an opportunity with any female better than Q_{ft}. Given that all males would be willing to mate with all females with $Q > Q_{ft}$ (i.e. males are indiscriminate over this range), these females should have a fixed threshold for accepting males as defined in A above. Thus Q_{opt} in equation (6.1) is Q_{mt} for females with $Q > Q_{ft}$. By an exactly analogous argument for the male's choice, Q_{opt} in (6.1) is Q_{ft} for all males with $Q > Q_{mt}$. Hence pairing should be random between all males of quality Q_m such that $Q_{mt} < Q_m < Q_{mmax}$ and females with quality Q_f in the range $Q_{ft} < Q_f < Q_{fmax}$. Since it is assumed for Fig. 6.5 that male investment in a pairing is rather less than female investment, Q_{mt} will be closer to Q_{mmax} than Q_{ft} is to Q_{fmax}.

Now consider females with $Q_f < Q_{ft}$. A fraction of best quality males will not accept such females, so these females must be less choosy. A female just below Q_{ft} (top graph) should have a threshold for accepting males that is a step below Q_{mt}; the interval of this step will be set by the effect of excluding males in the range Q_{mt} to Q_{mmax} from the range of potential mates. Similarly, a male just below Q_{mt} will be considerably less choosy than one just above Q_{mt} (lower graph); the step interval will here be greater than that for females because a relatively larger fraction of potential mates will be excluded. One possibility is that this effectively causes all males with $Q_m < Q_{mt}$ to be indiscriminate, in this case all females with $Q_f < Q_{ft}$ would have the same acceptance threshold and the population would consist of two types of female (highly choosy and less choosy) and two types of male (choosy and indiscriminate). The more interesting alternative occurs when the drop in male threshold (lower graph) does not cause a male with quality just below Q_{mt} to accept all females. When the optimal threshold for such a male is to accept females with $Q_f > Q_{fmin}$ there will be a range for both sexes over which the choice threshold is correlated with mate quality. In the case shown in Fig. 6.5, because of the investment asymmetry all females are discriminate to some degree (poorest quality females should only accept males with $Q_m > Q_{mz}$) whereas over a large range males of lower quality should be indiscriminate. If female mate quality varies much more than male mate quality, reverse conclusions can be obtained.

7

Mate choice in role-reversed species

MARION PETRIE

Why do females compete for males?

It is generally considered that males compete for females because their reproductive success is limited by the number of females which they can fertilise (Bateman, 1948; Trivers, 1972). Competition amongst females for males is unlikely to occur in a simple reversal of this situation because the superabundance of male sperm means that the accomplishment of fertilisation is never likely to limit female reproductive success. A situation in which male gametes were rare in comparison to female gametes would be at odds with the fundamental definition of the sexes (i.e. that males produce many small gametes and females a few large ones).

The work of Trivers (1972) has dominated theoretical discussions of the evolution of sex role-reversal. Trivers argues that 'the sex whose parental investment is greater than that of the opposite sex will become the limiting resource for that sex' and that this discrepancy in investment will lead to members of the lower-investing sex competing for access to members of the higher-investing sex. He defines parental investment as 'any investment by the parent in an individual offspring that increases the offspring's chance of surviving (and hence reproductive success) at the cost of the parent's ability to invest in other offspring'. Thus, he predicts that females will compete for males when male parental investment exceeds that of females. However, competition need not always occur in this way. For example, members of the higher-investing sex could be in competition for access to members of the lower-investing sex if, because of differential mortality, they were in short supply.

Theoretically, it should pay females to compete for males when the mates they acquire represent, or otherwise provide, an important *scarce* resource. This resource should contribute either directly or indirectly to their reproductive success in such a way that the benefits gained as a result of successful competition outweigh the costs incurred. These costs may not be simply energetic, they could also involve the risk of injury or death (Gosling & Petrie, 1981). It is important to emphasise that it is the scarcity of the resource which will lead to competition amongst females regardless of the relative investment made by the male to reproduction.

There are thus two main situations which could lead to female competition for mates: (1) Where there is variance in male quality and where there are fewer high quality males than females. And (2) where there is a shortage of available male partners and where males invest more in reproduction than by the provision of gametes. These two possibilities will be considered in turn.

Variance in male quality

The greater the variance in male quality the more likely it is that female competition will occur since there will be a greater *relative* fitness 'pay-off' for the female that successfully competes and secures a high-quality male (relative to females with low-quality males). Thus, there are two main questions to consider: (a) what constitutes a good quality male, and (b) what are the main sources of variance in male quality?

A good quality male is one that can contribute most to a female's reproduction. This contribution can take a number of forms. Males may help by:

(1) providing good genes that enhance the fitness of any offspring,
(2) providing the female with nutrients, as in the case of pre-copulatory food offerings,
(3) incubating eggs or tending them in other ways,
(4) brooding or feeding the young,
(5) defending the female or her young from predators, or
(6) defending a resource necessary for females for feeding, nesting or for successfully rearing their young.

With the exception of (1), the variation in the ability of males to perform these tasks can be of either genotypic or phenotypic origin.

If variance in male quality was purely heritable and, since high-quality mates (by definition) enhance a female's reproductive success, the genetic variance in male quality in the population should normally disappear after a few generations. All males would then be of similar high quality and the conditions favouring competition for males would also disappear. The following are possible ways in which genetic variance could be maintained in the population:

(1) There might be a fluctuating environment so that certain males are of poor quality only for restricted periods (Parker, 1979). In this case selection would not act continuously against males with poor quality genes.

(2) The recurrence of harmful mutations could result in a proportion of inferior or low-quality genotypes in the population.

(3) The preferred characteristic in males that enhances female reproductive success could have a cost to males of a higher risk of mortality at other times of the year (O'Donald, 1973). In this case the fitness of low- and high-quality males could be equal overall so that a variety of genotypes is maintained in the population.

(4) A variety of genotypes could also be maintained where females preferred more than one male characteristic and where the characteristics could not occur in the same males. Females would then be forced to choose between the two characteristics and, in the absence of any foreseeable advantage at the time of choice, both could persist in the population.

The amount of phenotypic variation between males will depend upon a variety of factors including developmental differences, however, phenotypic variation in the ability of males to perform a task is likely to increase with: (1) The proportion of their total reproductive effort that the task represents, given that there would be variation in the amount of resources males have available for reproductive effort. (2) The number of variables that affect a male's ability to perform a task. For example, a male's ability to defend a nest from predators may increase with its experience (age) and adult size. In this case, males that were both old and large would usually be rarer than males that had only one of these attributes. (3) Environmental variability. Where a male defends resources that are necessary for a female to reproduce, the spatial and temporal patterning of resources contribute to any variability in the resource-holding potential of males.

In systems where females compete with each other to obtain high quality males it would be surprising if they did not have the ability to assess male quality. Where males are defending resources or presenting pre-copulatory food offerings, a female can assess the quality of the resource directly. But, in situations where a good-quality male is one that can contribute most to care of the young, by incubation or feeding, a female must be able to assess a male, prior to mating, on the basis of its ability to perform a future task. In this case the most likely factors to affect a male's performance are its energy reserves or condition, and it seems reasonable to assume that a male's condition at the time of mating would correlate with its condition when caring for eggs or young. It might also pay a male to advertise his good qualities since he could potentially obtain more matings. Such advertisement by the male could also attract more competing females and thus increase the chance that the male would mate with one that was successful in intrasexual competition.

Empirical data on the adaptive significance of competition between females are rare, largely because of the rarity of the phenomenon. Aggressive interactions between females which determine access to mates have only been reported in a few species of insects (Smith, 1979; Gwynne, 1981), fish (Li & Owings, 1978*a, b*), anurans (Wells, 1978, 1981) and birds (Lack, 1968; Jenni, 1974; Emlen & Oring, 1977; Ridley, 1978). However, in the moorhen (*Gallinula chloropus*) there is some evidence that the function of female intrasexual competition is to secure access to high-quality males (Petrie, 1982*a, b*). In the Moorhen, pair formation occurs in winter flocks before the pairs leave to establish breeding territories. Females initiate courtship much more frequently than males. Aggressive interactions between females are common and typically occur when a female approaches a courting pair. These encounters sometimes lead to fighting with the opponents striking at each other with their sharply clawed feet (Fig. 7.1) and fights are more common between females than between males. The

Fig. 7.1. Fighting with the feet (shown in ii) in the moorhen (*Gallinula chloropus*) is normally preceded by a 'challenge' posture (shown in i). Redrawn from Wood (1974).

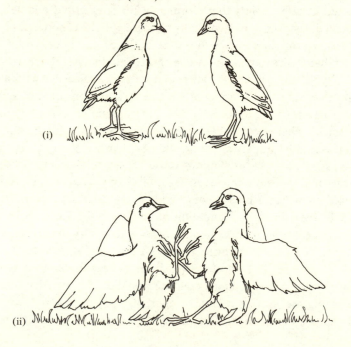

heaviest females tend to win most of their competitive interactions for males, and these females secure, and form pair bonds with, males that are in good condition (those with the largest fat reserves) (Fig. 7.2). As might be expected, those males without mates and territories are in significantly poorer condition than those that form pairs. Male Moorhens perform the majority of incubation and females with good-condition males can initiate more nesting attempts in a season and thus could potentially produce more young. These data suggest that females expend energy, and risk injury, in competition to obtain a 'high-quality', good-condition mate.

In a laboratory investigation of the mating behaviour of the Three-spined Stickleback, Li & Owings (1978a, b) noted that aggression between females occurred when females were kept alone and when they were with males. They found that when a subordinate female accepted a courting male in view of a dominant female, the latter usually disrupted the interaction. In this species, few male courtships lead to spawning and most are terminated by females. Li & Owings suggest that females are highly selective in their choice of males and, since many courtships were terminated after the male showed the female the nest, they argue that such selectivity may be based partly on characteristics of the nest. This hypothesis is supported by the high level of nest-directed disruptive behaviour by neighbouring males that occurs during courtship. Female competition in this species may determine preferential access to males with the best quality nest sites.

Fig. 7.2. The relationship between male condition and female weight in pairs of moorhens. Condition was measured using the index of body weight divided by (length in mm of tarsus + metatarsus)^3. The sample considers pairs from three breeding seasons. Where the same pair occurred more than once only those data collected in the first year were included.

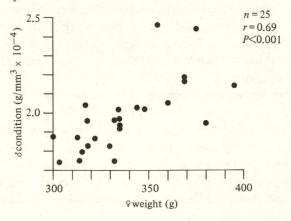

In the Red-winged Blackbird (*Agelaius phoniceus*) males establish territories and females are thought to choose their mates on the basis of territory quality. The fact that there is a concensus amongst females in their choice of territory is thought to result in polygyny with some males securing more than one female. However, within territories of a given quality, a female's reproductive success is reduced in relation to the number of females present and this may be the cause of the observed competition amongst females. Competition amongst female Red-winged Blackbirds thus occurs as females attempt to secure sole access to the best territories and, as a result, the largest harems are not always found on the preferred territories (Lenington, 1980).

Shortage of available male partners

A shortage of males in a population could occur if the sex ratio was skewed away from 50:50 either because of differential mortality or because some females have monopolised more than one male. Both events lead to situations where the number of available male partners is limited (Emlen & Oring, 1977).

Under what circumstances are females capable of monopolising more than one male? Emlen & Oring (1977) state that when the male performs most of the post-zygotic parental care the female is 'emancipated' and has the opportunity to increase her fitness by securing additional males to care for any further clutches; males sitting on eggs or caring for young in other ways are sexually unavailable and the operational sex-ratio thus becomes skewed with a shortage of males. In this case, the conditions favouring intrasexual competition amongst females would initially require the evolution of paternal care; this topic will be discussed in the next section.

One evolutionary pathway that could lead to polyandry has been suggested for the waders (Jenni, 1974). In some species, such as Temminck's Stint, *Calidris temminckii*, the female lays one clutch of eggs in a territory which is defended by the male. The male incubates this clutch whilst the female produces another clutch which she then incubates herself (Hilden, 1965). Such 'double-clutching' could lead to polyandry if the female left the first male to lay her second clutch for another male (as can occur in the Spotted Sandpiper, *Actitis macularia* (Hays, 1972; Oring & Knudson, 1972)). The basic difference in these two systems is the way in which the female apportions her energy reserves or reproductive effort. In the former strategy she maximises her reproductive success through incubation and in the latter she expends energy in competition for a second male which incubates the second clutch. These two strategies could be considered as alternatives since they can yield a similar number of clutches. However, the latter strategy could result in a higher relative fitness since a female that secures two males may prevent other females in the population from obtaining a mate at all, and since it may also be free to incubate an additional clutch itself.

Although it could be said that paternal care is a pre-requisite for polyandry, opportunities must also exist for females to gain subsequent matings after deserting one male. This point has been emphasised by Maynard Smith (1977). If all individuals in the population reproduced at the same time there would be few such opportunities (assuming a 50:50 sex ratio). Knowlton (1979) discusses the idea that reproductive synchrony is a sexual strategy adopted by one sex to reduce the chance of desertion by the other, an idea first suggested by Halliday (quoted in Krebs (1978)). Males could reduce the chance of desertion by delaying incubation until most other males in the population were also attending eggs.

Wells (1978) suggests that competition amongst females occurs in the Poison-arrow Frog (*Dendrobates auratus*) because there is a scarcity of males available to tend eggs. Males can only care for one clutch in the time it takes for females to lay many clutches. In Giant Water Bugs (*Abedus herberti*), males brood eggs that are attached to their backs by females. The space available on males can be a limited resource for a female since there are more gravid females in the population than males without eggs (Smith, 1979). Each female is capable of encumbering several males with eggs and, as a consequence, there is sometimes competition amongst females. Gwynne (1981) reports that female Mormon Crickets (*Anabrus simplex*) fight with each other when more than one approaches a singing male. These fights may be caused by competition for the limited supply of spermatophores produced by the male.

In the American Jacana (*Jacana spinosa*) females compete to obtain large territories which overlap smaller male territories. Those females that compete successfully obtain the largest territories and consequently gain exclusive access to most males. In this species the male performs all of the post-laying parental care, and females have more than one male incubating their clutches simultaneously. Some females have been reported to have as many as four males in their territories and thus have the chance of successfully producing four clutches (Jenni & Collier, 1972; Jenni, 1974).

In other bird species where both polyandry and sex role-reversal have been reported (see reviews by Jenni, 1974, and Ridley, 1978), it is tempting to assume that females which are successful in competition gain the most males. However, females could be competing for other scarce resources such as high-quality males and this seems a likely alternative explanation, especially in those species where an excess of males has also been reported. For example, the Variegated Tinamou (*Crypturellus variegatus*) shows sex role-reversal and sequential polyandry, but also has a sex ratio of four males to one female (Beebe, 1925).

So far the only form of female competition considered has been direct displacement of rivals. But, as in male intrasexual selection, it is possible that females could compete with each other through sexual advertisement, i.e. by being more attractive to males than their rivals.

The evolution of paternal care

Paternal care can occur only in those groups where the form of parental care allows male commitment. In the mammals, parental care may have become more restricted to females with the evolution of viviparity and lactation. (For a review of species showing paternal care see Ridley, 1978.) But why is paternal care a relatively rare phenomenon in those groups where this restriction does not apply? Trivers (1972) argued that the smaller gametic investment made by the male results in stronger selection by males to desert after fertilisation. However, it has been pointed out that past investment is not important and, rather, that it is the 'pay-off' to either sex from future reproduction that is responsible for the evolution of parental care as opposed to desertion (Dawkins & Carlisle, 1976). Under these circumstances it is not immediately obvious whether selection would favour male or female parental care.

The mode of fertilisation has been suggested as an important factor in determining which sex care for offspring. In fish, when fertilisation is external, parental care is usually performed by the male, and when internal, it is performed by the female (Maynard Smith, 1978; from data extracted from Breder & Rosen, 1966). Dawkins & Carlisle (1976) suggest that in a species with internal fertilisation there is a delay before egg deposition during which the male could desert, thus leaving the care to the female. Conversely, in a species with external fertilisation, eggs are released before sperm and there is time for the female to desert, leaving the care of the young to the male. This hypothesis does not explain the evolution of paternal care in birds although it may be an important explanation for the occurrence of paternal care in fish.

It has been suggested that with internal fertilisation paternity assurance is low and that this could lead to selection against paternal, as opposed to maternal, care (Trivers, 1972). Werren, Gross & Shine (1980) investigated this possibility using population genetics models and concluded that 'only in mating systems where a parental male "sacrifices" promiscuous matings can paternity influence the evolution of parental care'. For example, a corollary of a high certainty of paternity is that there are few opportunities for promiscuous matings and therefore a low cost to paternal care.

Maynard Smith (1977) uses game theory to explore the problem of conflict between the sexes over which should 'guard' the young and which should desert. He concludes that a situation where the male guards and the female deserts is favoured when the number of eggs laid by a female who deserts is very much greater than that of a female who guards. This could occur if parental care after laying is energetically expensive and if the female has a chance of re-mating. (It has often been suggested that paternal care evolves because it allows the female to lay more eggs; see Emlen & Oring (1977). However, any enhanced egg production could be a consequence rather than a cause of paternal care (Ridley, 1978).)

If females prefer to mate with males that are already incubating, or guarding eggs or young, then a male could gain more matings by performing parental care (Trivers, 1972) and it would thus pay a male to stay with fertilised eggs.

Could an element of male choice exist?

Male choice would be expected in any situation where the male makes any investment in reproduction (in addition to gametes) since discriminating males would be favoured by natural selection over indiscriminate ones if there was variability in the quality of females.

In many role-reversed species the male's major investment normally comes after egg laying (except in some species where the male provides pre-zygotic nourishment to the female at the time of mating) so it can be predicted that discrimination by males should occur after the eggs are laid and before the expense of any major reproductive effort. Whether the male then withholds his contribution should depend on his chances of securing a better female. If, however, females lay their eggs synchronously, males may not have the opportunity to desert one female to mate preferentially with another and they could then be forced to assess and choose between females at the time of mating. The intensity of selection for discrimination by males should depend upon the amount of variation in the quality of females, and any costs of searching by males.

A high-quality female is one that can contribute most to the reproductive success of a male. In many role-reversed species, where males perform all of the post-zygotic care, these females would be those that produce the most, or the largest, eggs or the female with the best genotype.

The sources of variability in the fecundity of females must be considered. If the amount of parental care that males perform is the main factor contributing to the variability in the number of eggs a female can lay, then it would not pay a male to discriminate between females on the basis of egg production. In many polyandrous species the number of eggs a female can lay does not appear to be limiting (Lack, 1968). In such cases, females may lay the number of eggs that a male can successfully rear and, in these circumstances, there would be little basis for male choice in relation to female egg production.

The idea that males may choose females on the basis of genetically determined traits suffers from the general problem that, normally, there is little additive genetic variance in fitness. However, there are ways in which genetic variance could be maintained in a population (see above). Theoretically, it should pay males to accept the results of competition between females since by mating with a highly competitive female a male ensures that any small genetic component in competitive ability is passed to his daughters, who will then gain better-quality, or more, mates. However, in species where polyandry occurs it may pay a male to select a subordinate female if such a female were to lay more eggs for him rather than compete to obtain a second male. A similar situation could occur where any reproductive effort expended in competition between females depletes reserves that could be spent in egg production. In these cases any costs incurred by not producing successful competitive daughters must also be considered.

Where the amount of care limits reproductive success, males may favour females who show more parental effort. Thus, although it could be said that female choice for caring males could lead to paternal care, the equivalent choice for caring females could result in care by both sexes; males could possibly withhold their contribution until the female has performed some parental duties.

Selection need not always operate in a way that favours discrimination by *all* males in a population. For example, in role-reversed species where females compete to obtain access to high-quality individuals, only the highest-quality males may have the opportunity to discriminate between females (Burley, 1977); if males of low quality reject a female they may not secure an alternative.

The only empirical data for the basis of male choice in a role-reversed species come from Gwynne's (1981) study of Mormon Crickets. Males sometimes withdraw without transferring a spermatophore in response to a coupling attempt by a female and Gwynne found that the mean weight of rejected females was significantly less than mated females. Heavier females can produce more eggs, and this suggests that males choose the more fecund individuals as mates.

Empirical data on the basis of male choice has, however, been recorded in some species which do not show role-reversal. For example, when two female Mottled Sculpins (*Cottus bairdi*) appear on a male's territory at the same time the male will court and mate with the largest female as larger females are more fecund (Downhower & Brown, 1981). Males are thought to prefer larger, more fecund females in Wood Frogs, *Rana sylvatica* (Berven, 1981), and in fresh water shrimps, *Asellus* spp. (Manning, 1975). Male Ring Doves (*Streptopelia risoria*) exhibit less courtship and more aggressive behaviour towards females that have recently associated with other males than towards females that have been isolated from other males. This difference in response may be related to the likelihood of cuckoldry (Erickson & Zenone, 1976; Zenone, Sims & Erickson, 1979). Burley & Moran (1979) obtained some evidence to suggest that captive male Feral Pigeons, *Columba livia*, prefer females with previous reproductive experience.

Summary

Competition amongst females for males is likely to occur when males represent, or provide, important scarce resources. There are two situations which could lead to female competition: (a) when there are a few high-quality males, and (b) where there is a shortage of available male partners.

A good quality male is one that can contribute most to a female's reproduction. This contribution can take a number of forms. There is some evidence to suggest that females compete for (a) good-condition males, (b) males with good nest sites, and (c) males with good territories.

Possible conditions leading to polyandry are discussed. In some polyandrous species, females that are successful in competition secure more than one male.

Possible factors favouring the evolution of paternal care are discussed.

The intensity of selection for discrimination by males should depend upon the amount of variation in the quality of females, and any costs of searching by males. Where males perform most of the parental care a high-quality female is likely to be most fecund or the one with the best genotype. Where the amount of parental care limits reproductive success, males may favour females who show more parental effort. There is some evidence that males prefer more fecund females.

Discussions with Tim Halliday helped during the initial stages of writing this chapter. I am also grateful to Pat Bateson and Morris Gosling for reading an earlier draft and making constructive comments.

References

Bateman, A. J. (1948). Intra-sexual selection in *Drosophila*. *Heredity*, **2**, 349–68.

Beebe, W. (1925). The variegated Tinamou, *Crypturellus variegatus variegatus*. *Zoologica*, **6**, 195–227.

Berven, K. A. (1981). Mate choice in the wood frog, *Rana sylvatica*. *Evolution*, **35**, 707–22.

Breder, C. M. & Rosen, D. E. (1966). *Modes of Reproduction in Fishes*. Natural History Press: New York.

Burley, N. (1977). Parental investment, mate choice and mate quality. *Proceedings of the National Academy of Sciences of the USA*, **74**, 3476–9.

Burley, N. & Moran, N. (1979). The significance of age and reproductive experience in the mate preferences of feral pigeons, *Columba livia*. *Animal Behaviour*, **27**, 686–98.

Dawkins, R. & Carlisle, T. R. (1976). Parental investment, mate desertion and a fallacy. *Nature*, **262**, 131–3.

Downhower, J. F. & Brown, L. (1981). The timing of reproduction and its behavioural consequences for Mottled sculpins, *Cottus bairdi*. In *Natural Selection and Social Behaviour*, ed. R. D. Alexander & D. W. Tinkle, pp. 78–95. Chiron Press: New York.

Erickson, C. J. & Zenone, P. G. (1976). Courtship differences in male ring doves: avoidance of cuckoldry? *Science*, **192**, 1353–4.

Emlen, S. T. & Oring, L. W. (1977). Ecology, sexual selection, and the evolution of mating systems. *Science*, **188**, 1029–31.

Gosling, L. M. & Petrie, M. (1981). The economics of social organisation. In *Physiological Ecology: An Evolutionary Approach to Resource Use*, ed. C. R. Townsend & P. Calow, pp. 315–45. Blackwells: Oxford.

Gwynne, D. T. (1981). Sexual difference theory: Mormon crickets show role-reversal in mate choice. *Science*, **213**, 779–80.

Hays, H. (1972). Polyandry in the spotted sandpiper. *Living Bird*, **11**, 43–57.

Hilden, O. (1965). Zur Brutbiologie des Temminckstrandläufers, *Calidris temminckii* (Leisl.). *Ornis Fennica*, **42**, 1–5.

Jenni, D. A. (1974). Evolution of polyandry in birds. *American Zoologist*, **14**, 129–44.

Jenni, D. A. & Collier, G. (1972). Polyandry in the American Jacana (*Jacana spinosa*). *Auk*, **89**, 743–65.

Knowlton, N. (1979). Reproductive synchrony, parental investment and the evolutionary dynamics of sexual selection. *Animal Behaviour*, **27**, 1022–33.

Krebs, J. R. (1978). Colonial nesting in birds with special reference to the Ciconiiformes. *Wading Birds Research Report*, No. 7. National Audubon Society.

Lack, D. (1968). *Ecological Adaptations for Breeding in Birds*. Methuen: London.

Lenington, S. (1980). Female choice and polygyny in red-winged blackbirds. *Animal Behaviour*, **28**, 347–61.

Li, S. K. & Owings, D. H. (1978a). Sexual selection in the three spined stickleback. I. Normative observations. *Zeitschrift für Tierpsychologie*, **46**, 359–71.

Li, S. K. & Owings, D. H. (1978b). Sexual selection in the three spined stickleback. II. Nest raiding during the courtship phase. *Behaviour*, **64**, 298–304.

Manning, J. T. (1975). Male discrimination and investment in *Asellus aquaticus* (L.) and *A. meridianus* Racovitsza (Crustacea: Isopoda). *Behaviour*, **55**, 1–14.

Maynard Smith, J. (1977). Parental investment – a prospective analysis. *Animal Behaviour*, **25**, 1–9.

Maynard Smith, J. (1978). The ecology of sex. In *Behavioural Ecology: An Evolutionary Approach*, ed. J. R. Krebs & N. B. Davies, pp. 159–79. Blackwells: Oxford.

O'Donald, P. (1973). Models of sexual and natural selection in polygamous species. *Heredity*, **31**, 145–56.

Oring, L. W. & Knudson, M. L. (1972). Monogamy and polyandry in the Spotted Sandpiper. *Living Bird*, **11**, 59–73.

Parker, G. A. (1979). Sexual selection and sexual conflict. In *Sexual Selection and Reproductive Competition in Insects*, ed. M. S. Blum & N. A. Blum, pp. 123–66. Academic Press: New York.

Petrie, M. (1982*a*). *Winter Flocking in Moorhens*. Ph.D. thesis, University of East Anglia.

Petrie, M. (1982*b*). Female moorhens compete for small fat males. (Submitted to *Science*.)

Ridley, M. (1978). Paternal care. *Animal Behaviour*, **26**, 904–32.

Smith, R. L. (1979). Paternity assurance and altered roles in the mating behaviour of a Giant Water Bug, *Abedus herberti* (Heteroptera: Belostomatidae). *Animal Behaviour*, **27**, 716–25.

Trivers, R. L. (1972). Parental investment and sexual selection. In *Sexual Selection and the Descent of Man, 1871–1971*, ed. B. Campbell, pp. 136–79. Aldine-Atherton: Chicago.

Wells, K. D. (1978). Courtship and parental behaviour in a Panamanian poison-arrow frog (*Dendrobates auratus*). *Herpetologica*, **34**, 148–55.

Wells, K. D. (1981). Parental behaviour of male and female frogs. In *Natural Selection and Social Behaviour*, ed. R. D. Alexander & D. W. Tinkle, pp. 184–97. Chiron Press: New York.

Werren, J. H., Gross, M. R. & Shine, R. (1980). Paternity and the evolution of male parental care. *Journal of Theoretical Biology*, **82**, 619–31.

Wood, N. A. (1974). The breeding behaviour and biology of the Moorhen. *British Birds*, **67**, 104–15 and 137–58.

Zenone, P. G., Sims, M. E. & Erickson, C. J. (1979). Male ring dove behaviour and the defense of genetic paternity. *American Naturalist*, **114**, 615–26.

8

Male–male competition and mate choice in anuran amphibians

ANTHONY ARAK

The social behaviour of frogs and toads (anuran amphibians) is currently receiving a great deal of attention from behavioural ecologists. Certain aspects of their mating behaviour make them particularly suitable for studying mechanisms of male–male competition and female choice. Their breeding aggregations are characterised by many individuals collecting in a relatively small area, so interactions can be observed frequently. Second, the animals are easily approached and observed and can be marked and recognised individually. Oviposition can be seen and external fertilisation makes it easy to determine which male fertilised the eggs. Finally, experimental manipulation of the vocal courtship displays of anurans can be carried out with relative ease.

Most species use vocal signals of some form during courtship, and their significance as species-isolating mechanisms has been extensively investigated (Bogert, 1960; Blair, 1964, 1968; Salthe & Mecham, 1974; Littlejohn, 1977). More recently, attention has focused on variability in signal properties *within* species and possible functions of vocal signals in male–male competition and female choice. It is possible to generate 'synthetic' vocalisations which are behaviourally equivalent to natural calls (Capranica, 1965; Loftus Hill & Littlejohn, 1971; Gerhardt, 1974). This enables the researcher systematically to vary specific parameters of the signal to test whether or not they are used as cues in assessment by males or mate choice by females.

In the first part of this chapter I describe the variety of behaviour adopted by males during mate-searching and attempt to find adaptive reasons for the differences between species. The function of alternative mate-acquisition strategies by males (see Dunbar, this volume) and behavioural variability in anuran mating systems are discussed in terms

181

of conflict between individual males for mating opportunities. The second part of the chapter takes a critical look at the role of female choice in anuran mating behaviour and discusses limitations of the methods used to test for it.

Male mate-locating behaviour

The methods that male anurans use to obtain females are remarkably diverse, both within and between species (for an excellent review, see Wells, 1977*b*). Between species, much of the variation in mating systems is explained by differences in duration of the breeding season. Those species in which mating and spawning occur over only a few hours or days – the 'explosive breeders' – form dense aggregations in which the males scramble for females (Fig. 8.1). Males typically approach and attempt to clasp any small objects moving nearby. Their motivation to mate is so strong that sometimes their attempts are misdirected against fish or floating debris. Struggles between males for the possession of females are common in explosive breeders.

In contrast, in those species with prolonged breeding seasons – of several months duration – territorial defence or lek-behaviour is the common pattern. Active searching and struggling for females is usually

Fig. 8.1. The breeding season of the European Common Toad (*Bufo bufo*) lasts for two weeks only. Like many other explosive breeders, males 'scramble' for females and attempt to dislodge amplectant males. Males have much reduced mating calls. (Photograph: D. C. Mackinder.)

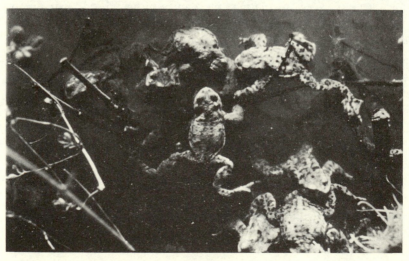

absent in prolonged breeders. Instead, males call from positions around or near the breeding pool and females approach stationary males (Fig. 8.2). Calling appears to have the dual roles of attracting females and maintaining a certain minimum distance between males. In some frogs the basic call has diversified into two distinct vocalisations: the 'advertisement' call, a long-range signal which serves to attract females and space out competing males, and the 'encounter' call which is used at short-range as the first stage in an aggressive encounter between males (Wells, 1977*b*, *c*; Littlejohn, 1977).

In other species, the advertisement call may carry separate messages to males and females. For example, in the Puerto Rican Frog, *Eleuthero-dactylus coqui*, males have a 'compound' advertisement call consisting of an introductory 'co' note followed by a longer 'qui' note. In experiments, females approach loudspeakers playing the normal call or the 'qui' note alone, but are not attracted to the 'co' note (Narins & Capranica, 1976). Males, on the other hand, will alternate calls with a playback of 'co' notes but ignore the 'qui' note. Males give only the 'co' note when challenging other males. This suggests that the 'co' note conveys an agonistic message to males and the 'qui' note serves to attract females.

Males of most prolonged breeders maintain individual distances at the

Fig. 8.2. The Natterjack Toad (*Bufo calamita*) is a prolonged breeder. Males call from the edge of temporary ponds for up to eight weeks. Females swim in the water behind the calling males for some time before approaching one. Amplexus is initiated when the female (left) nudges a calling male (right). (Photograph: A. Arak.)

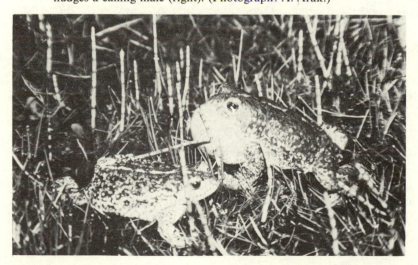

breeding site, resulting in regular spacing of males. Territorial behaviour is common, although it does not always involve site attachment or defence of resources needed by females. The males of many treefrogs defend calling sites on vegetation but move away to separate oviposition sites once paired with females. Males of some prolonged breeders call from the edge of water bodies and maintain regular spacing over the short-term, although individuals move frequently during the course of one night or between nights. Oviposition does not take place at calling sites. Frog choruses such as these resemble the 'lek' mating systems of some fish (Constanz, 1975), birds (van Rhijn, 1973; Wiley, 1973; Lill, 1974) and mammals (Buechner & Schloeth, 1965; Bradbury, 1977) since individual territories are non-resource based (see Wilson, 1975; Emlen, 1976). However, subtle variations of habitat suitability within chorus locations may make some calling sites better than others for attracting females. For example, females may be more likely to enter a chorus from a particular direction, or some sites may be better from the point of view of sound propagation (e.g. Fellers, 1979*a*; Greer & Wells, 1980). The term 'lek' should be reserved for cases where male clumping in space is greater than that required by the distribution of suitable calling or oviposition sites (K. D. Wells, personal communication).

Resource-based territoriality occurs in some anurans. Male Green Frogs (*Rana clamitans*) (Wells, 1977*a*, 1978), and Bullfrogs (*Rana catesbeiana*) (Howard 1978*a*, *b*, 1980, 1981) defend territories in which mating and spawning take place. In some dendrobatid frogs, males defend all-purpose territories throughout the entire year. Each territory includes a feeding site, spawning site and daytime shelter place (references in Wells, 1977*b*, 1980).

Evolutionary explanations for species differences

The different mate-locating tactics of explosive and prolonged breeders must be the result of different selection pressures acting on them. The reasons for some species having short breeding seasons and others having long ones are not known, although these differences are almost certainly due to differences in ecology between species. Factors such as the temporal pattern of rainfall and temperature, the permanence of breeding sites, variations in predator pressure at different times of the year and the co-occurrence of competing species all probably affect the length of the 'time window' within which successful development is possible. This, in turn, will influence the timing and the duration of the breeding season.

The duration of the breeding season has two main consequences. First, it determines the density of males at the breeding site. Male density is commonly much higher in explosive breeders than prolonged breeders. This is certainly clear in some families, such as the ranids and bufonids, which have representatives of both types (Table 8.1). Density is lower in the latter because the appearance of individuals at the breeding site is staggered in time. Also, on any given night, a proportion of the male population may be feeding away from the breeding site.

Second, arrival of females at the breeding pond is quite synchronous for species with short breeding periods and more asynchronous for prolonged breeders. Since females arrive at the breeding site over a much longer period of time in prolonged breeders, there are fewer females at the site on any one night. This is reflected in the heavily male-biased operational sex ratio (Emlen & Oring, 1977) of species with extended breeding seasons (Table 8.1).

The combination of a high male density and the relatively high proportion of females at the breeding site in explosive breeders favours active searching by males. As Wells (1977*b*) explains, 'the advantage of being first to encounter an incoming female probably outweighs the disadvantages of repeatedly clasping other males'. Moreover, high male densities probably mean that individual territories would not be economi-

Table 8.1. *Male density and operational sex ratio for some explosive and prolonged breeders*

Species	Duration of season (days)	Approximate number of males	Operational sex ratio (males:females)	Reference
Explosive breeders				
Rana sylvatica	10	300+	6:1	Howard, 1980
R. temporaria	10	90	2:1	Personal observation
Bufo bufo	15	350+	5:1	Davies & Halliday, 1979
B. americanus	7	200	4:1	Gatz, 1981*b*
B. typhonius	Several bursts of 1 day	80	2:1	Wells, 1979
Prolonged breeders				
R. catesbeiana	52	27	31:1	Howard, 1978*a*
R. clamitans	60	25	12:1	Wells, 1977*a*, 1978
Hyla crucifer	75	52	7:1	Gatz, 1981*a*
H. versicolor	75	41	5:1	Gatz, 1981*a*
H. rosenbergi	200	12	8:1	Kluge, 1981
B. americanus	56	20	6:1	Blair, 1943

Male numbers and operational sex ratio are mean *nightly* values. Where data from several years were given by the original authors, the samples from all years have been combined and averaged.

cally defensible. Conversely, for prolonged breeders the number of females at the breeding site at a given time is low, so a male is unlikely to improve his reproductive success by trying to maximise his encounter rate with other individuals. A male's success depends much more on his ability to attract females to his calling site and to maintain a considerable distance from other males.

Similar conclusions to those above are obtained by energetic arguments. In an explosive breeder, selection should favour a male expending considerable energy on obtaining the first mate, but relatively little should be invested in trying to get a second mate because the chances of success are so low. In a prolonged breeder, however, male mating effort should be spread more evenly throughout the breeding season because female arrival is to a large extent unpredictable. Data on weight loss by sexually active males of three anuran species provide some evidence that these expectations are borne out (Table 8.2). My observations show that male Common Toads (*Bufo bufo*) which search and fight for females lose weight at 3.3 times the rate of male Natterjack Toads (*B. calamita*), a species which calls to attract females. However, the breeding season of Natterjacks is twice as long as that of Common Toads, so that the overall difference in weight loss is just 1.64 times greater for male Common Toads. Although Common Toads make a greater total investment than Natterjacks, they have more time to replace their energy reserves before the next season. Constraints on the maximum amount of energy that can be allocated to mating effort must set limits to the sort of mate-locating tactics that can be adopted by a particular species. For example, imagine a male Natterjack who fights for females instead of calling. By the end of the breeding season he would have to invest 90% of his body weight to sustain his sexual activities. Clearly, such a level of investment would be impossible.

Life-history factors such as longevity and predation pressure may influence the total amount of mating effort invested per season. If the species is a long-lived one a male might be better off saving his resources

Table 8.2. *Energetics of mating behaviour for three different species*

Species	Behaviour	Days in pond	Daily weight loss (%)	Total weight loss (%)	Reference
Bufo bufo	Scramble	20	1.07	21.4	Personal observation
B. calamita	Calling	41	0.32	13.1	Personal observation
Rana clamitans	Territorial	60	0.175	10.5	Wells, 1978

until the following year when his chances of success might be greater. In short-lived species, male survivorship may be low regardless of the energy invested in mating, so selection will favour the maximum effort to obtain as many mates as possible during the first breeding season. Although so few data about life-history variables and the energetic costs of mating are available (but see MacNally, 1981), it is clear that both factors will influence the sort of mate-locating tactics adopted.

Mate-locating behaviour as evolutionarily stable strategies

The different mate-locating strategies adopted by explosive and prolonged breeders can be viewed as alternative evolutionarily stable strategies (*sensu* Maynard Smith, 1974). To illustrate this point, consider a mutant frog who adopts a calling strategy in an explosively breeding species. The mutant male would achieve little success, even if females responded to his advertisement calls, simply because they probably would be intercepted by searching males before reaching the calling mutant. Therefore, the active-searching strategy would be stable against invasion by the calling strategy. Similarly, consider a mutant male frog who adopts a searching strategy in a prolonged breeding species. Because of the low number of females at the breeding site, such a male probably would waste energy in fruitless encounters with other males and would rapidly become fatigued. It is difficult to imagine how such a mutant strategy could invade a population of calling males, unless the abundances of females increased. It is clear that the distinct strategies of males in explosive and prolonged breeders are the best solutions for securing matings, given the constraints imposed on male behaviour by the length of the breeding season and female arrival patterns.

Alternative male strategies
Explosive breeders

In some explosive breeders an interesting form of alternative mating behaviour occurs. In the Common Toad (*B. bufo*) and the Common Frog (*R. temporaria*), large males congregate around the communal spawn-site and attempt to dislodge paired males from females which have gone there to spawn. Small males, on the other hand, search for females away from the spawn site, often at the edges of the pond where unpaired females are arriving. However, the alternative strategies are not rigidly fixed in particular males; individuals move around the pond and switch between searching and struggling, but nevertheless, when the population is sampled it is found that there is a significant difference in male body size between those males searching at the spawn-site and those away from it (author's personal observations) (see Table 8.3).

Prolonged breeders

In some species that defend oviposition sites, a male's size relative to others in the population is an important influence on the type of mate-locating strategy which is adopted.

For example, in bullfrogs there are three patterns of male mating behaviour: territoriality, 'satellite' behaviour, and opportunism (Howard, 1978*a*, 1981). Large males call and defend territories, small males sit near a territorial male and attempt to intercept females attracted to the caller. Such satellite males do not call, but sit in a low posture, presumably to reduce the risk of being attacked by a territorial male. Opportunists are males who call from potential oviposition sites but do not defend such sites. If challenged, opportunistic males leave their calling sites and resume calling elsewhere. Usually opportunists are intermediate in size between territorial and satellite males.

Table 8.3. *Alternative mate-locating strategies adopted by male anurans*

Species	Mean size of males (mm)		Reference
	Strategy 1	Strategy 2	
Bufo bufo	Fight 65.8	Search 61.9**(*t*)	Personal observation
Rana temporaria	Fight 67.9	Search 62.9**(*t*)	Personal observation
B. calamita	Caller 69.6	Satellite 63.4***(*t*)	Personal observation
Hyla cinerea	Caller 53.1	Satellite 47.2	Garton & Brandon, 1975
H. crucifer	Caller 45.1	Satellite 43.0*(Sign)	Fellers, 1979; Gatz, 1981*a*
H. regilla	Caller 44.2	Satellite 43.9*(Sign)	Fellers, 1979; Gatz, 1981*a*
H. versicolor	Caller 46.5	Satellite 462*(Wilcox.)	Fellers, 1979; Gatz, 1981*a*
R. catesbeiana	Territorial 139.9	Satellite 112.8***(M–W U)	Howard, 1978*a*

Levels of significance for two-tailed tests: * $P < 0.1$; ** $P < 0.01$; *** $P < 0.005$. *t* refers to Student's *t*-test, Sign to sign test, Wilcox. to Wilcoxon test, and M–W U the Mann–Whitney U test.

Satellite behaviour may serve two functions in territorial species (Wells, 1977*a*). Satellite males may be attempting to intercept females approaching the territory owner, as in Bullfrogs, and/or they may be waiting for territories to become vacant when the owner becomes fatigued through prolonged defence. In Green Frogs, satellite males occasionally took over territories after the owners had abandoned them (Wells, 1977*a*, 1978).

The occurrence of alternative male strategies is particularly common in those species that call from positions removed from oviposition sites. Satellite behaviour is known to occur in *Hyla versicolor*, *H. chrysoscelis*, *H. squirella*, *H. regilla*, *H. crucifer*, *H. cinerea*, *H. microcephala*, *H. ebraccata*, *H. minuta* (Fellers, 1979*b*; Wells, 1977*b* and personal communication), and in several bufonids (Axtell, 1958; Brown & Pierce, 1967). It probably occurs in many other species whose mating systems have not been studied in detail.

In Green Treefrogs (*Hyla cinerea*) non-calling satellite males sit next to callers and attempt to intercept females (Perrill, Gerhardt & Daniel, 1978). Some males are consistent callers, whereas others are consistent satellites. Still others switch strategies frequently, sometimes in a single night. In experimental manipulations in which calling males were removed from caller-satellite associations, satellite males either began calling or became satellites on other calling males (Perrill, Gerhardt & Daniel, 1982). The tendency of a satellite male to begin calling after removal of a calling male could be suppressed by replacing the caller with a speaker playing conspecific calls.

When synthetic advertisement calls were played to calling males, some switched to satellite behaviour. However, the responses were not consistent between males or between different trials on one male. These experiments show that strategies are not fixed. Probably an individual male's strategy is determined by facultative responses to the proximity of other calling males. Differences in male body size account for some of the behavioural variability seen in nature: there is a weak but significant correlation between a male's body size and the percentage of times it is observed calling (Perrill *et al.*, 1982). Nevertheless, much of the variation in responses to the playbacks cannot be adequately explained by male size. Other factors such as differences in nutritional state, hormonal levels, previous outcomes of aggressive interactions and previous mating success are probably important in strategy choice.

In several species of toads with prolonged breeding seasons, non-calling males have been observed sitting near callers (e.g. *B. speciosus*, *B. cognatus*, *B. houstonensis*, *B. woodhouseii*, *B. valliceps* (references cited in Wells,

1977*b*) and *B. calamita* (author's personal observations)). Axtell (1958) noted that non-calling male *B. speciosus* are smaller than callers. He interpreted this as indicating that the smaller males with reduced calling abilities (i.e. lower intensity calls) were taking advantage of the larger males' abilities to attract females.

In Natterjack Toads (*B. calamita*) males call from the edge of temporary pools or rain-filled ditches. The spacing between males is not even. Males often sit in distinct groups of three or four individuals which I term 'call groups'. The distance between males within a call group is about 1–3 m, whereas the distance between neighbouring groups is 10–15 m (Mathias, 1971; personal observations). Within a call group some males call only occasionally and others act as non-calling satellites. The male in the group who calls most frequently usually is the largest male and most often is centrally situated within the group. The peripheral males usually are smaller and they call less frequently and less loudly than the central male. In a series of experiments I removed the main caller from a call group. In eight of 10 groups, the peripheral males dispersed within 15 min after the removal. In nine other groups, a peripheral male was removed, and in only one instance did any other males in the group disperse. These results support Axtell's (1958) hypothesis that small males exploit the superior ability of larger males to attract females. Further, large males most frequently moved away from a loudspeaker broadcasting synthetic calls, whereas small males stopped calling and oriented towards the loudspeaker (personal observations).

Functions of alternative strategies

In theory, alternative male strategies may be maintained by two means. First, it may be that the alternatives are equally successful and so each is able to persist in a population at some evolutionary stable ratio. Or second, it may be that one strategy is less successful than the other but it is able to persist in the population because it is the 'best of a bad job' given certain constraints on the individuals who adopt it (Bateson, 1976; Maynard Smith, 1978*a*; Dawkins, 1980).

An example of the first type of solution may be the 'caller' and 'satellite' strategies of Green Treefrogs discussed above (Maynard Smith, 1979; Davies, 1982). In the study by Perrill *et al.* (1978), callers and satellites achieved approximately equal reproductive success when females were released near caller-satellite associations. The strategy employed by males may be a mixed one such that all males spend, on average, the same proportion of time being a caller and a satellite.

The variance in male size in Green Treefrog populations is low since the species is quite small and short-lived. In contrast, in long-lived species there is considerable variance in male size, and small, young males frequently adopt less costly alternative strategies to obtain females. Sometimes this is reflected in the pattern of weight loss throughout the breeding season, with smaller males experiencing, on average, a lower percentage decrease in weight than larger males. This is known to be the case in Green Frogs (Wells, 1978) and Natterjack Toads (personal observations). These observations accord with the predictions of life history theory, that organisms which reproduce several times in their life should increase their yearly reproductive effort over the first few breeding seasons (Williams, 1966; Pianka & Parker, 1975; Stearns, 1976).

A proximate explanation of why small or young males should invest less is because they have a low probability of winning contests against larger or older males. Satellite male Natterjack Toads obtain fewer matings than callers. However, it is unlikely that a satellite could increase his reproductive success by calling since small males have weaker calls than large males. The satellite strategy is 'the best of a bad job' for a small male.

The advantages gained by small males in exploiting the ability of larger males to advertise efficiently are sufficient to explain the clumping of male toads into call groups. I suggest that this explanation may account for aggregation of males in choruses and the clumping of 'subordinate' males around 'dominants' in other animal species which form leks.

Behavioural variability in mating systems

There are two sources of behavioural variability in anuran mating systems. First, at a given time, behaviour may vary between individuals due to the existence of alternative mate-acquisition strategies. Second, a population's mating system may vary as the density of males changes at different times of the breeding season or between different study sites (Wells, 1977b).

In the Bullfrog, the typical mating system has separately been described as a lek system (Emlen, 1968, 1976) and as a territorial one (Howard, 1978a). In Emlen's study, females did not deposit spawn on males' territories but left the main chorus area before ovipositing. In Howard's study at the same pond females mated and spawned on individual males' territories. It is possible that Bullfrogs show a change from territorial to lek organisation with increasing density, because the costs of defending individual territories become prohibitively high as male density increases (Wells, 1977b; Howard, 1978a; Ryan, 1980a). However, there is some doubt as to whether the different results are meaningful due to the small number (six) of egg-masses found by Emlen.

The behaviour of male Natterjack Toads switches from calling from relatively stationary positions at low density, to active movement and clasping as density increases (personal observations). Such clasping behaviour can occasionally be witnessed at low male density when two males establish calling stations very near to each other, but as male density increases and males are forced to call closer and closer together, clasping becomes very frequent. Clasping interactions often follow the detection of movement of other toads near a calling male, and it is tempting to think that the behaviour is designed to capture females who are approaching a caller. Similar changes in male behaviour at different densities occur in *Bufo canorus* (Kagarise Sherman, 1980).

The opposite trend, a switch from active searching to stationary calling as density decreases, occurs in some species which normally breed at high density. In the Common Toad and the Common Frog males scramble for females at usual densities. However, at the beginning of the breeding season, whilst density is still low, some males call (Eibl-Eibesfeldt, 1950; personal observations).

What is the adaptive significance of these changes in mate-locating tactics? Alexander (1975) and Wells (1977b) suggested that the way in which males allocate their time between calling and searching is critically dependent on male density (see Fig. 8.3). At low density there is relatively little competition for the available females so it will pay all males to call. As male density increase some small males may do better by ceasing to call and attempting to intercept females approaching calling males. Further increases in density will favour the satellite strategy even more because satellites will be able to effectively patrol the periphery of the territories of several callers. However, when the risk of cuckoldry by satellite males becomes very great, callers will profit by spending an increasing proportion of their time searching for approaching females and chasing off satellite males. At very high densities, then, most males will be seen actively clasping other individuals.

Female choice

One of the biggest mistakes a female can make is to mate with a male of the wrong species. There is little doubt that female anurans possess mechanisms which enable them to prevent this. Evidence that females can discriminate between species on the basis of differences in male vocalisations has been documented by several authors (see reviews by

Bogert, 1960; Blair, 1964; Salthe & Mecham, 1974; Littlejohn, 1977). However, more recently 'female choice' has often been used in a narrower and more controversial sense. It has been suggested that females will benefit by choosing males in the population who possess 'good genes' (Trivers, 1972).

There are three main problems with the 'good genes' argument. First is the question of whether or not sufficient genetic variance can be maintained in the male population so that a female preference can persist. Under strong selection, any trait favoured by females should become rapidly fixed in a population leaving very little variance from which females might choose (Maynard Smith, 1978*b*). Under these circumstances, 'choosy' females might be selected against because the cost of being choosy is not offset by any further increase in offspring fitness (Parker, 1981, and this volume). An alternative view is that genetic variance may be maintained through environmental heterogeneity (MacKay, 1980), migration between locally adapted sub-populations (e.g. Felsenstein, 1976; Nevo, 1978; Slatkin, 1978), normal rates of mutation in polygenic characters (Lande,

Fig. 8.3. The proportion of callers:non-callers changes with male density. The height of the stippled area below the diagonal line represents the proportion of males who are calling. At low density it pays most males to call because there is not much vocal competition for the available females. As density increases some small males benefit by exploiting other males, as non-calling satellites. At still higher densities most males switch to searching to avoid being cuckolded by the satellite males. (Adapted from Alexander, 1975.)

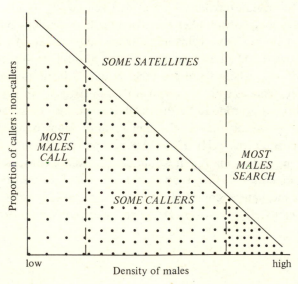

1976) or by a counter-balancing mechanism which favours the least attractive males (e.g. Cade, 1979). Measurements of heritability of fitness in real populations are lacking, apart from a few exceptions which suggest that fitness may have higher heritability than is usually assumed (Partridge, 1980; references in Andersson, 1982).

A second problem concerns whether females are capable of making discriminations between male phenotypic characters even if sufficient genetic variance exists. This is discussed at some length in the following sections. Finally, there may be an interpretative problem. In territorial species, males possess resources valuable to females as well as genes. In these species it is difficult to know what females are choosing – a male's genes or other resources which he possesses – such as a good territory or oviposition site.

Explosive breeders

Females have few opportunities to choose among potential mates in explosive breeders due to intense male–male competition (Wells, 1977b). It may, however, be possible for females to exercise some form of choice at low density, perhaps early in the breeding season before many males have arrived at the pond.

Davies & Halliday (1977) found that size-assortative mating occurred in a population of Common Toads. Since fertilisation success is greatest in those pairs which are well matched for size, they suggested that it may be advantageous for a female to mate with a male of about the same size. Potentially, females could exercise a form of mate-choice by influencing whether male–male competition takes place or not. If a female is paired with a desirable mate she may swim away from other males to avoid interference. If, however, she has been captured by an undesirable male, she could swim over to where there are other males to incite take-over attempts. However, females who become involved in struggles in regions of high male density, are prone to be drowned at the centre of a ball of struggling males, so it seems unlikely that this form of behaviour will be selected for in females. Davies & Halliday (1978, and personal communication) now view non-random mating in Common Toads as a consequence of male–male competition rather than female choice. Size-assortative mating is simply a mechanical consequence of the fact that only pairs well matched for size can resist take-overs by other males (see Wells, 1979).

Prolonged breeders

In territorial species, females benefit from choosing territories in which their offspring are most likely to survive and develop successfully. In Howard's (1978*b*) study of Bullfrogs, territories that were most favoured by females were those in which spawn predation by leeches was the lowest. Whether or not females take into account male quality as well as territory quality in territorial species is not known. Experimental changes of territory quality have not been carried out to ascertain which criteria females use.

In choosing territorial males, females may try to avoid being captured by satellite males in the territory. In both Green Frogs (Wells, 1977*a*) and Bullfrogs (Howard, 1981), females swim away when approached by silent males. Female Treefrogs appear actively to repel satellite males by shaking them off (Fellers, 1979*b*). What do females risk by mating with satellite males? In Bullfrogs and Green Frogs, females who mate with satellites stand to lose a good quality oviposition site because they are chased off by the territory owner (Howard, 1978*a*; Wells, 1977*a*). In Treefrogs which do not defend oviposition sites, discrimination against satellite males must occur for other reasons. No evidence suggests that callers and satellites differ genetically. It is quite possible that females avoid satellites for another reason: a satellite male who sits silently next to a caller may be a male of the wrong species.

Male Gladiator Frogs (*Hyla rosenbergi*) defend small water-filled basins on the forest floor and protect the eggs which the female oviposits there (Kluge, 1981). Females inspect a prospective mate's nest prior to pairing and sometimes reject males after inspection. Females also 'bump' males frequently during nest inspection, possibly to test how easily the prospective mate can be frightened from his territory. Males who are not easily frightened from their nests perhaps are more likely to provide effective parental care (Kluge, 1981). Thus it seems that both nest quality and male quality might be assessed by females.

Vocal cues in mate choice

In anuran species that do not defend oviposition sites females are unable to use the quality of a male's territory to judge his desirability as a mate (Wells, 1977*c*). Where females are simply attracted to calling males, the only information about males available to females is that contained in their vocal signals.

Some recent studies have claimed to find evidence for female choice of certain males based on differences in the properties of males' vocalisations. These studies fall roughly into two categories: (1) experiments that have shown females have frequency preferences, and (2) observations that suggest females prefer signals of high energy content. Since each category presents different problems I will discuss them in turn.

Frequency preferences

Ryan (1980*b*) has shown that female Leptodactylid Frogs, *Physalaemus pustulosus*, prefer advertisement calls of low frequency when given a choice between a low-frequency call and a high-frequency call. Because call frequency is inversely correlated with body size, females mate preferentially with large males. Females who mate with large males experience, on average, greater fertilisation success than those who mate with small males. This is due to more accurate juxtapositioning of the male and female cloacas during sperm emission (Ryan, in preparation). Also, larger males are either older or have grown faster than smaller males. Females may gain by mating with a large male because the benefits of rapid growth and/or survival will be passed on to offspring (if there is genetic heritability of these traits) (see Trivers, 1976).

Gerhardt (in press *a*) has pointed out that there may be other adaptive explanations for the frequency preferences of female anurans. Preferences for certain call properties could be the means by which females avoid heterospecific matings (which result in offspring of low viability) rather than a consequence of intraspecific mate choice. In situations where many species call together species-isolating mechanisms will be particularly important. Female Green Treefrogs (*H. cinerea*) show considerable frequency discrimination in choosing mates, but much of this discrimination is probably concerned with preventing mis-matings with males of two sympatric species, the Barking Treefrog (*H. gratiosa*) and the Squirrel Treefrog (*H. squirella*). These two species have calls with low-frequency peaks which are on either side of the frequency range of *H. cinerea*. Female Green Treefrogs, therefore, must choose calls which are approximately in the middle of the species range in order to prevent mating with the wrong species. Further, the discriminatory ability of females changes with temperature. At high temperatures females are able to discriminate between calls accurately and choose frequencies in the middle of the range, but under cooler conditions they choose calls at the bottom end of the frequency range. Hence, cool female Green Treefrogs are in danger of mating with male Barking Treefrogs, and in nature, they occasionally do so (Gerhardt & Mudry, 1980).

In anuran populations that are isolated from other species using vocal signals, females do not suffer the risk of mis-mating. Such populations, therefore, provide a useful situation in which to test ideas about intraspecific mate choice because female preferences are less likely to be concerned with species-recognition. I have tested frequency discrimination by female Natterjack Toads, a species which is isolated, in Britain, from other toads with mating calls. Female Natterjack Toads show no frequency preferences within the natural frequency range of the species. Moreover, females do not discriminate against calls which are *outside* the usual frequency range of the species (personal observations). I conclude that female Natterjacks are unable to choose certain males on the basis of natural differences in the frequency of their advertisement calls. The absence of sympatric species with similar calls means that females are not constrained to choose frequencies within the species range.

Female choice based on call properties of males is limited by the amount of information that can be transmitted in the anuran vocalisation under natural circumstances. In nature, many males take part in a chorus and call from different places within the habitat. To some extent the two-choice playback experiment is unrealistic because a female usually will be confronted by many calling males. On most occasions a female entering a chorus will have to pass several callers, before reaching the 'best' available male. The signals from those males nearest the female will be received at much higher intensities than those of distant males. If there is an evolutionary basis for preferring certain calls over others, we should expect females to choose preferred calls even when they are played back at much lower intensities than those of undesirable males. Further, interference by competing males is likely to lower the discriminatory ability of females in a real chorus. When female Green Treefrogs were given a choice between four signals with low-frequency peaks of 600, 700, 800 and 900 Hz played back simultaneously, they discriminated only against the 600 Hz call. In contrast to their performance in a two-choice trial, females did not prefer the 900 Hz call over the 700 Hz call. The results suggest that female discrimination is somewhat poorer in a complex acoustical situation than in a two-choice experiment (Gerhardt, in press *a*).

Information contained in vocalisations may be reduced in natural choruses because of the position of a calling male (Gerhardt, in press *b*). Males may call whilst floating in water, sitting on dry land, or from varying heights within bushes or trees. Such differences in the position of calling males can seriously affect the spectral composition of their calls (see Morton, 1975; Marten & Marler, 1977; Wiley & Richards, 1978). The high-frequency components of a call will suffer considerable excess attenuation when males call from water, or from positions near to the ground. Also, when both the source and the receiver are elevated then the relative amplitudes of the spectral components in the calls will change, because of interference between direct waves and waves reflected off the ground (Embleton, Piercy & Olson, 1976). It is therefore most likely that the variability of the environmental effects on spectral structure reduces the reliability of any information about the male encoded in the signal.

Preferences for calls of high energy content

A number of studies have shown that males who increase the total energy content of their vocalisations, either by calling more frequently, louder, or from areas with better sound transmission, achieve higher reproductive success (Whitney & Krebs, 1975a, b; Brattstrom, 1962; Fellers, 1979a, b; Greer & Wells, 1980). One interpretation of these results is that females prefer to mate with males who produce high energy output because it is an indication of high genetic fitness (see Andersson, 1982). An alternative explanation is that certain males attract more females simply because their calls are more likely to be heard or because they propagate further. Essentially, this is the distinction between 'active discrimination' and 'passive attraction' made by Parker (1982, and this volume). Although this distinction is a subtle one, it is not trivial. Active discrimination involves selection acting on males to increase (say) call loudness and on females to choose the loudest calls. Passive attraction, however, only involves selection on males. It does not matter whether females compare males or not; it will still pay males to call as loudly as possible.

In most studies, the mechanism responsible for differential male reproductive success seems more likely to be passive attraction. In Feller's (1979a) study of mate choice in the Grey Treefrog (*Hyla versicolor*), males who called from particular perches were most successful. Perches that were surrounded by little vegetation were the best places for effective sound transmission. Reproductive success was not correlated with any features of individual males other than their calling sites. Similarly, Greer & Wells (1980) showed that male *Centrolenella fleischmanni* calling from elevated sites obtained more mates than those calling from lower sites.

In the Pacific Treefrog (*H. regilla*) certain males in the population call more frequently than others and are more likely to initiate bouts of chorusing. Whitney & Krebs (1975a, b) termed these males 'chorus leaders'. In an artificial chorus of four loudspeakers, they found that females consistently prefer to approach speakers which initiate choruses rather than those which join in the chorus a few moments later. It is impossible to know, however, whether this is because females prefer chorus leaders because they possess good genes, or simply because their signal is more easily localised in a large chorus. If sound localisation is a problem in a large chorus, the obvious strategy for a male to employ is to start signalling before (or after) every other male to ensure that at least part of its signal is not interfered with by the calls of competing males.

In support of the active discrimination hypothesis, Fellers (1979*b*) showed that, when given a choice between calls, female Grey Treefrogs preferred the louder call. Female Natterjack Toads also prefer the louder call in a two-choice trial (personal observations). Loud calls may be more attractive to females than quiet ones because they act as better releasers of the phonotactic response due to a supernormal stimulus effect. It is easy to see how call loudness would then increase through evolutionary time through the Fisher (1958) effect. It is not necessary to assume an initial natural selection advantage to those males with the loudest calls, since stimulus summation is an adequate reason for the initial female preference for loud calls. A new mutant male who increases his call loudness will provide a supernormal releaser and will be preferred by females, in the same sense that Herring Gulls or Oyster Catchers prefer to incubate an abnormally large egg rather than a normal-sized one (Tinbergen, 1951, 1953). In fact the evolution and elaboration of ornaments and courtship displays in general, such as the peacock's tail and bird-song, initially may have depended upon their supernormal stimulus effects on females. The real problem to consider is whether what we observe at the present day is the result of a runaway selection process or merely the initial effect – a byproduct of the female's nervous system.

Structural and physiological design constraints

Supernormal stimulus effects have already been considered as possible design constraints affecting female preference. Another problem to consider is whether certain types of call are more localisable than others because of physiological limitations of the female's auditory system. For example, females might find it easier to localise low frequency calls rather than high ones, and calls of long duration rather than short calls. Functional explanations of female preference may be limited by *design constraints* inherent in the female anuran's auditory system (see Straughan, 1975; Feng, Gerhardt & Capranica, 1976; Littlejohn, 1977). To appreciate this, consider the problem that a female frog has in localising a sound source. For large vertebrates such as humans, the important cues which give directional information to the brain are sound intensity differences between each ear due to 'sound shadows' cast by the listener's head, and differences in time of arrival of the waves at each ear (Griffin, 1974). A frog, however, has a much smaller head than a human, so that differences in intensity and time differences between the ears are minute. The frog most probably relies on a mechanism known as a 'sound pressure gradient receiver' (Rheinlaender, Gerhardt, Yager & Capranica, 1979). An essential feature of this mechanism is that each tympanum receives sound from *both* ears simultaneously and compares the sound pressure between each side. Such a system is most effective when the wavelength of the sound is large in proportion to the dimensions of the tympanum. In other words, sounds of low pitch should be easier to localise than high-pitch sounds.

As in the case of call loudness, an initial preference for a certain frequency may result in a process of runaway selection through the Fisher (1958) effect. How, then, can we determine whether the preference arose as the result of a design constraint or whether it had some other selective value? Two approaches can be used. First, field experiments can be carried out to test the accuracy with which females localise and approach different types of call (see the methods of Rheinlaender *et al.*, 1979; Gerhardt, 1980). This method will immediately show whether there is any bias in the female's response. Second, by making broad comparisons across species, we can ask whether a preference for a certain call feature is a general phenomenon in anurans, or whether it depends on the species that is tested. If, for instance, we find that in all species females prefer low-frequency calls rather than high-frequency calls then it is a good reason to suspect the existence of a design constraint. If, however, some species prefer low-frequency calls and other species prefer high ones then there cannot be a common constraint and we should look for an adaptive explanation for the differences between species.

Another sort of constraint on female behaviour arises from the fact that anurans are ectothermic animals and their behavioural responses are temperature dependent. One function of the advertisement call of males is, most probably, to 'excite' the female and bring her into the proper physiological condition for mating. In female Natterjack Toads, the effectiveness with which it does so not only depends on the loudness of the stimulus but also on the ambient temperature. On very cold nights, the latency period prior to pairing was often very long, whereas on warm nights pairing sometimes occurred within a few seconds of the female entering the pond. In some instances, therefore, a female may fail to pair with a male, not because he is in any sense a 'bad' male, but simply because she has not had time to warm up.

For males, changes in temperature usually change some features of the advertisement call. In some species, the signal recognition mechanism of the female changes in a parallel fashion, so that the sender–receiver mechanisms are well coupled at all temperatures (e.g. Gerhardt, 1978). However, coupling is not always so efficient. As I have already mentioned, low temperatures cause significant changes in the frequency preferences of Green Treefrogs, but the frequency of the male's advertisement call does not change. The effects of temperature, therefore, may have important consequences on female preferences that do not have any obvious adaptive explanation. On the contrary, such consequences may be maladaptive in that the female is likely to mate with a male of another species.

Do females 'sample' several males?

A female would have to be very clever indeed to enter a pond and swim to the best male straight away. If there are advantages to females in choosing particular males, then we should expect to see females behaving in nature as if they are comparing several males before making a choice. Moreover, in a very complex acoustic environment, sequential 'sampling' rather than simultaneous comparison is probably necessary to discern differences between males.

In the Mottled Sculpin (*Cottus bairdi*), a freshwater fish, females visit several males at their nest sites before choosing to mate with one and spawn inside his nest. The observed patterns of male courtship success suggest that female Sculpins use very simple rules to choose a mate: they mate only with a male who is larger than or equal to the last male encountered (Brown, 1981). It is not known whether female frogs and toads use such simple rules to compare males, although the behaviour of some species is consistent with this interpretation (e.g. Duellman, 1966; Wells, 1977*a*, *c*; Fellers, 1979*a*, *b*; Howard, 1981).

Interpreting non-random mating

In most anuran populations which have been studied, non-random mating has been found (Table 8.4). This may take the form of size-dependent or size-assortative mating. Size-dependent mating means that male body size is an important determinant of mating success, so that, usually, larger than average-sized males in the population achieve the highest reproductive success. Size-assortative mating means that there is a significant correlation between the size of males and the size of females in mated pairs.

In a number of studies, non-random mating has been interpreted as *post facto* evidence for female choice, without much regard for alternative mechanisms (Licht, 1976; Davies & Halliday, 1977; Wilbur, Rubenstein & Fairchild, 1978; Fairchild, 1981). Non-random mating, however, is not sufficient evidence for female choice since it may come about through incidental effects, such as size-related patterns of arrival at breeding ponds (e.g. Flindt & Hemmer, 1968), or more likely, through male–male competition. Table 8.5 summarises the alternative mechanisms which could be responsible for non-random mating.

In some explosive breeders such as Common Toads and Common Frogs in which males fight for the possession of females, the mating pattern depends on male density at the breeding site (personal observations). In common frogs, size-assortative mating occurred in a population in which male density was high, but not in another population which had a much lower density of searching males. This was because in the high-density

Table 8.4. *Observed patterns of non-random mating in some anurans*

Species	Size dependent	Size assortative	Reference
Explosive breeders			
Rana sylvatica	Yes	No	Howard, 1980
R. temporaria			
Low density	No	No	Personal observation
High density	Yes	Yes	
Bufo bufo			
Low density	No	No	Personal observation
High density	Yes	Yes	Davies & Halliday, 1977, 1979
B. typhonius	Yes	No	Wells, 1979
B. americanus			
Low density	No	No	Wilbur *et al.*, 1978
High density	No	Yes	Licht, 1976
High density	Yes	No	Gatz, 1981*b*
Prolonged breeders			
Hyla cinerea	No	No	Gerhardt, in press *a*
H. crucifer	Yes	No	Gatz, 1981
H. versicolor	Yes	No	Gatz, 1981
H. marmota	Yes	No	Lee & Crump, 1981
Triprion petasatus	No	Yes	Lee & Crump, 1981
B. calamita	Yes	No	Personal observation
B. quercicus	Yes	No	Wilbur *et al.*, 1978
B. terrestris	No	No	Wilbur *et al.*, 1978
R. catesbeiana	Yes	Yes	Howard, 1978*a*
R. clamitans	Yes	No	Wells, 1977*a*

population struggles between searching males and pairs were frequent and many take-overs probably occurred. Experiments showed that size-assortative mating occurred because only those males who were well matched with females could resist take-over attempts. At low density, interactions between searching males and pairs were infrequent and take-overs were rare or absent.

Conclusions

This chapter is concerned with the extent to which adaptive explanations can be used to interpret sexual behaviour in different anuran species. For males, ecological factors affecting the length of the breeding season and the pattern of female arrival are important in shaping the sort of mate-locating behaviour adopted. In many anurans a great degree of behavioural flexibility is apparent and the extent to which each species can be said to have a 'typical mating system' is questionable. I view mating

Table 8.5. *Alternative explanations for size-dependent and size-assortative mating*

Observed mating pattern	Causes		
	Male–male competition	Female choice	Incidental effects
Size dependent	(1) Large males displace smaller ones from pairs (Davies & Halliday, 1979	Females prefer large males (Ryan, 1980*b*)	Large males have a thermal advantage over small ones (Flindt & Hemmer, 1968)
	(2) Large males control better territories than small ones do (Howard, 1978*a*)	Females prefer good territories (Howard, 1978*a*)	Large males produce calls which are easier to localise
	(3) Large males produce louder calls, they call more frequently or begin bouts of calling (Whitney & Krebs, 1975*a*, *b*)	Females actively avoid satellites (Wells, 1977*a*; Fellers, 1979; Howard, 1981)	
Size assortative	(1) Only well-matched pairs can resist take-over attempts successfully (Davies & Halliday, personal communication)	Older, experienced females are better at choosing large males (Howard, 1978*a*)	Different size-classes arrive at the breeding site at different times (Flindt & Hemmer, 1968)
	(2) Small females are more easily caught by satellites	Females prefer an optimum-sized male to increase their fertilisation success (Davies & Halliday, 1977)	An effect of combining samples from populations of different age structures

systems as a consequence of the way in which individuals interact in response to various ecological and social pressures. It is the collective behaviour of individuals which determines the mating system and not the other way round.

Much of the behavioural flexibility observed concerns how individuals apportion their time between searching and signalling. The way in which individuals do this can be best understood in terms of a game in which the best thing to do depends on what everyone else is doing. This applies to (1) the changes in behaviour that are observed as male density increases (as density increases switch from signalling to searching to avoid cuckoldry); and (2) the decision to call or to be a satellite (if there are few callers then call, if there are many callers become a satellite). A further complication is added to the game because all individuals are not identical. Male age/size influences the strategy decision in many species. Characteristically, large males adopt the strategy with the highest payoff and the highest cost, whilst small males go for the low payoff, low cost strategy. In those species which fight for females the rule used by males seems to be 'if big fight, if small search', and in those which call for females 'if big call, if small behave as satellite'. These simple rules serve only as illustrations, for in actual fact, male strategies are probably not phenotypically determined in such a hard and fast way. All individuals probably play a mixed strategy, but their thresholds for switching depend on size or condition.

Ryan, Tuttle & Taft (1981) suggest that the benefits of lower predation risk and higher mating probabilities associated with larger choruses are responsible for communal sexual displays in some frogs. I suggest an additional hypothesis which may explain grouping of males in some species. Males who are less effective advertisers could exploit males who are good advertisers by grouping around them and attempting to intercept females. Hence, neither predation nor female choice are necessary preconditions for communal display.

In the second part of the chapter I have critically reviewed the evidence that females prefer to mate with particular males in a population. Although females show definite preferences in a number of species, the reasons for such preferences are less clear. Wherever possible I have tried to point out the pitfalls in interpretation which can result from inadequate data or failure to test alternative hypotheses. These fall into three main categories:

(1) Non-random mating is necessary but not sufficient evidence for female choice. Male–male competition is an important force which generates non-random mating in a population. In calling species it is often

difficult to distinguish between differences in male mating successes that result from active discrimination by females and differences in success that result from differences in passive attraction. In fighting species, the effects of competition between males may render female choice impossible (Trivers, 1972; Wells, 1977*b*).

(2) Structural design constraints on the female's auditory system may bias her ability to localise certain sorts of call. Also, because anurans are ectothermic, levels of motivation, time to physiological responsiveness and the accuracy of coupling of sender–receiver mechanisms may be temperature dependent. These factors may affect female preferences and the readiness with which females will approach certain males.

(3) Even when active discrimination is proven there is the problem of which adaptive explanation to choose. Do females prefer certain males in the population, or are they merely trying to avoid mating with the wrong species? There is currently a tendency in behavioural ecology to adopt the most 'exciting' or most fashionable explanation for an observation at the expense of alternatives that are equally plausible (Gould & Lewontin, 1979). An approach that tests between alternatives is likely to be more fruitful in the future.

Summary

Male–male competition in anurans takes the form of scramble competition, territorial defence or calling in choruses. The type of mating system depends on the density of males and the operational sex ratio at the breeding site. Both these factors are affected by the duration of the breeding season. In all types of mating system there is a degree of behavioural variability; some males adopt alternative mate-acquisition strategies and switch behaviour according to male density. There is good evidence for female choice in a number of species but interpreting female choice is confounded by several factors, including species-isolating mechanisms, design constraints on the female's discriminatory ability, and intersexual selection.

I am grateful to Carl Gerhardt and Kent Wells for their kind hospitality during my visit to the United States. This chapter has benefited greatly from discussions with them. Also, I thank Pat Bateson, Nick Davies and Kent Wells for comments on an earlier draft, and Duncan Mackinder for help with the word processor. Malte Andersson and Mike Ryan provided unpublished manuscripts. This review was prepared whilst I was supported by a grant from the Natural Environment Research Council.

References

Alexander, R. D. (1975). Natural selection and specialized chorusing behaviour in acoustical insects. In *Insects, Science and Society*, ed. D. Pimentel, pp. 37–77. Academic Press: New York.

Andersson, M. (1982). Sexual selection, natural selection and quality advertisement. *Biological Journal of the Linnean Society*, **17**, 375–93.

Axtell, R. W. (1958). Female reaction to the male call in two anurans (Amphibia). *Southwestern Naturalist*, **3**, 70–6.

Bateson, P. P. G. (1976). Rules and reciprocity in behavioural development. In *Growing Points in Ethology*, ed. P. P. G. Bateson & R. A. Hinde, pp. 401–21. Cambridge University Press: Cambridge.

Blair, A. P. (1943). Population structure in toads. *American Naturalist*, **77**, 563–8.

Blair, W. F. (1964). Isolating mechanisms and interspecific interactions in anuran amphibians. *Quarterly Review of Biology*, **39**, 334–44.

Blair, W. F. (1968). Amphibians and reptiles. In *Animal Communication*, ed. T. A. Sebeok, pp. 289–310. Indiana University Press: Bloomington, Ind.

Bogert, C. M. (1960). The influence of sound on amphibians and reptiles. In *Animal Sounds and Communication*, ed. W. E. Lanyon & W. N. Travolga, pp. 137–320. American Institute of Biological Science: Washington.

Bradbury, J. W. (1977). Lek mating behaviour in the hammer-headed bat. *Zeitschrift für Tierpsychologie*, **45**, 225–55.

Brattstrom, B. H. (1962). Call order and social behaviour in the foam-building frog *Engystomops pustulosus*. *American Zoologist*, **2**, 394.

Brown, L. (1981). Patterns of female choice in mottled sculpins (Cottidae: Teleostei). *Animal Behaviour*, **29**, 375–82.

Brown, L. E. & Pierce, J. R. (1967). Male–male interactions and chorusing intensities of the Great Plains toad, *Bufo cognatus*. *Copeia*, 1967, 149–54.

Bucher, T. L., Ryan, M. J. & Bartholomew, G. A. (1980). The cost of croaking in a frog, *Physalaemus pustulosus* (Leptodactylidae). *American Zoologist*, **20**, 909.

Buechner, H. K. & Schloeth, R. (1965). Ceremonial mating behaviour in Uganda kob (*Adenota kob thomasi* Neumann). *Zeitschrift für Tierpsychologie*, **22**, 209–25.

Cade, W. (1979). The evolution of alternative male reproductive strategies in field crickets. In *Sexual Selection and Reproductive Competition in Insects*, ed. M. Blum & N. A. Blum, pp. 343–79. Academic Press: London.

Capranica, R. R. (1965). The evoked vocal response of the bullfrog: a study of communication by sound. *M.I.T. Research Monograph*, 33.

Constantz, G. D. (1975). Behavioural ecology of mating in the gila topminnow, *Poeciliopsis occidentalis* (Cyprinodontiformes: Poecilidae). *Ecology*, **56**, 966–73.

Davies, N. B. (1982). Behaviour and competition for scarce resources. In *Current Problems in Sociobiology*, ed. King's College Sociology Group, pp. 363–80. Cambridge University Press: Cambridge.

Davies, N. B. & Halliday, T. R. (1977). Optimal mate selection in the toad *Bufo bufo*. *Nature*, **269**, 56–8.

Davies, N. B. & Halliday, T. R. (1978). Deep croaks and fighting assessment in toads *Bufo bufo*. *Nature*, **274**, 683–5.

Davies, N. B. & Halliday, T. R. (1979). Competitive mate searching in male common toads *Bufo bufo*. *Animal Behaviour*, **27**, 1253–67.

Dawkins, R. (1980). Good strategy or evolutionarily stable strategy? In *Sociobiology: Beyond Nature/Nurture*, ed. G. W. Barlow & J. Silverberg, pp. 331–67. Westview Press: Boulder, Colorado.

Duellman, W. E. (1966). Aggressive behaviour in dendrobatid frogs. *Herpetologica*, **22**, 217–21.

Eibl-Eibesfeldt, I. (1950). Ein Beitrag zur Paarungsbiologie der Erdkrote (*Bufo bufo* L.). *Behaviour*, **2**, 217–36.

Embleton, T. F. W., Piercy, J. E. & Olson, N. (1976). Outdoor sound propagation over ground of finite impedance. *Journal of the Acoustical Society of America*, **59**, 267–77.

Emlen, S. T. (1968). Territoriality in the bullfrog, *Rana catesbeiana*. *Copeia*, 1968, 240–3.

Emlen, S. T. (1976). Lek organization and mating strategy in the bullfrog. *Behavioral Ecology and Sociobiology*, **1**, 283–313.

Emlen, S. T. & Oring, L. W. (1977). Ecology, sexual selection and the evolution of mating systems. *Science*, **197**, 215–23.

Fairchild, L. (1981). Mate selection and behavioural thermoregulation in Fowler's toads. *Science*, **212**, 950–1.

Fellers, G. M. (1979a). Mate selection in the gray treefrog, *Hyla versicolor*. *Copeia*, 1979, 286–90.

Fellers, G. M. (1979b). Aggression, territoriality, and mating behaviour in North American treefrogs. *Animal Behaviour*, **27**, 107–19.

Felsenstein, J. (1976). The theoretical population genetics of variable selection and migration. *Annual Review of Genetics*, **10**, 253–80.

Feng, A. S., Gerhardt, H. C. & Capranica, R. R. (1976). Sound localization behaviour of the green treefrog (*Hyla cinerea*) and the barking treefrog (*H. gratiosa*). *Journal of Comparative Physiology A*, **107**, 241–52.

Fisher, R. A. (1958). *The Genetical Theory of Natural Selection*. Dover Publications Incorporated: New York.

Flindt, R. & Hemmer, H. (1968). Beobachtungen zur Dynamik einer Population von *Bufo bufo* und *Bufo calamita*. *Zoologische Jahrbücher (Systematik)*, **94**, 162–86.

Garton, J. S. & Brandon, R. A. (1975). Reproductive ecology of the green treefrog, *Hyla cinerea*, in southern Illinois (Anura: Hylidae). *Herpetologica*, **31**, 150–61.

Gatz, A. J. (1981a). Size selective mating in *Hyla versicolor* and *Hyla crucifer*. *Journal of Herpetology*, **15**, 114–16.

Gatz, A. J. (1981b). Non-random mating by size in American toads, *Bufo americanus*. *Animal Behaviour*, **29**, 1004–12.

Gerhardt, H. C. (1974). The significance of some spectral features in mating call recognition in the green treefrog (*Hyla cinerea*). *Journal of Experimental Biology*, **61**, 229–41.

Gerhardt, H. C. (1978). Temperature coupling in the vocal communication system of the gray treefrog *Hyla versicolor*. *Science*, **199**, 992–4.

Gerhardt, H. C. (1980). Accuracy of sound localization in a miniature dendrobatid frog. *Naturwissenschaften*, **67**, 362–3.

Gerhardt, H. C. (in press a). Sound pattern recognition in some North American treefrogs (Anura: Hylidae): implications for mate selection. *American Zoologist*.

Gerhardt, H. C. (in press b). Mating call recognition in the green treefrog (*Hyla cinerea*): importance of two frequency bands as a function of sound pressure level. *Journal of Comparative Physiology A*.

Gerhardt, H. C. & Mudry, K. M. (1980). Temperature effects on frequency preferences and mating call frequencies in the green treefrog *Hyla cinerea* (Anura: Hylidae). *Journal of Comparative Physiology A*, **137**, 1–6.

Gould, S. J. & Lewontin, R. C. (1979). The spandrels of San Marco and the Panglossian paradigm: a critique of the adaptationist programme. *Proceedings of the Royal Society of London* B **205**, 581–98.

Greer, B. J. & Wells, K. D. (1980). Territorial and reproductive behaviour of the tropical American frog, *Centrolenella fleischmanni*. *Herpetologica*, **36**, 318–26.

Griffin, D. R. (1974). *Listening in the Dark: the Acoustic Orientation of Bats and Men.* Dover Publications: New York.

Howard, R. D. (1978*a*). The evolution of mating strategies in bullfrogs, *Rana catesbeiana. Evolution,* **32,** 850–71.

Howard, R. D. (1978*b*). Factors influencing early embryo mortality in bullfrogs. *Ecology,* **59,** 789–98.

Howard, R. D. (1980). Mating behaviour and mating success in woodfrogs, *Rana sylvatica. Animal Behaviour,* **28,** 705–16.

Howard, R. D. (1981). Male age–size distribution and male mating success in bullfrogs. In *Natural Selection and Social Behavior: Recent Research and New Theory,* ed. R. D. Alexander & D. W. Tinkle. Chiron Press: New York.

Kagarise Sherman, C. (1980). *A Comparison of the Natural History and Mating Systems of Two Anurans: Yosemite Toads* (Bufo canorus) *and Black Toads* (Bufo exsul). Ph.D. thesis, University of Michigan.

Kluge, A. G. (1981). The life history, social organization, and parental behaviour of *Hyla rosenbergi* Boulenger, a nest-building gladiator frog. *Miscellaneous Publications of the Museum of Zoology, University of Michigan,* no. 160, 1–170.

Lande, R. (1976). The maintenance of genetic variability by mutation in polygenic characters with linked loci. *Genetic Research,* **26,** 221–25.

Lee, J. C. & Crump, M. L. (1981). Morphological correlates of male mating success in *Triprion petasatus* and *Hyla marmota* (Anura: Hylidae). *Oecologia,* **50,** 153–7.

Licht, L. E. (1976). Sexual selection in toads (*Bufo americanus*). *Canadian Journal of Zoology,* **54,** 1277–84.

Lill, A. (1974). Sexual behaviour of the lek-forming white-bearded manakin (*Manacus manacus trinitatus*). *Zeitschrift für Tierpsychologie,* **45,** 225–55.

Littlejohn, M. J. (1977). Long-range acoustic communication in anurans: an integrated and evolutionary approach. In *The Reproductive Biology of Amphibians,* ed. D. H. Taylor & S. I. Guttman, pp. 263–94. Plenum Publishing Corporation: New York.

Loftus-Hill, J. J. & Littlejohn, M. J. (1971). Pulse repetition rate as the basis for mating call discrimination by two sympatric species of *Hyla. Copeia,* 1971, 154–6.

MacKay, T. F. C. (1980). Genetic variance, fitness, and homeostasis in varying environments: an experimental check of the theory. *Evolution,* **34,** 1219–22.

MacNally, R. C. (1981). On the reproductive energetics of chorusing males: energy depletion profiles, restoration and growth in two sympatric species of *Ranidella* (Anura). *Oecologia,* **51,** 181–8.

Marten, K. & Marler, P. (1977). Sound transmission and its significance for animal vocalizations I. Temperate habitats. *Behavioral Ecology and Sociobiology,* **2,** 271–90.

Mathias, J. H. (1971). *The Comparative Ecologies of Two Species of Amphibia* (Bufo bufo *and* Bufo calamita) *on the Ainsdale Sand Dunes National Nature Reserve.* Ph.D. thesis, University of Manchester.

Maynard Smith, J. (1974). The theory of games and the evolution of animal conflicts. *Journal of Theoretical Biology,* **47,** 209–21.

Maynard Smith, J. (1978*a*). Optimization theory in evolution. *Annual Review of Ecology and Systematics,* **9,** 31–56.

Maynard Smith, J. (1978*b*). *The Evolution of Sex.* Cambridge University Press: Cambridge.

Maynard Smith, J. (1979). Game theory and the evolution of behaviour. *Proceedings of the Royal Society of London* B **205,** 475–88.

Morton, E. S. (1975). Ecological sources of selection on avian sounds. *American Naturalist,* **109,** 17–34.

Narins, P. M. & Capranica, R. R. (1976). Sexual differences in the auditory system of the treefrog *Eleutherodactylus coqui. Science,* **192,** 378–80.

Nevo, E. (1978). Genetic variation in natural populations: pattern and theory. *Theoretical Population Biology*, **13**, 121–77.

Parker, G. A. (1982). Phenotype-limited evolutionarily stable strategies. In *Current Problems in Sociobiology*, ed. King's College Sociobiology Group, pp. 173–201. Cambridge University Press: Cambridge.

Partridge, L. (1980). Mate choice increases a component of offspring fitness in fruit flies. *Nature*, **283**, 290–1.

Perrill, S. A., Gerhardt, H. C. & Daniel, R. (1978). Sexual parasitism in the green treefrog, *Hyla cinerea*. *Science*, **200**, 1179–80.

Perrill, S. A., Gerhardt, H. C. & Daniel, R. (1982). Mating strategy shifts in male green treefrogs (*Hyla cinerea*): an experimental study. *Animal Behaviour*, **30**, 43–8.

Pianka, E. R. & Parker, W. S. (1975). Age specific reproductive tactics. *American Naturalist*, **109**, 453–64.

Rheinlander, J., Gerhardt, H. C., Yager, D. D. & Capranica, R. R. (1979). Accuracy of phonotaxis by the green treefrog (*Hyla cinerea*). *Journal of Comparative Physiology A*, **133**, 247–55.

Ryan, M. J. (1980*a*). The reproductive behaviour of the bullfrog (*Rana catesbeiana*). *Copeia*, 1980, 108–14.

Ryan, M. J. (1980*b*). Female mate choice in a neotropical frog. *Science*, **209**, 523–5.

Ryan, M. J. (in preparation). Sexual selection and communication in a neotropical frog, *Physalaemus pustulosus*.

Ryan, M. J., Tuttle, M. D. & Taft, L. K. (1981). The costs and benefits of frog chorusing behaviour. *Behavioral Ecology and Sociobiology*, **8**, 273–8.

Salthe, S. W. & Mecham, J. S. (1974). Reproductive courtship patterns. In *Physiology of the Amphibia*, ed. B. Lofts, vol. **2**, pp. 209–51. Academic Press: New York.

Slatkin, M. (1978). Spatial patterns in the distribution of polygenic characters. *Journal of Theoretical Biology*, **70**, 213–28.

Stearns, S. C. (1976). Life history tactics: a review of the ideas. *Quarterly Review of Biology*, **51**, 3–47.

Straughan, I. R. (1975). An analysis of the mechanisms of mating call discrimination in the frogs *Hyla regilla* and *H. cadaverina*. *Copeia*, **1975**, 415–24.

Tinbergen, N. (1951). *The Study of Instinct*. Clarendon Press: Oxford.

Tinbergen, N. (1953). *The Herring Gull's World*. Collins: London.

Trivers, R. L. (1972). Parental investment and sexual selection. In *Sexual Selection and the Descent of Man*, ed. B. Campbell, pp. 139–79. Aldine: Chicago.

Trivers, R. L. (1976). Sexual selection and resource accrual ability in *Anolis garmani*. *Evolution*, **30**, 253–69.

van Rhijn, J. G. (1973). Behavioural dimorphism in male ruffs *Philomachus pugnax* (L.). *Behaviour*, **47**, 153–229.

Wells, K. D. (1977*a*). Territoriality and male mating success in the green frog (*Rana clamitans*). *Ecology*, **58**, 750–62.

Wells, K. D. (1977*b*). The social behaviour of anuran amphibians. *Animal Behaviour*, **25**, 666–93.

Wells, K. D. (1977*c*). The courtship of frogs. In *The Reproductive Biology of Amphibians*, ed. D. G. Taylor & S. I. Guttman, pp. 233–62. Plenum Publishing Corporation: New York.

Wells, K. D. (1978). Territoriality in the green frog (*Rana clamitans*): vocalizations and agonistic behaviour. *Animal Behaviour*, **26**, 1051–63.

Wells, K. D. (1979). Reproductive behaviour and male mating success in a neotropical toad, *Bufo typhonius*. *Biotropica*, **11**, 301–7.

Wells, K. D. (1980). Behavioral ecology and social organization of a dendrobatid frog (*Colosthethus inguinalis*). *Behavioral Ecology and Sociobiology*, **6**, 199–210.

ıtney, C. L. & Krebs, J. R. (1975*a*). Mate selection in Pacific tree frogs, *Hyla regilla*. *Nature*, **255**, 325–6.

Whitney, C. L. & Krebs, J. R. (1975*b*). Spacing and calling in Pacific tree frogs *Hyla regilla*. *Canadian Journal of Zoology*, **53**, 1519–27.

Wilbur, H. M., Rubenstein, D. I. & Fairchild, L. (1978). Sexual selection in toads: the roles of female choice and male body size. *Evolution*, **32**, 264–70.

Wiley, R. H. (1973). Territoriality and non-random mating in the sage grouse, *Centrocercus urophasianus. Animal Behaviour Monographs*, **6**, 87–169.

Wiley, R. H. & Richards, D. G. (1978). Physical constraints on acoustical communication in the atmosphere: implications for the evolution of animal vocalizations. *Behavioral Ecology and Sociobiology*, **3**, 69–94.

Williams, G. C. (1966). *Adaptation and Natural Selection. A Critique of Some Current Evolutionary Thought*. Princeton University Press: Princeton.

Wilson, E. O. (1975). *Sociobiology: A New Synthesis*. Belknap Press: Cambridge, Massachusetts.

9

Mate choice in the European Rabbit

DIANA J. BELL

In the European Rabbit, *Oryctolagus cuniculus* L., ovulation, or the release of eggs from the ovaries, is induced by the act of copulation. A successful mating will be followed by a 30-day gestation period, but the corpora lutea will also continue to secrete progesterone if the eggs go unfertilised, causing the female to enter a 16–17 day pseudopregnancy during which she cannot conceive.

The 'costs' of an infertile mating, in terms of wasted parental investment, are therefore far greater for the female rabbit than the male. The relative 'cost' for a male may be illustrated by a report that the repeated mating of a single stud male over a six-hour period, resulted in 35 litters (Adams, 1972).

One might therefore expect a female to be relatively 'choosey' in her acceptance of a buck, and indeed predict that her 'choice' of mating partner be dictated by qualities such as the relative sexual and social status of courting males together, perhaps, with the relative 'quality' of the genes they can contribute to her offspring.

One of the main aims of this paper is to consider the possible criteria by which female European Rabbits may be able to assess the relative 'quality' of potential mates.

After presenting some general background information about the form of social organisation found in this species, I will then consider the evidence for, and functional significance of, intra-sexual competition within breeding groups since the question of which males and females finally reproduce together must be determined ultimately by some interaction of any system of female 'choice' with these processes of intra-sexual competition for access to important limited resources such as nesting warren, or oestrous female partners. Indeed it should become clear just how difficult it is, in practice, to dissociate these as separate systems. I will finally demonstrate the important role that scent signals have to play in mediating these social processes and propose certain androgen-dependent scents released by the male as possible criteria by which females may be able to assess the relative 'quality' of potential mating partners.

I have also tried to emphasise the need to view these processes of sexual selection in the context of the many other natural selection pressures acting on the species, from predators for example, since these may have been prime determinants of the form of social system to be found in the species today.

Social organisation in the European Rabbit

Studies of enclosed and free-living populations of European Wild Rabbit in Australia, New Zealand and the UK (Table 9.1) have found that the European Wild Rabbit lives in small territorial breeding groups. The area that is actively defended often constitutes only a small, warren-centred 'core area' within a larger home-range. These core territories have clearly defined boundaries which are actively patrolled and scent-marked, but members of adjacent breeding groups may show gradual movement out into 'communal' grazing pastures during the peak dawn/dusk feeding periods (Bell, 1980).

Breeding group size varies in relation to population density and the availability of 'burrowable' habitat (Table 9.1). Single male/female pairs have been reported in low density populations (Parer, 1977; Gibb, Ward & Ward, 1978) but in larger breeding groups the operational sex ratio is typically biased in favour of females.

'Satellite' individuals of either sex may also be present. These live in close proximity to particular breeding groups but fail to gain acceptance within the warren community, the satellite male being chased away from oestrous females by 'group' males, while satellite females are denied access to warren breeding sites by 'group' females.

Adults rarely move away from those warren groups where they first breed, so group composition shows considerable year-to-year stability (Myers & Poole, 1961; Dunsmore, 1974). In their ten-year population study, Gibb *et al.* (1978), for example, found that fewer than 5% of males and females over one year old shifted more than 100 yd between breeding seasons. Data concerning the dispersal of juveniles reveal a consistent pattern with females typically staying on to breed in their warren birth group while the sexually maturing males are often forced to migrate as a result of increasing hostility from adult males (Dunsmore, 1974; Parer,

1977). As a consequence, one might expect to find a high degree of relatedness between the females from the same breeding group.

Intra-sexual competition

Within the breeding groups hierarchical relationships are often reported between the adult males (Table 9.1). These may take the form of a complete linear ranking (Mykytowycz, 1958, 1960; Myers & Poole, 1959) or a single male dominant over several subordinates (e.g. Myers & Schneider, 1964). These dominance relationships appear to determine priority of access to oestrous females with the dominant males mating/

Table 9.1. *Social organisation of the European Wild Rabbit*

Source	Territorial	Breeding group size	Dominance hierarchies in breeding groups ♂	♀	Satellites[a]
Australia					
Myers & Poole (1959–61), E. 2-ac.	Yes[b]	♂ 1–5 ♀ 1–6	Yes	Never complete	Yes
Mykytowycz (1958–60), E. 1.75-ac.	Yes	♂ 1–5 ♀ 1–6	Yes	Yes	Yes
Myers & Schneider (1964), F.R.	Yes[b]	♂ 1–5 ♀ 1–6	Yes	Variable	Yes
Mykytowycz & Fullagar (1974), E. 82-ac.	Yes[b]	♂ 1–5 ♀ 1–6	1 ♂ dominant in each group	Variable	Yes
Parer (1977), F.R.	Day/night ranges < 30 m/> 100 m	Single pairs at low densities	—	—	—
New Zealand					
Gibb, Ward & Ward (1978), E. 21-ac.	Yes Day/night ranges	Single pairs at low densities	—	—	—
Great Britain					
Lockley (1964), E. 1-ac.	Yes	♂ 1–5 ♀ 1–6	Yes	Yes	Yes
Bell (1977), F.R.	Yes[b]	♂ 1–3 ♀ 1–4	Yes	Yes Variable	Yes

[a] Associated with some groups.
[b] With communal feeding grounds.
— No data.
F.R. Study population free-ranging.
E. 2-ac. Study population in 2-acre enclosure.

guarding different females as they enter oestrous but often returning to a preferred, 'regular', female partner between liaisons (Bell, 1980).

Relationships between adult females, however, appear to be more variable, ranging from apparently mutual toleration to similar linear hierarchies (Table 9.1). Existing data suggest that where competitive, hierarchical relationships do arise between females, the individuals concerned are competing for access to particular warren breeding sites.

The older experienced does initiate re-formation of breeding groups after the dry summers in S.E. Australia, for example, by 'selecting and defending particular burrows to which the older males then attach themselves...other members of the population are attracted to these selected warrens and hierarchical groups are formed after a series of aggressive interactions' (Myers & Poole, 1961). Mykytowycz & Fullagar (1973) similarly report that subordinate does were actively prevented from nesting in the warren area by females of the same group and therefore forced to drop their litters in isolated breeding 'stops' (see Mykytowycz, 1959, 1960; Mykytowycz & Gambale, 1965). It is also interesting to note that no evidence for female dominance hierarchies was found in studies where permanent warrens were not allowed to develop (Myers & Poole, 1959).

In general, however, females emerge as the more aggressive sex (Southern, 1948; Myers & Poole, 1961) and may actually fight to the death over possession of a burrow (Mykytowycz & Hesterman, 1975). Although rates of aggression increase in both sexes with increased population density (Myers, Hale, Mykytowycz & Hughes, 1971; Myers & Poole, 1961), this is primarily due to an increase in inter-group hostilities among the males, but intra-group fighting amongst the females (Myers, 1966).

Correlates of behavioural dominance

Reproductive success. Evidence for a positive relationship between social status and reproductive success in females is provided by both enclosed and free-living study populations. In Mykytowycz & Fullagar's (1973) five-year study of an enclosed population, for example, females were assigned a social rank of 1–4 on the basis of behavioural observations (Table 9.2). Of the 656 young which surfaced during four breeding seasons only 11% were of unknown maternity; 51% of the remaining 585 were produced by the 42 alpha females and only 7% attributed to the 57 females ranked 3 and 4. It is important to note that these were young which actually emerged from the nesting site so we do not know just when reproduction was failing in the subordinate females, i.e. whether they were losing litters pre-/post-natally or failing to mate. The authors also report that 'young born to dominant females were heavier and showed growth rates higher than those coevals born to second- and third-ranking females, at all ages between 30 and 150 days', and indeed a greater number of alpha females' young survived to the following breeding season.

Myers & Schneider (1964) provide analogous data on the relative productivity of known status females in a free-living population during a single breeding season (Table 9.3). Again the only aggressive acts reported were intrasexual. The dominant males repeatedly 'drove the subordinate

Table 9.2. *Reproductive success in relation to female social status in an enclosed population*

Social rank of mother ($N = 173$)	%	Number (and %) of young surfaced ($N = 585$)[a]
1	24.0	296 (51%)
2	43.0	247 (42%)
3 } 4 }	33.0	42 (7%)

Data collected over four breeding seasons.
[a] Of a total of 656 young surfaced, 11% were of unknown maternity. *Ranking system*: 1, dominant to all other females encountered; 2, dominant to some, but also lost some encounters; 3, interacted with others, but always subordinate; 4, subordinate, no social interaction. (After Mykytowycz & Fullagar, 1973.)

Table 9.3. *Warren group composition in free-living population, Adelaide, June 1961*[a]

Warren	Warren dwellers		Satellites	
	♂	♀	♂	♀
A	2	2	2	1
B	2	2	1	1
C	1	1	—	—
D	2	2	1	0
E	2	3	1	0
Total	9	10	5	2

[a] Population composition at outset of study.
(After Myers & Schneider, 1964.)

males away from oestrous females (178 observations)' and engaged in regular boundary 'pawscraping threat displays' (Bell, 1980) with associated satellite males. Overt aggressive acts between the dominant and subordinate females in warrens A and B were rarely observed, yet in both pairs the older, dominant female 'clearly had right of way'. The satellite female associated with warren A was similarly chased away in 79 observed attempts to enter the warren, yet she still managed to drop two litters in the warren and suckle them nightly while the resident does were away feeding. In both warrens A and B the warren-dwelling females produced more young than the associated satellites. Of the 92 young which surfaced on warrens A and B, the dominant and subordinate females were together responsible for 72 (78%) and the associated satellites 20 (22%).

In rabbits then, dominant does do not appear to enjoy the exclusive breeding rights reported for dominant females in other species (e.g. Rood, 1980). Their contribution to the gene pool of the subsequent generation may nevertheless be considerably greater than that of either the subordinate or satellite females. The short-term costs of playing a subordinate or satellite role in any one breeding season, in terms of reduced annual reproduction, must be balanced against the several benefits to be gained from warren group attachment/coloniality in this species (Table 9.4), and also the relative metabolic costs associated with subordinate/dominant status. We have recently found a positive correlation between metabolic

Table 9.4. *Some 'benefits' and 'costs' of coloniality in the European Rabbit*

Benefits	Costs
(1) Increased efficiency in detecting/deterring predators	(1) Increased chances of disease/parasite transmission
(2) Desirable changes in vegetation quality/ quantity through group foraging effects	
(3) Thermoregulatory costs reduced by 'huddling' above/below ground (Bell, 1977)	
(4) Some access to subterranean warren systems – as a refuge/ nesting site (cf. Alexander, 1974)	

rate and social status amongst groups of male rabbits organised in a stable social hierarchy, i.e. the costs of basal body maintenance appeared to be lower for the subordinate than for the high-ranking males (Bray & Bell, in press; see also Ely, 1981).

It is more difficult to establish the relationship between reproductive success and social status in male rabbits because of the usual problem of determining paternity of litters. Indeed blood group analysis has shown that litters of mixed paternity can occur (Stodart & Myers, 1964).

The relatively greater reproductive success of dominant does may be due to the interaction of a number of interrelated factors, namely:

(1) their earlier start to breeding – and therefore greater number of litters per season (Mykytowycz & Fullagar, 1973);

(2) their priority of access to best breeding warrens, and hence

(3) the appearance of their young under conditions of optimal climate and food availability, and low parasitic infestation (Mykytowycz & Fullagar, 1973; Myers, 1970; Mykytowycz, 1962);

(4) the possibility that the dominant females are mating with higher 'quality' males (see p. 220);

(5) a birth-site at the centre of colony activity may also afford greater protection of the dominant female's offspring, as a result of 'group vigilance' and the presence of the dominant male partner; and

(6) endocrine responses associated with the stress of subordinate status may also inhibit reproductive processes in low-ranking females (see Myers *et al.*, 1971).

Warrens. In the rabbit's ancestral areas around the western Mediterranean, warrens provide nesting sites for the highly vulnerable young and a refuge from high summer temperatures and large numbers of avian and ground predators (see, e.g., Delibes & Hiraldo, 1981). Climate and predation may therefore have been important selection pressures which favoured the evolution of a burrowing habit in this species.

Factors which may affect warren quality and/or availability and therefore give rise to intraspecific competition for particular warren systems are listed below:

(1) density/distribution of surface vegetation (as food and cover), water, predator species, conspecifics, and competing 'burrowing' species (see Lloyd & McGowan, 1968);

(2) local topography, e.g. susceptibility to flooding, angle to sun, etc.;

(3) substrate type/'burrowability'; and

(4) warren size – number of entrances, depth, length, width of tunnels.

In a detailed analysis of factors influencing the distribution of rabbit populations in Eastern Australia, Myers & Parker (1965) found 'gradients of favourability' both within and between major habitat types, e.g. raised, well-drained sites were at a premium in the wet subalpine/semitropical soils while the need for water dictated warren distribution in arid zone habitats (see also Rogers & Myers, 1979). There is also scattered evidence that warren productivity, in terms of number of young emerged, varies similarly in relation to many of those warren properties listed above.

In a four-year study of a New South Wales sand-dune population, for example, Wood (1980) found that the highly productive warrens were those either dug more deeply (down to 1.58 m) or dug in heavier inter-dune soils. These warrens suffered far less fox predation than those shallower warrens (maximum depth 0.66 m) dug in sandy soils (21 and 60% of litters respectively were dug out by foxes).

Young survival may also vary in relation to the frequency with which successive litters appear on a warren. Parer (1977) for example found that a litter's chances of surviving to 60 days were lower if another litter had been born in that same warren during the previous month. He suggests that the regular appearance of young somehow conditions predators to hunt there and indeed showed that feral cats killed proportionately more rabbits at warrens from which 15 or more young had emerged during a breeding season.

The adaptive significance of female behaviours such as fighting over warren access and indeed actual infanticide of unrelated young (Myers, 1964; Mykytowycz & Dudzinski, 1972) becomes apparent in that these will serve to regulate the appearance of young on a warren. Indeed, by manipulating the ratio of warren *usage* (littering frequency and number of adult occupants) to warren *size* (number of entrances, tunnel depth, length etc.) females may be increasing their reproductive fitness by maximising the chances of young survivorship.

One might further predict that the 'optimal' ratio of 'usage' to 'size' will vary in relation to the local external environmental pressures (predation, climate, vegetation cover, substrate, etc.) operating at that time.

Such female 'regulation' of littering frequency may clearly conflict with the interests of the promiscuously mating males who indeed counter with opposite strategies, policing fights between adult does (D. P. Cowan, personal communication; Southern, 1948; Dudzinski, Mykytowycz & Gambale, 1977) and protecting any youngsters under attack by a female (Mykytowycz & Dudzinski, 1972). A similar conflict of interests between the sexes occurs in another burrowing mammal, the Yellow-bellied Marmot (Downhower & Armitage, 1971). Male marmots maximise their reproductive success by acquiring a harem of two or three females while female success declines with increasing harem size. The 'compromise' system of one male to two females is the most common.

Scent-marking. Scent signals play a primary role in the communication system of the European rabbit. These originate from specialised skin glands and urine and may convey information about the individual identity, age, sex and reproductive status of the sender (see recent reviews by Bell, 1980, in press).

The chin, anal, inguinal and Harderian glands appear to be under androgenic control. The sexual dimorphism appears at sexual maturity and the glands are most active during the breeding season (Mykytowycz & Dudzinski, 1966). Testosterone replacement therapy reinstates their secretory activity in castrated males (Coujard, 1947; Strauss & Ebling, 1970).

The scent glands are largest and most active in those socially dominant individuals who are also responsible for most of the scent-marking activities performed within the breeding group (see Mykytowycz & Dudzinksi, 1966; Hesterman & Mykytowycz, 1968; Mykytowycz, 1965). Dominant males were responsible for 80% of those chin-marking acts recorded in a free-living colony of wild Rabbits on Skomer Island, off West Wales (Bell, 1980), for example, while the outcome of round-robin dominance tests with males of a Dutch-belted strain of domesticated rabbit could similarly be predicted from the relative frequency with which individuals chin-marked in previous isolation (Bell, 1981; also Black-Cleworth & Verberne, 1975).

Urine-marking may have similar status – signalling significance in the rabbit. Most of the conspecific and object-directed acts of urine-marking observed on Skomer Island were performed by dominant males, while laboratory tests suggested that urine released by dominant males may have similar male-aversive/female-attractant properties to those reported in mice and rats (Bell, 1981; Jones & Nowell, 1974; Krames, Carr & Bergman, 1969; Gawienowski, de Nicola & Stacewicz-Sapuntzakis, 1976). Sexually mature females spent longer investigating urine from high-frequency chin-marking, dominant males, for example, when this was paired against subordinate male urine in the context of two-choice arena test (Bell, 1981). Adult females also prefer to sniff and chin-mark dominant rather than subordinate males when these are presented in individual cages on opposite sides of a large arena (Bell, in preparation).

Further correlation analyses reveal that these socially dominant, high-frequency scent-marking males also have larger testes and higher levels of plasma testosterone (Bell, 1977, 1979). In the light of additional positive correlations reported between (a) testes weight and number of sperm released per ejaculate (Hafez, 1970), and (b) the levels of blood androgens and volume of gelatinous substance in semen, important for sperm transport (Kihlström & Degerman, 1963). I have earlier speculated that any androgen-dependent scents released by males may effectively provide a mechanism by which females may assess the relative fertility of potential mates (Bell, in press).

If the genetic correlation between testes weight and ovulation rate recently reported in mice and sheep (Land, 1973; Land, Carr & Lee, 1979) also exists in the rabbit, one could further speculate that an ability to discriminate males with large testes might increase the inclusive fitness of a female by firstly maximising the chances that her own ova will be fertilised and secondly increasing the testes size/ovulation rate in her sons and daughters.

The release of scent, in the form of urine, anal and chin-gland secretions, is a primary component of male courtship (Bell, 1977), while the rebuff of one male, and active 'solicitation' and sexual arousal of another by an oestrous doe might be regarded as active mate choice by that female (Bell, in press).

Summary

Mate 'choice' and reproductive success in the European Rabbit would appear to be primarily determined by those processes in intra-sexual competition whereby females compete for warren littering sites and males compete for access to oestrous females. It is suggested that scent signals play an important part in these processes, however. The release of male attractants by sexually receptive females (Bell, 1980, in press), may serve to intensify inter-male rivalry, in much the same way as the audible cries of the female elephant seal (Cox & Le Boeuf, 1977), while the release of androgen-dependent scents by the male may function to attract females and simultaneously intimidate rival males. The female preference for the odours of socially dominant over socially subordinate males found in laboratory tests suggests that male scents may also provide females with information about the relative 'quality' of potential mating partners. From an evolutionary standpoint it is important that we view these combined processes of sexual selection in the context of other natural selection pressures, e.g. from predators and climatic factors which have operated simultaneously on the species to determine the pattern of social organisation we see today.

References

Adams, C. E. (1972). The rabbit. In *UFAW Handbook on the Care and Management of Laboratory Animals*, 4th edn. Livingstone: Edinburgh.

Alexander, R. D. (1974). The evolution of social behaviour. *Annual Review of Ecology and Systematics*, **5**, 325–83.

Bell, D. J. (1977). *Aspects of the Social Behaviour of Wild and Domesticated Rabbits Oryctolagus cuniculus (L.)*. Unpublished Ph.D. Thesis, University of Wales.

Bell, D. J. (1979). Chemical communication and social status – some intercorrelations. Paper presented at *XVIth International Ethological Conference, U.B.C. Vancouver, 1979*.

Bell, D. J. (1980). Social olfaction in lagomorphs. *Symposium of the Zoological Society of London*, **45**, 141–64.

Bell, D. J. (1981). Chemical communication in the European rabbit: urine and social status. In *Proceedings of the World Lagomorph Conference, Guelph, 1979*, ed. K. Myers & C. D. McInnes. University of Guelph.

Bell, D. J. (in press). Lagomorph scents. In *Social Odours in Mammals*, ed. R. Brown & D. MacDonald. Oxford University Press: Oxford.

Black-Cleworth, P. & Verberne, G. (1975). Scent-marking, dominance and flehmen behaviour in domestic rabbits in an artificial laboratory territory. *Chemical Senses & Flavor*, **1**, 465–94.

Bray, G. C. & Bell, D. J. (1982). Physiological correlates of social status in the domestic rabbit, *Oryctolagus cuniculus* (L). In *Proceedings of the Third International Theriological Congress, 1982*, Helsinki. Helsinki University Press.

Coujard, R. (1947). Etudes des glandes odorantes du lapin et de leur influencement par hormones sexuelles. *Revue Canadienne de Biologie*, **6**, 3–14.

Cox, C. R. & Le Boeuf, B. F. (1977). Female incitation of male competition: a mechanism of mate selection. *American Naturalist*, **111**, 317–35.

Delibes, M. & Hiraldo, F. (1981). The rabbit *Oryctolagus cuniculus* as prey in the Iberian Mediterranean system. In *Proceedings of the World Lagomorph Conference, Guelph, 1979*, ed. K. Myers & C. D. McInnes. University of Guelph.

Downhower, J. F. & Armitage, K. B. (1971). The yellow-bellied marmot and the evolution of polygamy. *American Naturalist*, **105**, 355–70.

Dudzinski, M. L., Mykytowycz, R. & Gambale, G. (1977). Behavioural characteristics of adolescence in young captive European rabbits, *Oryctolagus cuniculus*. *Aggressive Behaviour*, **3**, 313–30.

Dunsmore, J. D. (1974). The rabbit in sub-alpine south-eastern Australia. I. Population structure and productivity. *Australian Wildlife Research*, **1**, 1–16.

Ely, D. (1981). Hypertension, social rank and aortic arteriosclerosis in CBA/J Mice. *Physiology and Behaviour*, **26**, 655–61.

Gawienowski, A. M., de Nicola, D. B. & Stacewicz-Sapuntzakis, M. (1976). Androgen dependence of a marking pheromone in rat urine. *Hormones and Behaviour*, **7**, 401–5.

Gibb, J. A., Ward, C. P. & Ward, G. D. (1978). Natural control of a population of rabbits, *Oryctolagus cuniculus* (L). for ten years in the Kourarau enclosure. *New Zealand Department of Scientific and Industrial Research Bulletin 223*.

Hafez, E. S. E. (1970). Rabbits. In *Reproduction and Breeding Techniques for Laboratory Animals*, ed. E. S. E. Hafez, pp. 275–97. Lea & Febiger: Philadelphia.

Hesterman, E. R. & Mykytowycz, R. (1968). Some observations on the odours of anal gland secretions from the rabbit *Oryctolagus cuniculus* (L). *C.S.I.R.O. Wildlife Research*, **13**, 71–81.

Jones, K. & Nowell, N. (1974). A comparison of the aversive and female attractant properties of urine from dominant and subordinate male mice. *Animal Learning & Behaviour*, **2**, 141–4.

Kihlström, J. E. & Degerman, G. (1963). Hormonally regulated cyclic variations in the sexual functions of the male rabbit. *Arkiv för Zoologie*, **15**, 357–8.

Krames, L., Carr, W. J. & Bergman, B. (1969). A pheromone associated with social dominance among male rats. *Psychonomic Science*, **16**, 11–12.

Land, R. B. (1973). The expression of female, sex-limited characters in the male. *Nature*, **241**, 208–9.

Land, R. B., Carr, W. R. & Lee, G. J. (1979). A consideration of physiological criteria of reproductive merit in sheep. Paper presented at the *Symposium on Selection Experiments in Animals, Harrogate*.

Lloyd, H. G. & McGowan, D. (1968). Some observations on the breeding burrows of the wild rabbit, *Oryctolagus cuniculus*, on the island of Skokholm. *Journal of Zoology (London)*, **156**, 540–9.

Lockley, R. M. (1964). *The Private Life of the Rabbit*. Andre Deutsch: London.

Myers, K. (1964). Influence of density on fecundity, growth rates and mortality in the wild rabbit. *C.S.I.R.O. Wildlife Research*, **9**, 134–7.

Myers, K. (1966). The effects of density on sociality and health in mammals. *Proceedings of the Ecological Society of Australia*, **1**, 40–64.

Myers, K. (1970). The rabbit in Australia. In *Proceedings of the Advanced Study Institute on Dynamics of Numbers in Populations* (Oosterbeek 1970), ed. P. J. den Boer & G. R. Gradwell, pp. 478–506. Centre for Agricultural Publishing & Documentation: Wageningen.

Myers, J., Hale, C. S., Mykytowycz, R. & Hughes, R. L. (1971). The effects of varying density and space on sociality and health in animals. In *Behaviour and Environment*, ed. A. H. Esser, pp. 148–87. Plenum Press: New York.

Myers, K. & Parker, B. S. (1965). A study of the biology of the wild rabbit in climatically different regions in Eastern Australia. I. Patterns of distribution. *C.S.I.R.O. Wildlife Research*, **10**, 1–32.

Myers, K. & Poole, W. E. (1959). A study of the biology of the wild rabbit, *Oryctolagus cuniculus* (L), in confined populations. I. The effects of density on home range and the formation of breeding groups. *C.S.I.R.O. Wildlife Research*, **4**, 14–26.

Myers, K. & Poole, W. E. (1961). A study of the biology of the wild rabbit, *Oryctolagus cuniculus* (L), in confined populations. II. The effects of season and population increase on behaviour. *C.S.I.R.O. Wildlife Research*, **6**, 1–41.

Myers, K. & Schneider, E. C. (1964). Observations on reproduction, mortality and behaviour in a small, free-living population of wild rabbits. *C.S.I.R.O. Wildlife Research*, **9**, 138–43.

Mykytowycz, R. (1958). Social behaviour of an experimental colony of wild rabbits, *Oryctolagus cuniculus* (L). I. Establishment of the colony. *C.S.I.R.O. Wildlife Research*, **3**, 7–25.

Mykytowycz, R. (1959). Social behaviour of an experimental colony of wild rabbits, *Oryctolagus cuniculus* (L). II. First breeding season. *C.S.I.R.O. Wildlife Research*, **4**, 1–13.

Mykytowycz, R. (1960). Social behaviour of an experimental colony of wild rabbits, *Oryctolagus cuniculus* (L). III. Second breeding season. *C.S.I.R.O. Wildlife Research*, **5**, 1–20.

Mykytowycz, R. (1962). Epidemiology of coccidiosis (*Eimeria* spp.) in an experimental population of the Australian wild rabbit, *Oryctolagus cuniculus* (L). *Parasitology*, **52**, 375–95.

Mykytowycz, R. (1965). Further observations on the territorial function and histology of the submandibular cutaneous (chin) glands in the rabbit *Oryctolagus cuniculus* (L). *Animal Behaviour*, **13**, 400–12.

Mykytowycz, R. & Dudzinski, M. L. (1966). A study of the weight of odoriferous and other glands in relation to social status and degree of sexual activity in the wild rabbit, *Oryctolagus cuniculus* (L). *C.S.I.R.O. Wildlife Research*, **11**, 31–47.

Mykytowycz, R. & Dudzinski, M. L. (1972). Aggressive and protective behaviour of adult rabbits *Oryctolagus cuniculus* (L) towards juveniles. *Behaviour*, **43**, 97–120.

Mykytowycz, R. & Fullagar, P. J. (1973). Effect of social environment on reproduction in the rabbit, *Oryctolagus cuniculus* (L). *Journal of Reproduction and Fertility (Supplement)*, **19**, 503–22.

Mykytowycz, R. & Gambale, S. (1965). A study of the inter-warren activities and dispersal of wild rabbits *Oryctolagus cuniculus* (L), living in a 45-acre paddock. *C.S.I.R.O. Wildlife Research*, **10**, 111–23.

Mykytowycz, R. & Hesterman, E. (1975). An experimental study of aggression in captive European rabbits, *Oryctolagus cuniculus* (L), with appendix on method of multivariate analysis of data by Dudzinski, M. L. & Edwards, C. B. H. *Behaviour*, **52**, 104–23.

Parer, I. (1977). The population ecology of the wild rabbit, *Oryctolagus cuniculus* (L) in a Mediterranean-type climate in New South Wales. *Australian Wildlife Research*, **4**, 171–205.

Rogers, P. M. & Myers, K. (1979). Ecology of the European wild rabbit, *Oryctolagus cuniculus* (L), in Mediterranean habitats. *Journal of Applied Ecology*, **16**, 691–703.

Rood, J. P. (1980). Mating relationships and breeding suppression in the dwarf mongoose. *Animal Behaviour*, **28**, 143–51.

Southern, H. N. (1948). Sexual and aggressive behaviour in the wild rabbit. *Behaviour*, **1**, 173–94.

Stodart, E. & Myers, K. (1964). A comparison of behaviour, reproduction and mortality of wild and domestic rabbits in confined populations. *C.S.I.R.O. Wildlife Research*, **9**, 144–59.

Strauss, J. S. & Ebling, F. J. (1970). Control and function of skin glands in mammals. *Memoirs of the Society of Endocrinology*, **18**, 341–71.

Wood, D. H. (1980). The demography of a rabbit population in an arid region of New South Wales, Australia. *Journal of Animal Ecology*, **49**, 55–79.

IV: NON-RANDOM MATING

10

Non-random mating and offspring fitness

LINDA PARTRIDGE

Introduction

My aim in this chapter is to review the ways in which mating that is non-random with respect to genotype may affect offspring fitness. The genotypes of parents may affect their own ability to provide for their offspring as well as the genotypes of the offspring. I will discuss the effects of parental genotypes only in respect of their effect on offspring genotypes.

A large part of the empirical evidence presented in this chapter comes from work on the Genus *Drosophila*. The narcotic effects on ethologists of this otherwise admirable taxonomic group are well known, but I hope that the information provided is sufficiently important to overcome the problem.

Various patterns of non-random mating have been postulated to increase offspring fitness, although it is important to bear in mind that non-random mating may also incur costs (see Parker, this volume). For example, a tendency not to mate with close relatives is likely to be a consequence of dispersal or mate choice, both of which may be costly. Many of the benefits of non-random mating may be purely phenotypic (see Parker, this volume). For example, large males may be better able than small ones to protect a female from being damaged by other males during mating.

It is also important to bear in mind that the history of a population can have an important effect on the consequences of the current mating pattern. For example, in a population with a history of strong inbreeding, non-random mating may have very little consequence for offspring genotypes.

I have organised the rest of the chapter into four sections each dealing with one form of non-random mating. These are: variation in individual mating success, inbreeding, assortative mating and frequency-dependent mating success. For each of these forms of non-random mating I have discussed the mechanisms which could affect offspring fitness, and I have also mentioned any important fitness consequences which are not the result of an effect on individual offspring fitness.

Variation in individual mating success
Introduction
Many studies have shown that there can be considerable variation in mating success between individuals, especially between males (e.g. Bateman, 1948; Gibson & Guiness, 1980; Thornhill, 1981). Such variation means that some individuals may never mate while others may mate many times (Le Boeuf, 1974).

Could this sort of non-random mating produce offspring of higher fitness than those that would be produced by random mating? Fitness comprises various components such as viability (zygote to adult survival), mating success and fertility. For an individual with higher than average mating success to produce offspring of higher than average net fitness, the offspring fitness components must be affected in one of two ways. First, mating success itself could be inherited, males with high mating success tending to produce sons with high mating success; for these sons to have higher *total* fitness than average, genetic variation producing high mating success should not also correspondingly lower some other fitness component. A correlation between the mating success of fathers and sons is the basis of Fisher's (1930) runaway process of sexual selection. Second, there could be a positive correlation across individuals between mating success and the net score on the other fitness components; in other words, individuals with high mating success could also be more viable or fertile and would then produce offspring that scored highly on other fitness components as well as mating success. Both of these suggestions involve two related assumptions. First, they assume that net fitness is inherited. Second, they assume particular sorts of correlations between different fitness components; in the first case a non-negative or sufficiently low negative correlation and in the second case a positive correlation between mating success and the net score on other fitness components. These two assumptions will be examined in turn.

Fitness heritability?
Population genetics theory suggests that fitness should not be heritable in a population at genetic equilibrium under natural selection

(Falconer, 1981). Genetic variation for individual fitness may *exist* in equilibrium populations, but such fitness variation should not be *heritable*. Heterozygous advantage can maintain genetic variation in populations at equilibrium under selection, and there will be fitness variation between genotypes, but this variation will not be heritable. However, this conclusion has recently been disputed. Borgia (1979) suggested that, if heterozygous advantage occurs at a single locus with two alleles, then a mutant female which recognised and mated with heterozygous males would leave more progeny than females mating at random. This would occur, he suggested, because heterozygous males would leave a higher proportion of heterozygous (and hence fitter) progeny than would homozygous males; all matings involving heterozygous males produce one half heterozygous progeny irrespective of the genotype of the female and, unless the two homozygotes have equal fitness so that they are present at equal frequency in the population, females which mated with the two types of homozygous males in the proportions in which they occurred in the population would on average leave progeny less than half of which were heterozygous. This is true, but Borgia (1979) has ignored the relative proportions of the two unequally fit homozygotes in the progeny. If these are taken into account, then a mutant female which mated with heterozygous males would leave no more surviving progeny after one generation than females which mated with one type of homozygous male or both homozygous males in the proportions in which they occurred. This conclusion is derived in Appendix 1. Strictly speaking, this conclusion is valid only for a rare mutant for female choice of heterozygotes invading a large randomly mating population behaving deterministically. With inbreeding the conclusion no longer applies (Hill & Robertson, 1968). Also, if females 'know' their own genotype then, for example, *aa* females could produce entirely heterozygous offspring by mating with *AA* males. The assumption that females know their own genotype may be unrealistic and is discussed later (see *Inbreeding and outbreeding*).

Thus the outcome of constant selective forces is zero fitness heritability. However, it is important to realise that this analysis ignores the importance of factors such as mutation, migration from other populations and changes in selection over time. All of these factors could alter the conclusion that fitness heritability should not occur.

The effects of naturally occurring new mutations have been studied in *Drosophila* in the laboratory, using a technique where single chromosomes extracted from completely homozygous flies are allowed to accumulate new mutations over several generations. During this period the chromosomes are kept heterozygous with chromosomes carrying mutant markers and many inversions. These inversions suppress recombination, and the new mutations, many of them partially recessive, are to some extent protected from the effects of selection during the time that they accumulate. The chromosomes are then made homozygous, and their effects on fitness components can be compared with the effects of chromosomes from the original inbred stock. In general, new mutations made homozygous have deleterious effects on viability, and the viability of heterozygotes is also reduced to a lesser extent (Mukai, Chigusa, Mettler & Crow, 1972; Ohnishi, 1977a, b; Simmons & Crow, 1977). The effects of naturally-occurring new mutations on *total* fitness have not been studied, although the effects on total fitness of mutations induced by chemicals have been studied, and they have a deleterious effect both when homozygous and heterozygous.

Theoretical studies show that a genetic equilibrium can be set up by a mutation/selection balance. This results in low frequencies of deleterious mutations in populations, the exact frequency of a particular mutation depending upon its effect on fitness, degree of dominance and the mutation rate (Crow & Kimura, 1970). Lande (1976) has considered the effect of mutation on characters affected by genetic variation at many loci. He concluded that mutation could be a potent force in maintaining genetic variability and heritability in such characters. There is considerable evidence that a mutation selection balance may occur in natural populations. Studies on wild *Drosophila* populations show that alleles with both mildly and severely deleterious homozygous effects on viability are present (Simmons & Crow, 1977). The deleterious alleles present in wild populations seem to differ from the newly arisen mutations studied in the laboratory in that their effects when heterozygous are less marked; in other words, the deleterious effects on fitness of new mutations are more dominant than those of the mutations found in wild populations. This difference probably reflects the action of selection because low frequency alleles will be mostly present in the heterozygous condition, so that an allele with a marked effect when heterozygous is likely to be more readily eliminated by selection than a more recessive allele. Alleles with deleterious homozygous effects on *total* fitness have also been found in natural populations (Simmons & Crow, 1977). Their heterozygous effects have not been studied. This is particularly unfortunate in the present context, because most of the fitness variation caused by these deleterious mutations in natural populations may occur through their heterozygous effects, because mutations present at low frequency in a population are rarely homozygous. Mukai & Yamaguchi (1974) have shown that alleles which are lethal when homozygous are probably eliminated from wild *D. melanogaster* populations mainly by their effects on heterozygotes, because the homozygous lethals never reach a sufficient frequency for their homozygous effects to be significant. Whether this is also true for mutations with less drastic homozygous effects is not known.

Thus the indications are that deleterious mutations can accumulate to some extent in natural populations. To understand fully the implications of this for fitness heritability, we need to know the frequencies and fitnesses of homozygotes and heterozygotes for such mutations. Unfortunately this information is not yet available for any population.

Disruptive selection could also produce some fitness heritability. If different local populations are genetically adapted to local circumstances, then gene flow between such locally adapted populations could result in progeny with heritable low fitness. For example, Jain & Bradshaw (1966) have studied grasses adapted to living on the contaminated soil found on heavy-metal mines. Wind-blown pollen can be transferred from the resistant grass on the mine to the non-resistant population down wind of the mine, producing progeny with some alleles conferring heavy-metal resistance. These partially resistant progeny are less fit than non-resistant forms in soil which is not contaminated. Disruptive selection and gene flow are probably common in nature (see *Inbreeding and outbreeding*).

Temporal variation in selective forces could also result in some fitness heritability. It is known that different genotypes may be favoured at different times of year and that at any one time a population may therefore consist of a mixture of genotypes of unequal fitness (e.g. Dobzhansky, Ayala, Stebbins & Valentine, 1977; Berry, 1977).

Thus it seems very likely that there is some fitness heritability in natural populations, but its extent is uncertain. Quite high heritabilities for ecologically important traits such as the timing of reproduction have been demonstrated in the Great Tit (Van Noordwijk, Van Balen & Scharloo, 1980).

Association between different fitness components

Associations between different fitness components have been little studied, and the evidence so far is mildly contradictory. Ideally we should like to know how the heritable variation in natural populations affects all fitness components and hence total fitness; we do not yet have this information. It is important to realise that it is *genetic* correlations, in other words correlations produced by genetic variation which are important in this context; purely phenotypic correlations are not relevant.

Some studies, all with *D. melanogaster* in the laboratory, have shown positive or non-negative correlations between fitness components.

Brittnacher (1981) found no significant correlation between male mating success and either viability or adult female weight (which is closely correlated with female fecundity) when he compared different chromosome homozygotes. In outbred flies I have found that adults allowed to mate non-randomly produce more viable offspring than do adults mated at random. If variation in male mating success was responsible for the non-random mating then these results may indicate an association between male mating success and offspring fitness (Partridge, 1980). Watanabe & Oshima (1973) and Watanabe & Ohnishi (1975) have found a weak correlation between viability and a measure of fertility in flies made homozygous for different chromosomes.

Other studies have suggested negative correlations between certain fitness components. In *D. melanogaster* a selection experiment revealed a negative correlation between fertility early and late in life in females (Rose & Charlesworth, 1981*a*, *b*) and a study of chromosome homozygotes and heterozygotes revealed a negative correlation between female fertility and rate of development (Hiraizumi, 1961). Another study of chromosome heterozygotes showed that new mutations and the existing genetic variation in a population can have different effects on the relationship between different fitness components. New mutations which lower viability tend also to lower other fitness components, while those existing mutations found in fly populations which have a deleterious effect on viability have a compensatory positive effect on other aspects of fitness (Simmons, Preston & Engels, 1980). The implication of this finding is that standing genetic variation which lowers viability may be very nearly neutral so far as overall fitness is concerned. One weakness of all the *Drosophila* studies where viability and overall fitness are studied is that the two characters are not studied under exactly the same conditions, and it is possible that doing so might alter the conclusions.

One consistent point to emerge from the studies with *Drosophila* is that male mating success is a very important component of fitness. Studies with flies carrying visible mutants have shown that male mating success can overshadow the effects of other fitness components in laboratory cage populations (Prout, 1971; Bundgaard & Christiansen, 1972) and in wild populations (Anderson *et al.*, 1979). Brittnacher (1981) has shown that chromosome homozygosis has a more drastic effect on male mating success than on viability or female fertility.

It is not easy to assess the implications of these results. If total fitness is heritable in real populations, then the correlations between each fitness component and the rest cannot be entirely negative. As we have seen, the extent of fitness heritability in real populations is uncertain. Clearly more work is needed.

Female choice?

Variation in male mating success could be a result of female choice and competition among males. Female preference for particular male phenotypes is a very rarely documented phenomenon and its general occurrence is uncertain (Halliday, this volume). What are needed are more studies investigating the possible involvement of female choice. These could then be followed by studies of the fitness consequences of preferred male traits and their genetic basis. Fisher (1930) and Lande (1981, described in Arnold, this volume) have pointed out that theoretical models of sexual selection do not lead to the conclusion that evolution will necessarily occur towards female preference for male traits leading to high fitness under natural selection. Any role of female choice in mediating fitness consequences of variation in male mating success is therefore uncertain. Parker's idea (this volume) of passive choice may be an important one in this context, because it does not rely on discrimination between different male phenotypes by females. In species where males call to attract females, these may move up a sound gradient or, in species where males approach and court females, these may have a fixed probability of accepting any courting male. Males that call loudly and frequently or males that search effectively and persistently court females would then be favoured. Any fitness consequences of variation in male mating success may well be mediated by these or other forms of intrasexual competition between males.

There are three other immediate ways in which the phenotype of a mate may be important to females. First, in species that store sperm, it may pay a female to mate with a male that is likely to transfer a lot of sperm. The female might then take longer to run out of sperm, and if mating is dangerous this would be beneficial. I know of no empirical evidence that females choose males that are likely to transfer a lot of sperm, but there is some evidence that male courtship intensity is related to the amount of sperm that is transferred in the ensuing copulation in newts (Halliday & Houston, 1978) and butterflies (Rutowski, 1979). Second, seminal feeding of females by males has been reported in butterflies (Boggs & Gilbert, 1979; Boggs & Watt, 1981). It is not yet known if this type of feeding is widespread, but where it occurs some males may produce more nutrients than others, and females could benefit by mating with males that transfer more nutrients. There is as yet no evidence that females can recognise such males before mating, but there is some evidence that females re-mate more quickly after mating with a male that has transferred a small spermatophore (Rutowski, 1980; Boggs, 1981). Third, some males may be better able than others to protect females during mating. Borgia (1981) found that copulating pairs of Dungflies were better able to fly away from an artificial disturbance if the male was large. Large males were also better able to protect their females from disturbance by other males while mating and ovipositing. Borgia obtained evidence that females behaved in a way which increased the likelihood that they would be mated by large males.

On the longer term, the phenotype of a male may affect his parental ability in those species where males play a role in parental care, and male resources such as food or territory are also important criteria used by females when choosing a mate (Thornhill, 1981; Zimmerman, 1971).

Inbreeding and outbreeding
The genetic effects of inbreeding

Inbreeding is the mating of individuals related by ancestry. All members of the same species are related by ancestry if their pedigrees are traced back far enough. Dioecious organisms each have two parents, four grandparents, eight great-grandparents etc. In some past generation the number of individuals required to provide separate ancestors for all the present individuals would have been larger than the real population size. Any pair of conspecifics must therefore be related to each other through one or more common ancestors in the more or less remote past; and the smaller the past size of the population, the less remote are the common ancestors or the greater their number (Falconer, 1981). Pairs mating at random are therefore more closely related to each other in small populations than in large ones. If, within a population, relatives tend to mate with each other more often than expected under random mating, then there will be stronger inbreeding than that attributable solely to population size, because by definition relatives are more closely related by ancestry than are randomly chosen members of the population. Thus inbreeding results from non-random mating produced by sub-division of species into more or less discrete populations between which there is restricted gene flow and by a tendency for relatives within a population to mate.

Crow & Kimura (1970), Falconer (1960) and Hartl (1980) all provide clear accounts of the genetic consequences of inbreeding. The essential genetic result of the sharing of a common ancestor by two individuals is that they may both carry a replicate of a single allele present in the ancestor; and if they mate they may each pass one of these replicates to their offspring. Two such alleles present in an offspring are identical by descent, and the individual is hence homozygous for that allele. The inbreeding coefficient is the probability that the two alleles at a locus in an individual will be identical by descent from a single allele in some specified earlier generation. As we have seen this probability is higher both for individuals from small populations with random mating and in individuals from lineages where relatives tend to mate. This means that, other things being equal, inbreeding will tend both to increase homozygosity in an originally outbred population and to maintain homozygosity in a continuously inbred population. Other things will often not be equal; selection, mutation and gene flow can all modify the outcome of a particular pattern of inbreeding (Falconer, 1981).

Inbreeding also tends to hold together existing combinations of alleles at different loci. This happens because genetic recombination, which would tend to break up existing allelic combinations at different loci, can occur only between two loci which are both heterozygous. Inbreeding reduces heterozygosity and with it the opportunity for recombination. In the extreme case, where all loci become homozygous, no recombination at all can occur, and the existing allelic combination will be transmitted within each inbred lineage.

Inbred and outbred matings can have numerous effects. I shall deal first with the beneficial effects of inbreeding (and the detrimental effects of outbreeding) and second with the detrimental effects of inbreeding (and the benefits of outbreeding).

The benefits of inbreeding

There are four main ways in which inbreeding can produce benefits. In the first two cases the benefits arise because of an effect on offspring fitness components other than the mating pattern itself. In the second two cases benefits arise directly from the mating pattern, in one case because of reduced costs of mate finding, in the other because of an inclusive fitness effect.

First, epistatic interactions may be important in determining fitness. This means that particular combinations of alleles at different loci are favoured so that there may be adaptive peaks (Wright, 1931, 1960) produced by different, highly fit allelic combinations. These combinations, once created, might be disrupted by random mating and recombination. Relatives are more likely to have the same allelic combinations at different loci than are randomly chosen individuals, and inbreeding would tend to hold these combinations together, provided that the fittest combinations are not heterozygous. Some hermaphrodite plants and animals habitually inbreed by self-fertilization and the predicted homozygosity is observed (Selander & Hudson, 1976; McCracken & Selander, 1980; Clegg, Allard & Kahler, 1972; Allard, Babbel, Clegg & Kahler, 1972). Lineages homozygous for different allelic combinations can co-exist, possibly indicating the existence of alternative adaptive peaks. In these selfing forms, natural selection has been said to act to structure the genome into highly interacting co-adapted gene complexes which are not disrupted by recombination (Hedrick, Jain & Holden, 1978) although there is no direct evidence that this is so.

Existing combinations of alleles are also held together by apomictic parthenogenesis where reproduction is by mitosis, so that offspring are genetically identical to their one parent. This type of reproduction produces asexual clones which, like natural inbred lineages, have been said to contain highly co-adapted gene complexes, although in this case there is no necessary increase in homozygosity (Herbert, 1974a, b).

The potential importance of this benefit of inbreeding must depend partly upon the ubiquity and magnitude of epistatic interactions affecting fitness. These are considered widespread by some authors (e.g. Lewontin, 1974; Wright, 1970; Templeton, Sing & Brokaw, 1976; Ohta, 1980). The data are at present inadequate to say whether different co-adapted gene complexes are indeed held together by inbreeding in natural populations. Some habitual inbreeders do show hybrid vigour when crossed which suggests that inbreeding may not create the fittest possible allelic combinations.

Second, members of the same local population are likely to be adapted to the same set of local circumstances. If offspring tend to encounter the same environments as their parents, either because of philopatry (Greenwood, 1980; Shields, in press) or habitat selection (Partridge, 1978), then mating within the same local population would help to maintain the adaptation in the offspring, because gene flow from other differently adapted populations would be prevented. Strictly speaking it is assortative mating in respect of the characters producing local adaptation which is important here. Inbreeding will achieve this assortative mating only in as much as relatives are adapted to the same conditions. Many studies of disruptive selection (e.g. Maynard Smith, 1966; Jain & Bradshaw, 1966) confirm that assortative mating can achieve local adaptation. In plants, self-fertility can be associated with strong disruptive selection caused by the occurrence of toxic heavy metals near mines (Antonovics, 1968). Apomictic parthenogenesis can also maintain local adaptation because here gene flow from adjacent populations is prevented by asexual reproduction. Recent studies of forest-living moths (Mitter, Futuyma, Schneider & Hare, 1979; Schneider, 1980) have shown that moths of the same species living on different tree species and on different individual trees differ in their time of hatching in such a way that the larvae appear at the same time as the leaves. Local adaptation is maintained by very low dispersal together with apomictic parthenogenesis. Sexual forms of the same moth species do not show the same degree of local adaptation.

Third, outbreeding may also incur either hazards associated with dispersal from the natal area and establishment in a new one (Bengtsson, 1978) or the costs of active mate choice (see Parker, this volume). These costs may reduce the number of offspring produced by outbreeders. Conversely, inbreeding may lower these costs. Inbreeding could be especially beneficial where mate finding is difficult because of low population densities. Ghiselin (1969) has suggested that hermaphroditism and selfing may be adaptive under these circumstances.

Fourth, inbreeding can increase inclusive fitness if one sex competes for mates. Thus, if males compete for mates, then a female will increase the mating success of a male relative, and hence her own inclusive fitness, by mating with him (Maynard Smith, 1978*b*; Smith, 1979; Packer, 1979; Parker, this volume). Under these circumstances there may be a conflict between the sexes over mating, because selection may favour inbreeding by one sex but not the other (Smith, 1979; G. Parker, this volume). If there is competition between related males for matings with their female relatives, there will be selection for a female-biased sex ratio (Hamilton, 1967). This happens because a parent which produces more females will leave more grandchildren because mate competition between male relatives will reduce their reproductive potential. An association between inbreeding, local mate competition and a skewed sex ratio is frequently seen in species with haplo-diploid sex determination (Hamilton, 1967; Alexander & Sherman, 1977; Cowan, 1979; Waage, 1982). Maynard Smith (1978*a*) has suggested that skewed sex ratios are rare in species with other methods of sex determination because in these species variation in the sex ratio of offspring may not be heritable, so that natural selection for a skewed sex ratio would not be effective.

The benefits of outbreeding

It has generally been found in laboratory studies that an artificially imposed increase in the extent of inbreeding results in a decline in many aspects of offspring fitness (see Falconer, 1981). Inbred matings in natural populations of species that usually outbreed can have a similar effect

(Packer, 1979; Greenwood, Harvey & Perrins, 1978; but see Van Noorwijk & Scharloo, 1981). This inbreeding depression has been attributed to the increase in homozygosity which accompanies inbreeding. Homozygosity may decrease fitness in two ways which are related to the processes maintaining polymorphisms in the original population. First, if the polymorphisms were maintained by single locus heterosis, then an increase in homozygosity would automatically reduce fitness. Second, if the polymorphisms were not maintained by selection, but instead reflected the presence of low-frequency deleterious recessive alleles in the population, then homozygosity for these deleterious recessives would produce lowered fitness. We have already seen that there is evidence that many natural populations do carry considerable genetic variation in the form of deleterious recessive alleles. The role of a mutation/selection balance in producing this sort of polymorphism has already been discussed. There are some examples of single locus heterosis notably that of sickle cell anaemia (Allison, 1954) and also others involving known gene products (Koehn, 1969; Frelinger, 1972). The general importance of single locus heterosis is very hard to evaluate because of the difficulty of eliminating the effects of loci closely linked to those under study. Berger (1976) has reviewed these problems and the evidence for single locus heterosis for enzyme variants. Recent work with *Drosophila* (MacKay, 1980, 1981) has strongly suggested that heterozygotes may be at an advantage to homozygotes in variable environments. Previous studies have tended to estimate fitnesses under constant conditions and MacKay's suggestion warrants further studies. Whatever the reasons for inbreeding depression, its existence implies that there is a cost to inbreeding in habitual outbreeders. In nature, persistent strong inbreeding should result in the loss of recessive deleterious alleles from the population by a process of inter-clonal selection. In support of this, there is some evidence that habitually selfing forms do show less hybrid vigour than do inbred lines derived from outbreeders (Mather, 1973).

Like asexual reproduction, strong inbreeding leads to the loss of potential for genetic recombination. Strong inbreeding will therefore lead to the same disadvantage as apomictic parthenogenesis, whatever these may be. A geographical survey of inter- and intraspecific variation in plants (Levin, 1975) has shown that mechanisms which reduce recombination, including apomictic parthenogenesis and selfing, are found particularly in weeds, colonising forms, plants from transient and temperate habitats and populations at the edge of the species range. Recombination-reducing mechanisms are rarely found in tropical plants. A similar geographical survey has been made for animals (Glesner & Tilman, 1978). These authors did not survey selfing, but apomictic parthenogenesis showed a very similar ecological distribution to that in plants, being associated with high latitudes, xeric conditions, disturbed habitats and maritime areas. The authors of both these surveys suggested that recombination is an adaptation for life in biologically complex environments; organisms in these environments are under pressure to evolve continuously in the face of evolutionary advances in their predators, pathogens and competitors. Recombination is, they suggested, an adaptation to facilitate this continuous evolution. There are numerous precise genetic models of how recombination may facilitate evolution (e.g. Maynard Smith, 1978*b*, 1980; Hamilton, 1980). Inbreeding may therefore entail some loss of potential for evolution. Predominantly inbreeding forms may outcross occasionally, and this would to some extent alleviate the loss of evolutionary potential caused by inbreeding (Maynard Smith, 1978*b*).

Conclusions

There may be an element of positive feedback in the consequences of inbreeding and outbreeding. Once outbreeding is adopted, deleterious recessives can accumulate and inbreeding becomes more costly. Once inbreeding is adopted, deleterious recessives are lost, locally adapted and co-adapted gene complexes can be created and these will be destroyed by outbreeding.

There is a large array of theoretical costs and benefits associated with various degrees of inbreeding, but it is difficult to evaluate their relative importance in producing the patterns of inbreeding and outbreeding seen in nature. The largest selective forces acting on inbreeding and outbreeding seem to stem from inbreeding depression and the inclusive fitness effect outlined in *The benefits of inbreeding*. These two forces act in opposition, because both inbreeding depression and the inclusive fitness benefits are greatest for matings between close relatives. The fact that most plants and animals are not strongly inbred (Maynard Smith, 1978*b*) suggest that the single most important factor setting the limit to inbreeding is inbreeding depression and the empirical evidence for inbreeding depression is overwhelming. The effects of epistasis therefore seem to be relatively unimportant and indeed the evidence for the existence of different co-adapted gene complexes in the same population is weak. Local adaptation may be an important force setting the limits to outbreeding (see *Assortative mating*).

What are needed are studies in natural populations of the fitness consequences of various degrees of inbreeding. In such studies it will be important to know both the past and the present size of the populations being studied because the size of the population will affect the overall relatedness and genetic variability of its members.

Assortative mating

Mating is assortative when it occurs between certain phenotypes more often than expected under random mating. Positive assortment (simply called assortative mating), refers to a tendency for phenotypically similar individuals to mate, while negative assortment (called disassortative mating) involves the mating of phenotypically unlike individuals. If the phenotypic traits involved in assortment are heritable then the particular pattern of assortment in a population will have consequences for the pattern of genetic variation. In general, assortative mating tends to increase the genetic variation between individuals while disassortative mating tends to decrease it (Mather, 1973). In the extreme case, assortative mating within an originally interbreeding population may lead to sympatric speciation (Bush, 1969; Tauber & Tauber, 1977a, b). Inbreeding and assortative mating differ in that, when compared with random mating, inbreeding involves mates which are genetically similar at all variable loci, while in assortative mating mates are similar only at those loci affecting variation in the traits for which assortment occurs. In practice, the two processes are often confounded, because inbreeding will involve assortative mating for those traits in respect of which relatives tend to be similar.

Assortment need not imply that animals 'know' their own phenotype. In some species, variation between individuals in mating preference has been demonstrated and in these cases the phenotype preference is established by experience of parents or siblings (Bateson, 1978, 1980, this volume; Cooke, Finney & Rockwell, 1976; Cooke, 1978; Cooke & Davies, this volume).

One possible benefit of assortative mating has already been discussed (see inbreeding and outbreeding) namely the possibility that assortative mating can maintain local adaptation in progeny. The benefits of both local adaptation and avoidance of extreme inbreeding may be achieved by a balance between assortative and disassortative mating. Bateson (1978, 1980, this volume) has described such a system of mate choice in Japanese Quail, and it would be interesting to know whether local differentiation occurs in this species in the wild. Bateson's findings point to slight weaknesses in the traditional view of assortment as being only either positive or negative. Quail choose an intermediate level of dissimilarity in a mate and similarly subtle patterns of assortment may occur in nature. Quite detailed knowledge of criteria used in mate choice and of their pattern of variation would be necessary to detect such assortment. A combination of assortative mating and dispersal could also achieve both local adaptation and inbreeding avoidance. For example, White-crowned Sparrows have local song dialects and, while both sexes disperse after fledging, they tend not to move into areas where the song dialect is different from the one in their natal area (Baker & Mewaldt, 1978, 1981; Petrinovich, Patterson & Baptista, 1981). There are some genetic differences between populations with different dialects (Baker, 1975), but whether these differences are concerned with adaptation to local conditions is not known.

Individuals with similar feeding specialisations have sometimes been found to mate assortatively. For example, Oystercatcher pairs share the same prey specialisation and feeding technique more often than would be expected if birds paired at random with respect to their feeding specialisation (Norton-Griffiths, 1968). The specialisations are learned from both parents by young birds which can take three years to achieve adult feeding efficiency. In this instance it may be important to mate assortatively if the young can learn only one feeding skill efficiently. It is not known how the non-random mating in Oystercatchers is achieved; it may be that birds with the same prey specialisation are more likely to encounter one another because they will tend to co-occur in areas where their prey type is abundant.

In Oystercatchers genetic differences between birds may not be related to the different feeding specialisations because cross-fostered birds acquire the feeding specialisation of the foster parents. In a rather similar example, genetic differences may well be involved; assortative mating has been reported in Darwin's Medium-billed Ground Finch (*Geospiza fortis*) (Boag & Grant, 1978). These finches pair assortatively for bill size (and several other size measures), and in this species bill size is known to be heritable and related to diet (Boag & Grant, 1978, 1981; Grant *et al.*, 1976). Assortatively mated pairs had greater success in fledgling young than did pairs showing no assortment, but the reason for this was not clear (Boag & Grant, 1978).

In one case offspring fitness seems to be unaffected by assortment. Cooke & Davies (this volume) have demonstrated assortative mating for colour in the Lesser Snow Goose, but assortment does not result in an increase in the number of surviving young. The colour polymorphism in these birds seems to be controlled by a single locus and originally the two colour morphs were allopatric. They have subsequently become sympatric, with colour morph frequency differences between different breeding populations. Assortative mating may be a consequence of early learning of family appearance, originally selected because it prevented hybridisation with other species.

Disassortative mating seems to be uncommon. Relatively subtle disassortative mating of the type reported by Bateson (1978, 1980, this volume) may be common. A classic example of disassortative mating was found in the moth *Panaxia dominula* by Sheppard (1952) and another example has been found in Feral Pigeons in Britain. These birds are polymorphic for colour, there being four morphs which mate disassortatively (Murton, Westwood & Thearle, 1973). The causes and consequences of the negative assortment in these examples are not understood.

Frequency-dependent mating success

Male mating success is often negatively frequency-dependent, a phenomenon sometimes known as the 'rare male effect'. Negatively frequency-dependent mating success has been found in *Drosophila* species (Petit, 1951, 1954, 1958; Ehrman, 1967; Ehrman & Spiess, 1969; Spiess & Spiess, 1969; Spiess & Ehrman, 1978) and has also been reported in a parasitic wasp (Grant, Snyder & Glessner, 1974), the Two-spot Ladybird (Muggleton, 1979; O'Donald & Muggleton, 1979), a flour beetle (Sinnock, 1970) and the Guppy (Farr, 1977). The relevance of these studies to the natural situation is unclear because most have been done in the laboratory with inbred strains, or with mutants very rarely seen in nature or with geographical strains which do not normally meet. A few studies (e.g. Ehrman, 1966; Spiess, 1968) have been done in the laboratory with naturally occurring genetic variants which are found together in nature, and one study has been done in nature (Muggleton, 1979; O'Donald & Muggleton, 1979). Thus although frequency-dependent male mating success may well occur regularly in nature, more evidence is needed on this point.

Discussions of the adaptive significance of negatively frequency-dependent mating success have suggested that it will result in outbreeding because, by choosing a rare male as a mate, a female with a common genotype will mate disassortatively (Farr, 1977; Grant, Burton, Contoreggi & Rothstein, 1980; Lewontin, 1974; Lacy, 1979; Averhoff & Richardson, 1974). Disassortative mating will result in offspring with higher levels of heterozygosity and so perhaps greater fitness than offspring produced by random mating. However, there is no empirical evidence that males with locally rare genotypes produce fitter than average offspring. Moreover, there is a major theoretical difficulty with the suggestion; genotypes may be rare because their overall fitness is low. Rare genotypes of low fitness could be produced by recurrent deleterious mutation or by gene flow from other populations adapted to different local conditions. It is therefore not at all obvious that a general female preference for rare males would be adaptive. Furthermore, as pointed out by Lewontin (1974), the levels of polymorphism found in natural populations mean that any male is 'rare' if all its loci are considered. This difficulty could be overcome if variation at only a few loci is responsible for the rare male effect, but numerous single gene mutants as well as purely phenotypic variation (Ehrman, 1966; Dal Molin, 1979) seem to produce the effect. A closer examination of the evidence therefore seems worthwhile.

An important question is that of female choice or preference: does frequency-dependent mating success occur because females prefer to mate with males that are rare? The empirical evidence on this point is equivocal. Nearly all the studies of frequency-dependent mating success are discussed by their authors in terms of female preference for rare males, but usually on the basis of inadequate evidence. To show choice or preference it is necessary to show that females behave differently towards different types of male. This means that the behaviour of females towards different types of male must be observed directly with a view to discovering whether or not female behaviour is responsible for mediating differences in male mating success. This sort of evidence is not available from most rare-male experiments, which have been done with groups of males and females and have taken the mere existence of frequency-dependent mating success as evidence for female choice in favour of rare males. Unfortunately, if groups of females and males are used, then a 'rare-male effect' can arise from fixed female preferences for particular male types irrespective of their frequency (see below). If single females or groups of females are tested with groups of males, then competition between males can generate frequency-dependent male mating success (see below). Thus evidence based only on the pattern of matings observed is not adequate to demonstrate female preference for rare males.

Two other sets of evidence have been cited as demonstrating a role for female preference in mediating the rare male effect. In *Drosophila* and the wasp *Nasonia* (formerly *Mormoniella*) experiments have been performed where air which has first been blown over males of one of the genotypes used in the mating tests is then passed over the flies in the mating chamber (Ehrman, 1966, 1969, 1970; White & Grant, 1977). The general finding has been that the rare genotypes in the mating chamber lose some or all of their advantage if the air blown into the mating chamber has first been blown over males of that genotype. This sort of experiment does not demonstrate that female preference is affected by the experimental manipulation; it could equally be the males that are affected. Direct evidence of an effect on female behaviour is needed. The second sort of evidence comes from experiments with *Drosophila* using single females and groups of males (Spiess & Schwer, 1978; Spiess & Kruckeberg, 1980). In these experiments, a male with a particular genotype was less likely to mate with a female if a male of the same genotype had been the first to court that female. In general, the likelihood that males of a particular genotype will be the first to court a female will depend upon the frequency of these males in the population. Therefore a female tendency to avoid mating with males of the same genotype as that of the first male to court her would automatically generate a rare male effect. On the basis of detailed observations of both male and female behaviour, Spiess & Kruckeberg (1980) suggested that female behaviour was responsible for mediating the rare male effect which they found when they varied the frequency of males which were allowed to court single females. Unfortunately, however, we have not been able to replicate Spiess & Kruckeberg's results in this laboratory (Partridge & Gardner, in press).

The evidence for female choice of rare males is therefore not overwhelming and other possible explanations for the rare-male effect deserve consideration. If individual females vary in the nature or degree of their mating preferences for particular sorts of male, then this can generate a rare male effect (Charlesworth & Charlesworth, 1975; O'Donald, 1977, 1980). If a constant proportion of females prefer to mate with one of the male morphs while another constant proportion prefers the other male morph and the rest mate at random, then each of the male morphs, when rare, will mate relatively more often than the other. O'Donald (1980) has successfully fitted models involving such frequency-independent female mating preferences to several sets of rare male data. This alone does not prove that a mixture of fixed female mating preferences is responsible for the rare male effect in these cases. What is now needed is a study of the mating preferences of individual females; do some females consistently prefer one male morph while other females prefer another? This question could be answered by examining repeated matings by individual females courted by a mixture of male morphs. If the identity of the female has a consistent effect on the mating success of the different male morphs, then a detailed study of male and female behaviour should be made. It is not obvious why selection would favour a mixture of female mating preferences in a single population.

Competition between males for females can also generate a rare male effect for two different reasons.

One model has been developed by Ewing (1978) and is based on an idea put forward by Haldane (1931, 1932) and extended by Milkman (1973). Ewing (1978) considered competition between two populations with different distributions of male mating ability. He showed that frequency-dependent mating may occur if truncation selection is applied to the mixed population so that only a certain proportion of the total male population can mate. In particular, if the variance of male mating ability is different in the two strains, then frequency-dependent mating success will always appear. The direction and extent of this frequency-dependence will depend upon the quantitative and qualitative differences in male mating ability between the strains, the intensity of male competition for females and the stage in the experiment at which the data are analysed. The results obtained by Ewing (1978) using two outbred strains of *Drosophila melanogaster* (Pacific and EDTA-adapted Pacific) accorded well with the predictions of the model. Male size seemed to be a very important variable underlying male mating ability. When raised under conditions of low larval competition, Pacific flies were larger than EDTA flies, and experiments using the two strains raised in this way showed a rare-male effect. Two groups of flies of the Pacific stock made phenotypically large or small by varying the degree of larval competition showed a rare-male effect, while flies of the two different stocks made the same size by adjusting larval competition did not show a rare-male effect. Male size and mating success are strongly correlated in *D. melanogaster* (Ewing, 1961, 1978). Ewing's (1978) results therefore suggest that a difference between strains in male mating ability may be important if the rare male effect is to appear, and his model suggests that it is variance in male mating ability which is especially important. His mechanism will automatically produce a rare-male effect if there is this difference in mating ability between the strains and it is not easy to rule it out as a possible explanation for any set of results. A rare-male effect between strains of identical mating ability could not be explained by this model. Where differences in mating ability occur, then detailed information of timings of individual matings is needed to rule out the mechanism or to determine its magnitude, and this information is not provided in most sets of data.

Competition between males may also produce a rare-male effect if males of one strain compete particularly with each other and less with males of the other strain. Petit & Nouaud (1976) have shown that *D. melanogaster* males of different strains can differ in the position from which they court females. Males therefore compete mainly with others of the same strain for space near females. How general such an effect may be can only be discovered by direct observations of behaviour, but where it occurs it is likely to generate a rare-male effect, because the intensity of competition between males for space near females will depend strongly upon the frequency of their own strain.

Thus a rare-male effect can be produced by at least three biological mechanisms other than female preference for males that are rare. In addition to these complicating variables there have been a number of serious problems with experimental design and statistical analysis in this field (Ewing, 1978). The rare-male effect can appear as an experimental artefact of wing clipping as a technique for marking flies (Bryant, Kence & Kimball, 1980; Kence, 1981) and as an artefact of some methods of analysis (Goux & Anxolabehere, 1980). Unexplained negative results are found with some strains (Markow, 1978; Markow *et al.*, 1980; Pot, Van Delden & Kruijt, 1980; Partridge & Gardner, in press). It is not yet clear under exactly what circumstances frequency-dependent male mating success will appear, although the experiments of Ewing (1978) provide a promising working hypothesis. A new set of experiments is needed, examining in detail the different possibilities listed above. Once the rare-male effect is better understood and its possible occurrence in nature better documented, it will be easier to assess whether or not it has any consequences for offspring fitness.

Conclusions

Variation in individual mating success is fairly well documented, but we have little idea of its genetic consequences, if any. It is therefore at present not possible to say whether female choice in favour of males with high heritable fitness could be favoured by selection. It is quite possible that, in species where a male contributes only gametes to the female, most of the variation in male mating success is attributable to intrasexual competition. Of course in many species the male contributes more than gametes: he may help protect the female from other males and predators during or after mating, provide resources or help in parental care, and all of these features could favour female choice.

Probably the most clearly documented case of a consequence of the mating pattern for offspring fitness is inbreeding depression. Local adaptation may pose selection against mating with a genetically very dissimilar individual, the extreme of which would be interspecific hybridisation. It is interesting that it is in this context that we have some of the clearest evidence for female and male choice, based on a balance between assortative and dissortative mating, the criteria for which are set by early experience of parents and siblings.

Frequency-dependent mating success is a well-documented but poorly understood phenomenon. It is not clear that female choice is involved, and the mechanisms producing the effect require further study.

Random-mating with respect to genotype is a common assumption of many population genetics models. It would be very interesting to know how common random mating really is in natural populations.

Summary

The fitness consequences for offspring of four sorts of non-random mating are discussed.

Variation in individual mating success may affect offspring fitness if individuals with high mating success produce offspring either with high mating success or a high score on other fitness components. For this to occur, net fitness must be heritable. Mutation, disruptive selection and changes in selective forces over time could all produce some fitness heritability in natural populations. It is not clear what the extent of fitness heritability is in natural populations nor how it relates to variation in mating success. More work is needed on this form of non-random mating since it is a very common one.

Inbreeding and outbreeding can have a major effect on offspring fitness. Inbreeding is associated with inbreeding depression. On the other hand it maintains adaptation to local conditions, it may hold co-adapted gene complexes together and it can improve the inclusive fitness of females by increasing the mating success of their male relatives. Outbreeding has the opposite effects and has the long-term effect of maintaining the potential for recombination. Most species are not strongly inbred, and it seems likely that inbreeding depression is the main selective force acting to set a limit to inbreeding. The limit to outbreeding may be set by selection for local adaptation.

Assortative mating is a fairly common finding while disassortative mating is less common and the selective forces producing it are less well understood. Assortative mating may maintain local adaptation.

Frequency-dependent mating success is a commonly reported but poorly understood phenomenon. It can be produced as a result of competition between males of different genotypes without any involvement of female choice, and the evidence for an involvement of female choice is very weak. Its importance in nature and its effects on offspring fitness are unclear.

I am extremely grateful to Philip Ashmole, Pat Bateson, Brian Charlesworth, Alastair Ewing, Arthur Ewing, Vernon French, John Maynard Smith and Geoff Parker for their suggestions for improvement of the manuscript.

References

Alexander, R. D. & Sherman, P. W. (1977). Local mate competition and parental investment in social insects. *Science*, **196**, 494–500.

Allard, R. W., Babbel, G. R., Clegg, M. T. & Kahler, A. L. (1972). Evidence for coadaptation in *Avena barbarata*. *Proceedings of the National Academy of Sciences of the USA*, **69**, 3043–8.

Allison, A. C. (1954). Protection afforded by the sickle-cell trait against subtertian malarial infection. *British Medical Journal*, **1**, 290–4.

Anderson, W. W., Levine, L., Olvera, O., Rowell, J. R., de la Rosa, M. E., Salceda, V. M., Gaso, M. I. & Guzmán, J. (1979). Evidence for selection by male mating success in natural populations of *Drosophila pseudoobscura*. *Proceedings of the National Academy of Sciences of the USA*, **76**, 1519–23.

Antonovics, J. (1968). Evolution in closely adjacent plant populations. V. Evolution of self-fertility. *Heredity*, **23**, 219–38.

Averhoff, W. W. & Richardson, R. H. (1974): Pheromonal control of mating patterns in *Drosophila melanogaster*. *Behavior Genetics*, **4**, 207–25.

Baker, M. C. (1975). Song dialects and genetic differences in white-crowned sparrows (*Zonotrichia leucophrys*). *Evolution*, **29**, 226–41.

Baker, M. C. & Mewaldt, L. R. (1978). Song dialects as barriers to dispersal in white-crowned sparrows, *Zonotrichia leucophrus nuttali*. *Evolution*, **32**, 712–22.

Baker, M. C. & Mewaldt, L. R. (1981). Response to "Song dialects as barriers to dispersal: a re-evaluation". *Evolution*, **35**, 189–90.

Bateman, A. J. (1948). Intra-sexual selection in *Drosophila*. *Heredity*, **2**, 349–68.

Bateson, P. (1978). Sexual imprinting and optimal outbreeding. *Nature*, **273**, 659–60.

Bateson, P. (1980). Optimal outbreeding and the development of sexual preferences in Japanese Quail. *Zeitschrift für Tierpsychologie*, **53**, 231–44.

Bengtsson, B. O. (1978). Avoiding inbreeding: at what cost? *Journal of Theoretical Biology*, **73**, 439–44.

Berger, E. (1976). Heterosis and the maintenance of enzyme polymorphism. *American Naturalist*, **110**, 823–39.

Berry, R. J. (1977). *Inheritance and Natural History*. Collins: London.

Boag, P. T. & Grant, P. R. (1978). Heritability of external morphology in Darwin's finches. *Nature*, **274**, 793–4.

Boag, P. T. & Grant, P. R. (1981). Intense natural selection in a population of Darwin's finches (Geospizinae) in the Galapagos. *Science*, **214**, 82–5.

Boggs, C. L. (1981). Selection pressures affecting male nutrient investment at mating in heliconiine butterflies. *Evolution*, **35**, 931–40.

Boggs, C. L. & Gilbert, L. E. (1979). Male contribution to egg production in butterflies: evidence for transfer of nutrients at mating. *Science*, **206**, 83–4.

Boggs, C. L. & Watts, W. B. (1981). Population structure of pierid butterflies. IV. Genetic and physiological investment in offspring by male *Colias*. *Oecologia*, **50**, 320–4.

Borgia, G. (1979). Sexual selection and the evolution of mating systems. In *Sexual Selection and Reproductive Competition in Insects*, ed. M. S. Blum & N. A. Blum, pp. 19–80. Academic Press: New York.

Borgia, G. (1981). Mate selection in the fly *Scatophaga stercoraria*: female choice in a male-controlled system. *Animal Behaviour*, **29**, 71–80.

Brittnacher, J. G. (1981). Genetic variation and genetic load due to the male reproductive component of fitness in *Drosophila*. *Genetics*, **97**, 719–30.

Bryant, E. H., Kence, A. & Kimball, K. T. (1980). A rare-male advantage in the housefly induced by wing clipping and some general considerations for *Drosophila*. *Genetics*, **96**, 975–93.

Bundgaard, J. & Christiansen, F. B. (1972). Dynamics of polymorphisms. I. Selection components in an experimental population of *Drosophila melanogaster*. *Genetics*, **71**, 439–60.

Bush, G. L. (1969). Mating behavior, host specificity and the ecological significance of sibling species in frugivorous flies of the genus *Rhagoletis* (Diptera: Tephritidae). *American Naturalist*, **103**, 669–72.

Charlesworth, D. & Charlesworth, B. (1975). Sexual selection and polymorphism. *American Naturalist*, **109**, 465–70.

Clegg, M. T., Allard, R. W. & Kahler, A. L. (1972). Is the gene the unit of selection? Evidence from two experimental plant populations. *Proceedings of the National Academy of Sciences of the USA*, **69**, 2474–8.

Cooke, F. (1978). Early learning and its effect on population structure. Studies of a wild population of snow geese. *Zeitschrift für Tierpsychologie*, **46**, 344–58.

Cooke, F., Finney, G. H. & Rockwell, R. F. (1976). Assortative mating in lesser Snow Geese (*Anser caerulescens*). *Behavior Genetics*, **6**, 127–40.

Cowan, D. P. (1979). Sibling matings in a hunting wasp: adaptative inbreeding? *Science*, **205**, 1403–5.

Crow, J. F. & Kimura, M. (1970). *An Introduction to Population Genetics Theory*. Harper Row: New York.

Dal Molin, C. (1979). An external scent as the basis for a rare-male mating advantage in *Drosophila melanogaster*. *American Naturalist*, **113**, 951–4.

Dobzhansky, T., Ayala, J. J., Stebbins, G. L. & Valentine, J. W. (1977). *Evolution*. W. H. Freeman & Co.: San Francisco.

Ehrman, L. (1966). Mating success and genotype frequency in *Drosophila*. *Animal Behaviour*, **14**, 332–9.

Ehrman, L. (1967). Further studies on genotype frequency and mating success in *Drosophila*. *American Naturalist*, **101**, 415–24.

Ehrman, L. (1969). The sensory basis of mate selection in *Drosophila*. *Evolution*, **23**, 59–64.

Ehrman, L. (1970). Simulation of the mating advantage of rare *Drosophila* males. *Science*, **167**, 905–6.

Ehrman, L. & Spiess, E. B. (1969). Rare type mating advantage in *Drosophila*. *American Naturalist*, **103**, 675–80.

Ewing, Arthur, W. (1961). Body size and courtship behaviour in *Drosophila melanogaster*. *Animal Behaviour*, **9**, 93–9.

Ewing, Alastair, W. (1978). *An Investigation Into Selective Mechanisms Capable of Maintaining Balanced Polymorphisms*. Ph.D. Thesis, Portsmouth Polytechnic.

Falconer, D. S. (1981). *Introduction to Quantitative Genetics*. Longman: London.

Farr, J. A. (1977). Male rarity or novelty, female choice behaviour and sexual selection in the guppy, *Poecilia reticulata* Peters (Pisces: Peociliidae). *Evolution*, **31**, 162–8.

Fisher, R. A. (1930). *The Genetical Theory of Natural Selection*. Oxford University Press: Oxford.

Frelinger, J. A. (1972). The maintenance of transferrin polymorphism in pigeons. *Proceedings of the National Academy of Sciences of the USA*, **69**, 326–9.

Ghiselin, M. T. (1969). The evolution of hermaphroditism among animals. *Quarterly Review of Biology*, **44**, 189–208.

Gibson, R. M. & Guiness, F. E. (1980). Differential reproduction among red deer (*Cervus elaphus*) stags on Rhum. *Journal of Animal Ecology*, **49**, 199–208.

Glesner, R. R. & Tilman, D. (1978). Sexuality and the components of environmental uncertainty: clues from geographic parthenogenesis in terrestrial animals. *American Naturalist*, **112**, 659–73.

Goux, J. M. & Anxolabehere, D. (1980). The measurement of sexual isolation and selection: a critique. *Heredity*, **45**, 255–62.

Grant, B., Burton, S., Contoreggi, C. & Rothstein, M. (1980). Outbreeding via frequency-dependent mate selection in the parasitoid wasp, *Nasonia* (= *Mormoniella*) *vitripennis* Walker. *Evolution*, **34**, 983–92.

Grant, B., Snyder, G. A. & Glesser, S. F. (1974). Frequency-dependent mate selection in *Mormoniella vitripennis. Evolution*, **28**, 259–64.

Grant, P. R., Grant, B. R., Smith, J. N. M., Abbot, I. J. & Abbott, L. K. (1976). Darwin's finches: population variation and natural selection. *Proceedings of the National Academy of Sciences of the USA*, **73**, 257–61.

Greenwood, P. J., Harvey, P. H. & Perrins, C. M. (1978). Inbreeding and dispersal in the great tit. *Nature*, **271**, 52–4.

Greenwood, P. J. (1980). Mating systems, philopatry and dispersal in birds and mammals. *Animal Behaviour*, **28**, 1140–62.

Haldane, J. B. S. (1931). A mathematical theory of natural and artificial selection. Part VII. Selection intensity as a function of mortality rate. *Proceedings of the Cambridge Philosophical Society*, **27**, 131–6.

Haldane, J. B. S. (1932). *The Causes of Evolution.* Longman S. Green and Co.: London, New York, Toronto.

Halliday, T. & Houston, A. (1978). The newt as an honest salesman. *Animal Behaviour*, **26**, 127–4.

Hamilton, W. D. (1967). Extraordinary sex ratios. *Science*, **156**, 477–88.

Hamilton, W. D. (1980). Sex versus non-sex versus parasite. *Oikos*, **35**, 282–90.

Hartl, D. L. (1980). *Principles of Population Genetics.* Sinauer: Sunderland, Massachusetts.

Hedrick, P., Jain, S. & Holden, L. (1978). Multilocus systems in evolution. In *Evolutionary Biology*, vol. **11**, ed. M. K. Hecht, W. C. Steere & B. Wallace, pp. 101–84. Plenum Press: New York and London.

Herbert, P. D. N. (1974a). Enzyme variability in natural populations of *Daphnia magna* II. Genotypic frequencies in permanent populations. *Genetics*, **77**, 323–34.

Herbert, P. D. N. (1974b). Enzyme variability in natural populations of *Daphnia magna* III. Genotypic frequencies in intermittent populations. *Genetics*, **77**, 335–41.

Hill, W. G. & Robertson, A. (1968). The effects of inbreeding at loci with heterozygous advantage. *Genetics*, **60**, 615–28.

Hiraizumi, Y. (1961). Negative correlation between rate of development and female fertility in *Drosophila melanogaster. Genetics*, **46**, 615–24.

Jain, S. K. & Bradshaw, A. D. (1966). Evolutionary divergence among adjacent plant populations. I. The evidence and its theoretical analysis. *Heredity*, **21**, 407–41.

Kence, A. (1981). The rare-male advantage in *Drosophila:* a possible source of bias in experimental design. *American Naturalist*, **117**, 1027–8.

Koehn, R. K. (1969). Esterase heterogeneity: dynamics of a polymorphism. *Science*, **163**, 943–44.

Lacy, R. C. (1979). Adaptiveness of a rare male mating advantage under heterosis. *Behavior Genetics*, **9**, 51–5.

Lande, R. (1976). The maintenance of genetic variability by mutation in a polygenic character with linked loci. *Genetic Research Cambridge*, **26**, 221–35.

Lande, R. (1981). Models of speciation by sexual selection on polygenic traits. *Proceedings of the National Academy of Sciences of the USA*, **78**, 3721–5.

Le Boeuf, B. J. (1974). Male–male competition and reproductive success in elephant seals. *American Zoologist*, **14**, 163–76.

Levin, D. A. (1975). Pest pressure and recombination systems in plants. *American Naturalist*, **109**, 437–51.

Lewontin, R. C. (1974). *The Genetic Basis of Evolutionary Change*. Columbia University Press: New York & London.

MacKay, T. F. C. (1980). Genetic variance, fitness and homeostasis in varying environments: an experimental check on the theory. *Evolution*, **34**, 1219–22.

MacKay, T. F. C. (1981). Genetic variation in varying environments. *Genetic Research Cambridge*, **37**, 79–93.

Markow, T. A. (1978). A test for the rare male advantage in coisogenic strains of *Drosophila melanogaster*. *Genetic Research Cambridge*, **32**, 123–7.

Markow, T. A., Richmond, R. C., Mueller, L., Sheer, I., Roman, S., Laetz, C. & Lorenz, L. (1980). Testing for rare male advantages among various *Drosophila melanogaster* genotypes. *Genetic Research Cambridge*, **35**, 59–64.

Mather, K. (1973). *Genetical Structure of Populations*. Chapman & Hall: London.

Maynard Smith, J. (1966). Sympatric speciation. *American Naturalist*, **100**, 637–50.

Maynard Smith, J. (1978a). Optimization theory in evolution. *Annual Review of Ecology and Systematics*, **9**, 31–56.

Maynard Smith, J. (1978b). *The Evolution of Sex*. Cambridge University Press: Cambridge.

Maynard Smith, J. (1980). Selection for recombination in a polygenic model. *Genetic Research Cambridge*, **35**, 269–77.

McCracken, G. F. & Selander, R. K. (1980). Self-fertilization and monogenic strains in natural populations of terrestrial slugs. *Proceedings of the National Academy of Sciences of the USA*, **77**, 684–8.

Milkman, R. (1973). A competitive selection model. *Genetics*, **74**, 727–2.

Mitter, C., Futuyma, D. J., Schneider, J. C. & Haire, J. D. (1979). Genetic variation and host plant relations in a parthenogenetic moth. *Evolution*, **33**, 777–90.

Muggleton, J. (1979). Non-random mating in wild populations of polymorphic *Adalia bipunctata*. *Heredity*, **42**, 57–65.

Mukai, T., Chigusa, S. I., Mettler, L. E. & Crow, J. F. (1972). Mutation rate and dominance of genes affecting viability in *Drosophila melanogaster*. *Genetics*, **72**, 335–55.

Mukai, T. & Yamaguchi, O. (1974). The genetic structure of natural populations of *Drosophila melanogaster*. XI. Genetic variability in a local population. *Genetics*, **76**, 339–66.

Murton, R. K., Westwood, N. J. & Thearle, R. J. P. (1973). Polymorphism and the evolution of a continuous breeding season in the pigeon, *Columbia livia*. *Journal of Reproduction and Fertility Supplement*, **19**, 563–77.

Norton-Griffiths, M. (1968). *The Feeding Behaviour of the Oystercatcher* Haematopus ostralegus. D. Phil. Thesis, University of Oxford.

O'Donald, P. (1977). Mating advantage of rare males in models of sexual selection. *Nature*, **267**, 151–4.

O'Donald, P. (1980). *Genetic Models of Sexual Selection*. Cambridge University Press: Cambridge.

O'Donald, P. & Muggleton, J. (1979). Melanic polymorphism in ladybirds maintained by sexual selection. *Heredity*, **43**, 143–8.

Ohnishi, O. (1977a). Spontaneous and ethyl methanesulfonate induced mutations controlling viability in *Drosophila melanogaster*. II Homozygous effect of polygenic mutations. *Genetics*, **87**, 529–45.

Ohnishi, O. (1977b). Spontaneous and ethyl methanesulfonate induced mutations controlling viability in *Drosophila melanogaster*. III Heterozygous effects of polygenic mutations. *Genetics*, **87**, 547–56.

Ohta, A. (1980). Coadaptive gene complexes in incipient species of Hawaiian *Drosophila*. *American Naturalist*, **115**, 121–32.

Packer, C. (1979). Inter-troop transfer and inbreeding avoidance in *Papio anubis*. *Animal Behaviour*. **27**, 1–36.

Partridge, L. (1978). Habitat selection. In *Behavioural Ecology*, ed. J. R. Krebs & N. B. Davies. Blackwell: Oxford.

Partridge, L. (1980). Mate choice increases a component of offspring fitness in fruit flies. *Nature*, **283**, 290–1.

Partridge, L. & Gardner, A. Failure to replicate the results of an experiment on the rare male effect in *Drosophila melanogaster*. *American Naturalist*, In press.

Petit, C. (1951). Le rôle de l'isolement sexual dans l'évolution des populations de *Drosophila melanogaster*. *Bulletin biologique de la France et de la Belgique*, **85**, 392–418.

Petit, C. (1954). L'isolement sexual chez *Drosophila melanogaster*. Etude du mutant white et de son allélomorphe sauvage. *Bulletin biologique de la France et de la Belgique*, **88**, 435–43.

Petit, C. (1958). Le déterminisme génétique et psychophysiologique de la compétition sexuelle chez *Drosophila melanogaster*. *Bulletin biologique de la France et de la Belgique*, **92**, 248–329.

Petit, C. & Nouaud, D. (1976). Ecological competition and the advantage of the rare type in *Drosophila melanogaster*. *Evolution*, **29**, 763–76.

Petrinovich, L., Patterson, T. & Baptista, L. F. (1981). Song dialects as barriers to dispersal: a re-evaluation. *Evolution*, **35**, 180–8.

Pot, W., Van Delden, W. & Kruijt, J. P. (1980). Genotypic differences in mating success and the maintenance of the alcohol dehydrogenase polymorphism in *Drosophila melanogaster*. No evidence for overdominance or rare genotype mating advantage. *Behavior Genetics*, **10**, 43–58.

Prout, T. (1971). The relation between fitness components and population prediction in *Drosophila*. 1. The estimation of fitness components. *Genetics*, **68**, 127–49.

Rose, M. R. & Charlesworth, B. (1981a). Genetics of life history in *Drosophila melanogaster*. I. Sib analysis of adult females. *Genetics*, **97**, 173–86.

Rose, M. R. & Charlesworth, B. (1981b). Genetics of life history in *Drosophila melanogaster*. II. Exploratory selection experiments. *Genetics*, **97**, 187–96.

Rutowski, R. L. (1979). The butterfly as an honest salesman. *Animal Behaviour*, **27**, 1268–76.

Rutowski, R. L. (1980). Courtship solicitation by females of the checkered white butterfly, *Pieris protodice*. *Behavioral Ecology and Sociobiology*, **7**, 113–17.

Schneider, J. C. (1980). The role of parthenogenesis and female aptery in microgeographic, ecological adaptation in the fall cankerworm, *Alsophila pometaria* Harris (Lepidoptera: Geometridae). *Ecology*, **61**, 1082–90.

Selander, R. K. & Hudson, R. O. (1976). Animal population structure under close inbreeding: the land snail *Rumina* in southern France. *American Naturalist*, **110**, 695–718.

Sheppard, P. M. (1952). A note on non-random mating in the moth *Panaxia dominula* (L). *Heredity*, **6**, 239–41.

Shields, W. M. (In press). Optimal inbreeding and the evolution of philopatry. *The Ecology of Animal Movement*, ed. I. R. Swingland & P. J. Greenwood. Oxford University Press: London.

Simmons, M. J. & Crow, J. F. (1977). Mutations affecting fitness in *Drosophila* populations. *Annual Review of Genetics*, **11**, 49–78.

Simmons, M. J., Preston, C. R. & Engels, W. R. (1980). Pleiotropic effects on fitness of mutations affecting viability in *Drosophila melanogaster*. *Genetics*, **94**, 467–75.

Sinnock, P. (1970). Frequency dependence and mating behaviour in *Tribolium castaneum*. *American Naturalist*, **104**, 469–76.

Smith, R. H. (1979). On selection for inbreeding in polygynous animals. *Heredity*, **43**, 205–11.

Spiess, E. B. (1968). Low frequency advantage in mating of *Drosophila pseudoobscura* karyotypes. *American Naturalist*, **102**, 363–79.

Spiess, E. B. & Ehrman, L. (1978). Rare male mating advantage. *Nature*, **272**, 188–9.

Spiess, E. B. & Kruckeberg, J. F. (1980). Minority advantage of certain eye color mutants of *Drosophila melanogaaster*. II. A behavioral basis. *American Naturalist*, **115**, 307–27.

Spiess, E. B. & Schwer, W. A. (1978). Minority advantage of certain eye color mutants of *Drosophila melanogaster*. I. Multiple choice and single female tests. *Behavior Genetics*, **8**, 155–68.

Spiess, L. D. & Spiess, E. B. (1969). Minority advantage in interpopulational matings of *Drosophila persimilis*. *American Naturalist*, **103**, 155–72.

Taubert, C. A. & Tauber, M. J. (1977*a*). Sympatric speciation based on allelic changes at three loci: evidence from natural populations in two habitats. *Science*, **197**, 1298–9.

Tauber, C. A. & Tauber, M. J. (1977*b*). A genetic model for sympatric speciation through habitat diversification and seasonal isolation. *Nature*, **268**, 702–5.

Templeton, A. R., Sing, C. F. & Brokaw, B. (1976). The unit of selection in *Drosophila mercatorium*. I. The interaction of selection and meiosis in parthenogenetic strains. *Genetics*, **82**, 349–76.

Thornhill, R. (1981). *Panorpa* (Mecoptera: Panorpidae) Scorpionflies: systems for understanding resource-defense polygyny and alternative male reproductive efforts. *Annual Review of Ecology and Systematics*, **12**, 355–86.

Van Noordwijk, A. J. & Scharloo, W. (1981). Inbreeding in an island population of the great tit. *Evolution*, **35**, 674–88.

Van Noordwijk, A. J., Van Balen, J. H. & Scharloo, W. (1980). Heritability of ecologically important traits in the great tit (*Parus major* L.). *Ardea*, **68**, 193–203.

Waage, J. K. (1982). Sib-mating and sex ratio strategies in scelionid wasps. *Ecological Entomology*, **7**, 103–12.

Watanabe, T. K. & Ohnishi, S. (1975). Genes affecting productivity in natural populations of *Drosophila melanogaster*. *Genetics*, **80**, 807–19.

Watanabe, T. K. & Oshima, C. (1973). Fertility genes in natural populations of *Drosophila melanogaster*. II. Correlation between productivity and viability. *Japanese Journal of Genetics*, **48**, 337–47.

White, H. C. & Grant, B. (1977). Olfactory cues as a factor in frequency-dependent mate selection in *Mormoniella vitripennis*. *Evolution*, **31**, 829–35.

Wright, S. (1931). Evolution in Mendelian populations. *Genetics*, **16**, 97–159.

Wright, S. (1960). Physiological genetics, ecology of populations and natural selection. In *Evolution after Darwin*, ed. S. Tax, pp. 429–75. University of Chicago Press: Chicago, Illinois.

Wright, S. (1970). Random drift and the shifting balance theory of evolution. In *Mathematical Topics in Population Genetics*, ed. K. Kojima. Springer-Verlag: New York.

Zimmerman, J. L. (1971). The territory and its density dependent effect in *Spiza americana*. *Auk*, **88**, 591–612.

Appendix

Proof that, given a locus at equilibrium under heterozygous advantage, female choice based on male genotype will not affect the average fitness of the progeny produced

Assume a single locus with two alleles and heterozygous advantage with genotypes and fitnesses as follows:

Genotypes	AA	Aa	aa
Fitnesses	$1-S_1$	1	$1-S_2$

Assume that selection occurs between the time of zygote formation and mating.

Let the frequency of A be p and of a, q.

Females do not know their own genotype. An average female will transmit an A gamete with probability p and an a gamete with probability q. We can now consider the mean fitness of the offspring produced by an average female mating with each of the three male genotypes.

(a) *Heterozygous Aa males*

		Male gametes	
		$\frac{1}{2}A$	$\frac{1}{2}a$
Female	pA	AA	Aa
gametes	qa	aA	aa

We can now multiply the offspring genotypes by their frequencies and fitnesses.

Expected
offspring $= \frac{1}{2}p(1-S_1)+\frac{1}{2}p+\frac{1}{2}q+\frac{1}{2}q(1-S_2)$　　　　(10.1)
fitness

(b) *Homozygous AA males*

		Male gametes
		A
Female	pA	AA
gametes	qa	Aa

Expected
offspring $= p(1-S_1)+q$ (10.2)
fitness

(c) *Homozygous aa* males

		Male gametes
		a
Female	*pA*	*Aa*
gametes	*qa*	*aa*

Expected   (10.3)
offspring $= p+q(1-S_2)$
fitness

In a population at genetic equilibrium under heterozygous advantage:

$$p = S_2/(S_1+S_2), \quad q = S_1/(S_1+S_2)$$

Substituting these values for p and q in the expressions (10.1), (10.2) and (10.3) above, in all three cases gives an expected offspring fitness of:

$$(S_1+S_2-S_1 S_2)/(S_1+S_2) = 1 - S_1 S_2/(S_1+S_2)$$

For an average female, the expected fitness of offspring is therefore the same for all three genotypes of mate, and the female can therefore not improve her expected offspring fitness by mate choice.

11

Optimal outbreeding

PATRICK BATESON

Finding a compatible partner is an important part of mate choice. Members of different species do not make good mates. At the other pole, too much inbreeding can also reduce reproductive success. For many years it was supposed that, providing the two extremes were avoided, choice of mate was influenced by all the other factors that are known or assumed to be important (see Halliday, this volume). However, even within the species excessive outbreeding may be costly for a variety of reasons (Bateson, 1980; Shields, 1983). This means that the balance between too much inbreeding and too much outbreeding may have to be struck more carefully than was previously supposed. In this chapter I shall review briefly the possible costs of both inbreeding and outbreeding, then consider ways in which animals might achieve the optimal balance when choosing a mate, and how their actual preferences can be measured. Finally, I shall return to some of the evolutionary implications of optimal outbreeding.

The balance

Fifty years ago Sewall Wright (1933) wrote: 'The most general conclusion is that evolution depends on a certain balance among its factors... A certain amount of crossbreeding is favorable but not too much'.

A useful way of representing the optimal balance between inbreeding and outbreeding was suggested by Bischof (1972) and Alexander (1977) and is redrawn in Fig. 11.1. Inbreeding has costs, outbreeding has costs, and natural selection is presumed to have operated on mechanisms involved in mate choice to minimise both sets of costs. The outcome of selection, the argument continues, will have been a preference for a mate that is not too closely related and not too distantly related.

A similar idea derives from the possibility that inbreeding may have benefits as well as costs (e.g. Smith, 1979). Providing the costs fall off more rapidly with the decline in the closeness of relationship between mates than do the benefits an optimal mate should be one that maximises the benefits relative to the costs. The difference between the two ways of expressing the balance is more apparent than real since losing a benefit of inbreeding is equivalent to gaining a cost from outbreeding. We can, therefore, prepare two lists, one for the costs of inbreeding and one for the costs of outbreeding.

Two such lists are given in Table 11.1 and Partridge (this volume) considers the issues in greater detail in her chapter. Some of the entries in the lists relate to the costs and benefits of sexual reproduction. This is because, in genetic terms, inbreeding approximates to asexual reproduction and outbreeding maximises the advantages of sexual reproduction. Since considerable theoretical disagreement revolves around the supposed advantages of sex, it follows that some of the entries in Table 11.1 are controversial. For instance, one disputed idea is that because the recombination arising from sexual reproduction increases the differences between offspring, sexual reproduction is advantageous in a variable environment,

Fig. 11.1. Hypothetical costs of inbreeding and outbreeding arising from choosing mates of different degrees of relatedness. The optimal mate is one in which the combined costs of mating are at a minimum. The optimum is not necessarily at the point of intersection of the lines.

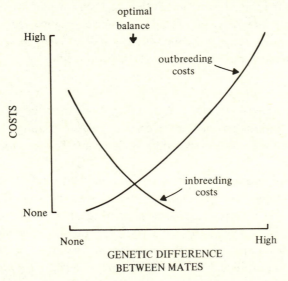

the point being that one or other of the offspring is likely to be able to cope with the prevailing conditions. Maynard Smith (1978) attempted to model this intuitively reasonable proposal and concluded that such a consequence of sexual reproduction would only have selective advantages under very special and rather implausible changes in environmental conditions from one generation to the next.

Maynard Smith accepted Williams' (1975) suggestion that sexual reproduction could reduce competition between offspring. However, he was concerned about what would happen when genes at different loci influenced the organism's character adapted to a particular environment. Would not this mean that the habit of sexual reproduction would fail to spread? I am not sure that this is necessarily the case. If an animal mates with a fairly close relation, it might be able to reduce the costs of breaking up co-adapted complexes of genes while at the same time gaining benefits from having somewhat variable offspring. The possibility needs careful modelling to see whether it could work in principle.

Another of Maynard Smith's (1978) arguments is also worth developing

Table 11.1. *The hypothetical disadvantages of inbreeding and outbreeding*

Costs of inbreeding
    1 Deleterious genes more likely to be fully expressed.
    2 Beneficial interactions (heterozygous advantage or over-dominance) between different alleles at same genetic locus lost.
    3 Offspring insufficiently variable for one or other to cope with a varying environment.
    4 Offspring more like each other and so compete more intensely.

Costs of outbreeding
    1 Genes required for adaptation to particular environment lost or suppressed.
    2 Co-adapted gene complexes broken up by recombination.
    3 In polygynous species advantage of having extra-closely related offspring lost and parental genes less well represented in next generation.
    4 Infection from pathogens carried by mate more likely.
    5 Travelling into another population costly and dangerous.
    6 Acquired skills useful in one environment not appropriate in another.
    7 Mismatch of habits acquired by mates in different environments disrupts parenting.

Note: In any one species only a sub-set of these costs would be likely to operate.

in relation to the notion of optimal outbreeding. Suppose that a gene increasing the likelihood of animals' outbreeding means that the majority of the offspring are less well adapted to the environment than those animals lacking the gene. Nevertheless, a few offspring from outbreeding parents are better adapted than all those of inbreeding parents. In such circumstances, the gene influencing the habit of outbreeding could increase in frequency by the so-called 'hitch-hiking effect'. It is the successes that matter, not the failures. Maynard Smith (1978) believed such an effect played an important role in the evolution of sexual reproduction but made the following comment: 'It explains why some recombination (either a little, or 50%) should be favoured over no recombination. It does not as yet explain why a lot of recombination should be favoured over a little.' (p. 123). Here again, a resolution could be that those pairs that outbreed a lot have a lower overall reproductive success than those that outbreed only slightly. If so, a gene making the difference between a slight amount of outbreeding and a lot would be crucial and could spread through the population.

Dawkins (1979) has criticised the arguments that individuals should tend to inbreed because this brings extra-close relatives into the world. He regards this as one of the numerous misunderstandings of kin selection. The error is found, for instance, in Thiessen & Gregg (1980). Dawkins argued that if an individual female refrains from mating with her brother, he is free to mate with some other female. So an outbreeding female gains a nephew or niece with co-efficients of relationship of a quarter, plus a normal offspring of her own with a co-efficient of relationship of a half. This would match the single super-offspring of the female who mated with her brother, and had a co-efficient of relationship with her of three-quarters. Dawkins, accepted, however, the views of Parker (1979) and Smith (1979) that the kin selection argument could apply in polygynous species. If variance in male reproductive success is high and many males do not mate, a female, by mating with her brother, may not deprive him of the chance to mate with another female. Most probably, the mating that his sister gives him is the only one he will get. A female does not deprive herself of an independent nephew or niece by mating with her brother, and she does bring into the world an offspring that is very closely related to her and, therefore, particularly likely to transmit her special adaptations and with them the habit of mating with brothers.

Some of the genetic costs of inbreeding are short-lasting in evolutionary terms. The probability of damaging genes being expressed goes up, of course, as inbreeding takes place. But once fully revealed, they are eliminated from the population and fitness rises once again. Other costs are more subtle and often more stable (Maynard Smith, 1978). Different alleles at the same locus may interact in a beneficial way giving advantage to the heterozygote. Alternatively, the developmental process called dominance may suppress the damaging effects of certain alleles in the heterozygous condition but not their beneficial pleiotropic effects which maintain the allele in the population even in its homozygous form. Whatever the explanation for stable inbreeding depression, it clearly would lead to a selection pressure for some outbreeding. But how much?

Hybrid vigour is so dramatic when it occurs that it seems to make the arguments for outbreeding depression implausible. Nevertheless, some empirical evidence supports the view that outbreeding too much can carry genetic costs in certain species. Turkington & Harper (1979) asexually propagated Clover (*Trifolium repens*) in a glasshouse and then transferred the plants back into the original grass sward from which each type came. Each clover-type made significantly more growth when transplanted back into the particular part of the sward from which its type was taken. The suggestion is that each type of clover was particularly well adapted to local conditions. It is only a presumption, of course, that if each type had been outcrossed by sexual reproduction, local adaptations would have been lost. Nonetheless, the experiment suggests that tests of outbreeding depression should be made in the natural environment where the benefits of co-adapted gene complexes can be revealed. Price & Waser (1979) have performed such a field experiment with another plant. They found that in the Mountain Delphinium (*Delphinium nelsoni*) the largest number of seedlings was produced by crosses between plants that were 10 m apart. Plants that were selfed and those that were crossed with plants 1000 m away, gave rise to significantly smaller numbers of seedlings. This is direct evidence for both inbreeding and outbreeding depression, but unquestionably a great many more such studies are needed before strong conclusions can be drawn.

In animals direct evidence for the genetic costs of outbreeding is still relatively slender, although the examples of naturally-inbred populations are starting to multiply (e.g. Cowan, 1979; van Noordwijk & Scharloo, 1981). Some of the studies of humans suggest that fecundity is related to the similarity between spouses. For example, in one study the more alike the humans were on 17 out of 19 measures of the body (such as forearm length, height, and ear length), the more children they had (Thiessen & Gregg, 1980, Table 3). Although most correlations were positive, each correlation coefficient was very low and could, of course, be explained by shared associations between the measures and a third variable such as social class. A more compelling example of the costs of outbreeding in humans is provided by the distribution of incompatible blood groups. For instance, the r complex is very infrequent in Chinese people but common in Europeans (Mourant, Kopec & Domaniewska-Sobozak, 1976). This means that a rhesus-negative Chinese woman with a rhesus-positive European husband is likely to have 'blue' babies after her first child. This would more than counteract any effects of hybrid vigour on the couple's life-time reproductive success.

It will be apparent from the list in Table 11.1, that not all the costs of outbreeding are genetic in character. If and when they operate, they further complicate the interpretation of laboratory breeding experiments aimed at settling whether or not outbreeding can be costly. For instance, two unrelated individuals in the laboratory may produce many offspring and, because they share adjoining cages and common antibodies, incur no cost from being exposed to pathogens carried by the other. It could be a very different story in the natural environment. Similarly, the advantage of using skills acquired for dealing with the local environment could counteract the genetic advantage of moving into another area prior to breeding. Yet the non-genetic advantage could not be assessed in a laboratory experiment. Nor could the various costs of movement (Bengtsson, 1978), such as increased risks from predation. Clearly, we have to be very cautious in jumping to conclusions about just where the balance between inbreeding and outbreeding is likely to be struck.

Finally, it is worth emphasising that the opposed selection pressures may generate more than one optimal solution. For instance, multiple optima could arise if the variability of a population is not linearly related to the degree of inbreeding. It is known that members of a partly inbred population of mice (*Mus domesticus*) can be *more* variable than outbred mice (Festing, 1976). Such effects could generate multiple optima if, say, variability in characteristics influences the strength of the opposed selection pressures.

Mechanisms of optimal outbreeding

If an animal has to choose a mate that is neither a close relative nor totally unrelated to it, what mechanisms could it use? Of the various types of explanation that have been offered, two are likely to be very important. The first proposes that prior to mating, members of one sex move away from the area where they were hatched or born. Providing they do not move too far, their mates are likely to bear some relationship to themselves and so optimal outbreeding could be achieved. The second possibility is that animals are able to recognise close kin and, on the assumption that external appearance is a measure of genotypic similarity, choice of a mate that looks, sounds, or smells, a bit different but not too different from close kin, will also result in optimal outbreeding. These two explanations are not mutually exclusive. Some species could employ both mechanisms. The evidence certainly suggests that both are found in the animal kingdom.

First, in many species of bird and mammal, one sex moves out of the natal area prior to breeding (review in Greenwood, 1980). In most species of birds, females move away although there are exceptions such as the Snow Goose (*Anser coerulescens*) in which the male is unlikely to return to the natal area (Cooke, this volume). In most species of mammal, the males are more likely to move away but here again, there are exceptions such as the Chimpanzee (*Pan troglodytes*) (Pusey, 1980). The costs of travel can be quite considerable and usually the distance travelled by the sex that moves is not great. The net effect of restricted movements in one direction and returns by offspring in the next generation could be an overall population that was quite highly inbred. An important question remains whether such a system would be sufficiently finely tuned to preserve the optimal balance between inbreeding and outbreeding. Also, as Greenwood (1980) notes, explanations other than those in terms of inbreeding avoidance are possible for sex differences in dispersal.

Recognition of kin, the other suggested mechanism for optimal outbreeding, could be done in one of two ways. Conceivably the genes that influence an animal's external appearance also directly influence its ability to recognise another animal very much like itself without the involvement of any learning process. More plausibly, the animal learns the characteristics of close kin, or failing that itself, and recognises novel individuals that are similar. Some studies which have been cited in support of the first possibility (e.g. Harvey, 1980) are open to alternative explanations. Wu, Holmes, Medina & Sackett (1980) found that Stump-tail Macaques (*Macaca nemestrina*) preferred novel half-siblings to novel non-siblings in choice tests, although the authors admitted that each monkey might generalise to kin having learned its own characteristics – a process that has already been described in Domestic Chicks (*Gallus gallus*) (Salzen & Cornell, 1968). Indeed, the data given in Wu *et al.*'s paper suggest that the monkeys' ability to discriminate depended on experience since preference for kin was only pronounced in the older monkeys.*

* Wu *et al.* (1980) wrongly discounted the age effect by correlating age with the ratio of time spent near kin to the total time near both stimulus animals and empty cages. This method failed to show a significant correlation. Their reason

Another set of results that is sometimes used as evidence for unlearnt kin recognition mechanisms, comes from studies of genetic variation in the histo-compatibility complex, and its effects on mate choice in male mice (Yamazaki *et al.* 1976, 1978). In some of the experiments males preferred to mate with females differing only in one allele from those of the same genotype as themselves. However, interpretation is complicated because in other experiments males preferred females of their own genotype to those differing by one allele, and in yet others a particular strain of female was preferred over the other by males of both the same genotype and of the other genotype (Andrews & Boyse, 1978; Yamaguchi, Yamazaki & Boyse, 1978). It is possible to make sense of these apparently conflicting data (Bateson, 1979). But the issue in question here is whether they provide any support for the notion of unlearnt recognition of particular genotypes. I think not.

Even though a single allele can affect mate choice, the particular way in which that gene influences recognition has not been examined. If a gene influences the odour of the females, the males may have been exposed to the distinctive odour of sisters when young. Alternatively, the gene may also influence the odour of the males themselves. It remains an open question whether, by self-stimulation or exposure to members of kin of the same genotype, the male mice have acquired a standard against which the odour of females is compared. Furthermore, a growing body of evidence suggests, not only that rodents learn the characteristics of their immediate kin (D'Udine & Alleva, this volume; Dewsbury, 1982) but so do animals in many other taxonomic groups (e.g. Linsenmair & Linsenmair, 1972; Buckle & Greenberg, 1981; Waldman, 1981).

At present no firm evidence supports the view that optimal outbreeding depends on an unlearnt recognition of kin. By contrast, a mounting body of evidence indicates that mating preferences are influenced by early experience with particular individuals who are usually close kin. That this might be the case in humans was first suggested by Westermarck (1891). He believed that satisfying sexual relationships are not formed between

for correlating age with the ratio, rather than with the measure they had already used to demonstrate a preference for kin, was because it controlled for (hypothetical) age differences in mobility. However, using time spent near kin divided by time spent near kin and non-kin – a measure of kin preference which also takes account of age differences in mobility – a clear age-difference can be demonstrated. Dividing the sample in half, the eight younger monkeys had a mean score of 0.48 ± 0.11, and the eight older monkeys had a mean score of 0.77 ± 0.06. The chance level is 0.50 and the older monkeys had a significantly stronger preference for kin than the younger ones ($t = 2.34$, $P < 0.05$).

people who have spent their childhood together. Over the years support has accumulated for his view (e.g. Spiro, 1958; Talmon, 1964; Wolf, 1966; Shepher, 1971) and examples from animal studies have started to multiply.

Aberle *et al.* (1963) noted an example of what they called 'asexual imprinting' in Canada Geese (*Branta canadensis*). They wrote as follows:

> The luckless breeder who takes a male and a female from the same brood to raise geese is doomed to disappointment: the pair will not mate even if no other partners are available. If, however, two members of the same brood are separated before hatching occurs and are subsequently re-introduced to each other, having been raised with different families, they may become mates (p. 259).

I have argued that the disinclination to mate with members of the opposite sex familiar from early life, far from being a separate phenomenon, is part of sexual imprinting (Bateson 1978a, b). As will become apparent, I now think I was wrong to imply that a single learning process is involved. Anyway, in order to understand what happens when a choice of mate occurs, it is helpful to borrow a psychological principle that has been used in the study of aesthetics and perceptual classification (see McClelland & Clarke, 1953; Berlyne, 1960). This states that the most attractive object is one that differs somewhat, but not too much, from a familiar standard. When the principle is applied to the effects of early experience on sexual preferences, it has a satisfying effect of bringing together ideas about mating within the species with those about the avoidance of inbreeding.

The optimal discrepancy hypothesis is shown in Fig. 11.2. Bischof (1972), when considering human mating preferences, proposed a rather similar model. One difference is that his graph of mating preferences plotted against relatedness is symmetrical with maximum inbreeding being avoided as much as hybridisation with another species. The model shown in Fig. 11.2 suggests that, while mating with a parent, sibling or offspring is less preferred than mating with a more distant relative, it is more preferred than mating with another species. Another difference between the models is that Bischof thought that sexual imprinting involves learning the general characteristics of the species, but that at maturity previous attachment to mother and siblings is replaced by active detachment and exploration. I proposed that sexual imprinting sets the standard (or standards) of what immediate kin look like and the animals subsequently prefer to mate with an individual who looks slightly different. Therefore, my model suggests a much finer tuning of sexual preferences than does Bischof's.

Experiments with Japanese Quail (*Coturnix coturnix*) have suggested

that their sexual preferences are, indeed, sharply tuned (Bateson, 1980).
The birds were reared in pseudo-families (groups of individuals not
necessarily related to each other) for the first 30 days after hatching and
then socially isolated until they were sexually mature. They were then given
choices between a familiar member of the opposite sex that had been in
their pseudo-family, and a novel member of the opposite sex drawn at
random from the colony. The stimulus birds were placed behind one-way
screens so that when a test bird spent more time near one of the stimulus
birds than the other, it was unambiguously making the choice. The results
showed that adult male and female Japanese Quail were likely to approach
a member of the opposite sex which they had not seen before, in preference
to one with which they grew up. However, they only did this if the group
in which they were reared when young, contained a particular number of
the opposite sex: two females in the case of males and three males in the
case of females. I explained the result in terms of the likelihood of the novel
member of the opposite sex being slightly different from those with which
the birds grew up. If the number of individuals of the opposite sex was
small, a novel one was likely to be unacceptably strange, and if the number
was high, any novel bird from a limited laboratory stock was likely to

Fig. 11.2. The postulated relationship between the sexual response to
an individual and its degree of novelty relative to familiar objects
which would be kin in natural conditions (Bateson, 1978*b*). A positive
response means sexual approach, and a negative response could mean
escape.

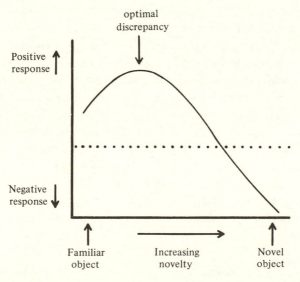

resemble one or other of the familiar birds. These results drew attention to some of the ambiguities in two-way choice tests.

When animals are given choices between two objects, the results of the experiment could depend critically on how different the familiar and novel objects are from each other. The point is illustrated in Fig. 11.3. Depending on how similar the novel object was to the familiar, the same animal might appear either to show a preference for the novel or for the familiar. As we have seen, superficially conflicting results were obtained in experiments with Japanese Quail (Bateson 1978*b*, 1980). Also two studies of female Zebra Finches (*Taeniopygia guttata*) have suggested that when given choices between very close relatives and non-kin, they prefer to approach and mate with close relatives (Miller, 1979; Slater & Clements, 1981). As Slater & Clements (1981) point out, it is not clear whether the female finches would have preferred slightly more distant relatives if given the choice. Uncertainty about how to interpret the result will remain until such experiments have been done.

If the experiments on optimal discrepancy were to move forward, two improvements in technique were desirable. First, it was essential to find a way of placing the stimulus animals used in the choice test on a continuum of increasing dissimilarity from the familiar. Secondly, the true nature of the preference curve was most likely to be revealed if the test animals were given choices between many stimulus animals ranged along the continuum.

With these points in mind, I have used Japanese Quail with pedigrees that were known for at least four generations (Bateson, 1982). It was possible, therefore, to test all birds with a variety of members of the opposite sex that were of different degrees of relationship, but of the same

Fig. 11.3. An illustration of the ambiguities of a two-choice experiment in which the position of the most preferred mate is unknown relative to the familiar and novel test animals.

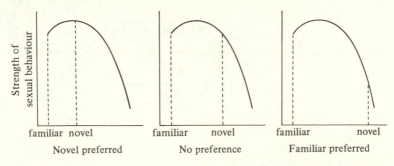

age. On the basis of a study with Bewick's Swans (*Cygnus columbianus*) (Bateson, Lotwick & Scott, 1980), I assumed that genetically related birds would look more alike than unrelated birds. Later I confirmed that the similarity in plumage between Japanese Quail was proportional to the genetic relatedness between them (Bateson, in preparation).

The apparatus used to test the quail was inspired by the work of Sonnemann & Sjölander (1977) who gave female Zebra Finches multiple choices between males. Their apparatus had inward-facing stimulus cages which would have made the use of one-way screens difficult. Since I wanted to use one-way screens, I reversed the arrangement so that the stimulus cages faced outwards and the test bird was able to move freely from one window to the next in the dark, outer part of the apparatus (see Fig. 11.4). In principle, the quail might have been trapped by the first individual they

Fig. 11.4. Apparatus used for testing preferences of adult Japanese Quail. Stimulus birds are put singly in the inner compartments which are painted white and lit from above. The outward-facing windows are fitted with one-way screens. A test bird can move freely round the black unlit outer part of the apparatus. A pedal in front of each window automatically records a test bird's proximity to the window (Bateson, 1982).

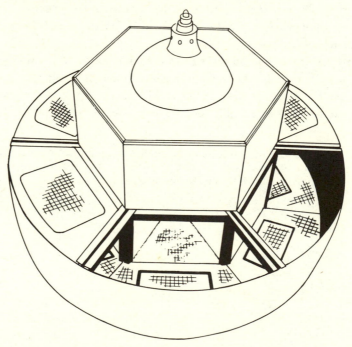

saw and might have stayed in front of one window, but in practice this did not happen.

Since I wanted to minimise the variation within the rearing groups, the quail were reared with true siblings instead of unrelated individuals as in the earlier experiments. They were isolated 30 days after hatching and testing started at 60 days when the quail were sexually mature. Fig. 11.5 (from Bateson, 1982) shows the mean percentage duration spent in front of each category of stimulus bird by both adult males and females. The males were slightly more ready than females to spend time near a third-cousin of the opposite sex. However, the most striking part of the result is that a first-cousin is preferred by both sexes over both familiar and novel siblings and also unrelated birds. Clearly, the birds' sexual preferences were very finely tuned – a result that had been predicted from the earlier experiments. Furthermore, when true siblings were used in the rearing groups (Bateson, 1982), the number of members of the opposite sex in each group was not an important source of variation in the results as it had been in the previous experiment (Bateson, 1980). This was presumably because siblings looked alike and therefore provided similar standards.

Fig. 11.5. The mean percentage time spent by adult Japanese Quail near members of the opposite sex that were either familiar siblings (Sib.), novel siblings, novel first-cousins, novel third-cousins, or novel unrelated individuals. The males ($n = 22$) are shown as triangles and the females ($n = 13$) as circles (Bateson, 1982).

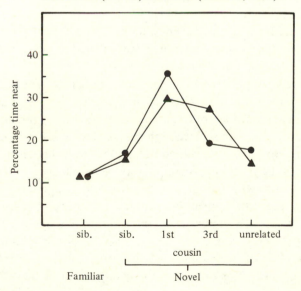

A difficulty about generalising from such laboratory work is that the conditions of rearing and testing the animals are vastly different from the natural world of the wild-living animal. It would not be surprising, for instance, if the effect of restricted experience in both the Quail and Zebra Finch studies was that the birds were more ready to escape from novelty than would be the case in free-living birds. The emphasis on preferences for mating with close-kin could be misleading. Given such uncertainties, it is encouraging that McGregor & Krebs (1982) have found that in wild-living Great Tits (*Parus major*) the mates of females have songs that are slightly different but not too different from the females' fathers.

How could finely tuned sexual preferences arise from early experience? At least four types of explanation might be offered.

(1) *The punishment hypothesis.* Numerous competitions for food and other resources in early development meant that individuals encountered during that period were associated with punishment and, therefore, have become slightly aversive.

(2) *The frustration hypothesis.* Attempts at full-blown sexual behaviour with members of the opposite sex are frustrated in early life by lack of adequate sexual apparatus, or lack of co-operation on the part of the other sex. The individuals with which such frustration is associated, are avoided in later life.

(3) *The sexual boredom hypothesis.* Attempts at sexual behaviour were successful in the sense that copulation was complete. The birds are less strongly aroused by individuals with which they previously mated and, when adult, respond more strongly to others.

(4) *The aesthetic hypothesis.* Responsiveness to the familiar was reduced by mere exposure and consequently individuals that differed slightly from the known standards are most attractive.

Quail do not have reduced preferences for familiar members of their own sex (Bateson, unpublished), a result which makes the first hypothesis less plausible. The second and third hypotheses require careful observation of the young birds prior to isolation and, though contradictory, neither can be totally discounted. However, I do not consider either to be very likely and most favour the last hypothesis. A simple way of producing a finely tuned preference displaced away from the familiar, could be to superimpose habituation on imprinting. Filial imprinting is known to restrict preferences to the familiar (see Bateson, 1979) and sexual imprinting could operate in exactly the same way. Habituation, by contrast, reduces responsiveness to the familiar. The net effect of superimposing one learning process on the other is shown in Fig. 11.6. Not only does the combination of the two learning processes produce a sharply peaked preference for something a bit different from the familiar, it suggests direct ways of experimentally manipulating preferences by influencing one or other of the learning processes.

What happens to the population?

Learning about close kin and choosing a mate that looks a bit different, seem to provide an effective way of striking a balance between inbreeding and outbreeding. However, there is a problem which needs to be thought about clearly. If, in each generation, animals mate with a first-cousin, the population is bound to get more and more inbred (see Baker & Marler, 1980). What is the merit of a mechanism that merely delays a damaging consequence? The answer hinges on whether the visual similarity between close kin and the most preferred mate remains constant irrespective of the degree of inbreeding of the population. If that is the case an interesting safety valve would seem to be built into the optimal discrepancy mechanism. The point can be clarified by considering Fig. 11.7.

Fig. 11.6. A possible way in which a preference for a mate, differing slightly from familiar members of the opposite sex, might be generated. In the idealised case shown here, all the animals along a graded continuum initially have the same value. Imprinting reduces responsiveness to the novel and habituation reduces responsiveness to the familiar. The shaded part represents the area under the resulting preference curve.

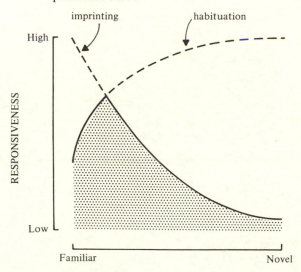

In a totally inbred population all individuals will be identical. In an outbred population individuals sharing common parents (siblings) would be more like each other than those sharing two common grand-parents (first-cousins). In the simplest case considered in Fig. 11.7 where the individual chooses a mate slightly different from its one sibling of the opposite sex, the number of immediate forebears shared with a preferred mate will vary with how inbred a population is. Mating with kin, however, closely related, increases the frequency of gene loci that are homozygous in offspring, so optimal discrepancy mating will make the population more inbred as Baker & Marler (1980) argued. Nevertheless, the move towards complete homozygosity, which is asymptotic even in matings between siblings generation after generation (Crow & Kimura, 1970), would be slowed down considerably in a species employing an optimal discrepancy system. If the population became too inbred, a member of it might be unable to find a mate that was sufficiently dissimilar to its siblings. This might provide the trigger for members of one or other of the sexes to move out of the natal area in search of optimally discrepant mates. What is promising about this line of thought is that it begins to provide ways of explaining variation in patterns of mating and the probability of dispersal in terms of the genetic structure of the population.

Fig. 11.7. The postulated relationships between the inbredness of a population and the likely differences in appearance between an individual and three other members of the population (sibling, first-cousin, and unrelated). If the individual is familiar with its one sibling (in this simplified case), the most preferred mate is shown by the dashed line.

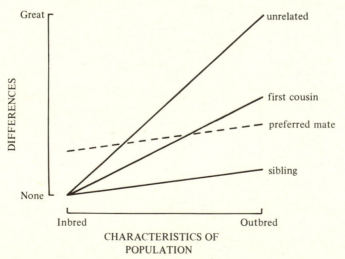

A different point relates to evolutionary theories that have accumulated around the idea that sexual imprinting might influence speciation. Many theoreticians have explored the possibility that, by being imprinted with parents and preferring to mate with an individual looking like the parents, two morphs of the same species could become reproductively isolated from each other (reviewed by Immelmann, 1975). All this work took as axiomatic the classical view of imprinting that the preferred mate closely resembles the individual to which the bird was exposed early in life. However, the evidence that birds choose mates differing somewhat from familiar individuals suggests that the assumption may have been wrong. Scudo (1976) foresaw some of the complications that would be introduced by assortative mating that was neither wholly positive nor wholly negative. Now that we have some data suggesting where the balance may be struck, the theories for speciation by imprinting need to be re-worked.

Conclusion

The evidence for optimal outbreeding is still relatively meagre. Furthermore, many of the proposals for selection pressures, that supposedly lead to the evolution of optimal outbreeding mechanisms, are the product of little more than guess work. Nonetheless, the ideas have had an invigorating effect on studies of sexual imprinting in birds in particular and the ontogeny of sexual preferences generally. The classical view of Konrad Lorenz (1935) that sexual imprinting was concerned with species recognition held sway until the last year or two and, indeed, a whole book of essays was recently devoted to the topic of species recognition (Roy, 1980). The idea that first and foremost mating preferences are based on kin recognition is, of course, much more in line with modern evolutionary theory. Nevertheless, it might still have been the case that so long as birds avoided close kin and members of other species, they showed no further restriction of their sexual preferences. While some species may yet prove to have rather broad preferences, we have seen that the sexual preferences of Japanese Quail are remarkably finely tuned by their early experience and the same is probably true for the Zebra Finch (Slater & Clements, 1981) and the House Mouse (D'Udine & Alleva, this volume). These findings give greater weight to the view that finding a mate of an optimum degree of relatedness is of great importance, at least to some animals. To test this idea properly requires field experiments of outbreeding depression. These experiments are not easy to do but at least we now have good reasons for making the effort.

A brief comment is required on the term 'optimal inbreeding' which

Shields (1982) uses instead of the one I coined. The justification for the change seems to be that since some populations are markedly inbred, 'optimal inbreeding' characterises mating in such organisms more satisfactorily. To be set against this, it would be highly misleading to suggest that *all* populations are inbred. Furthermore, since the notion that inbreeding is 'bad' is so deeply ingrained in many people's minds, it seems wiser to preserve 'optimal outbreeding' which represents the more congenial departure from conventional thought. Nonetheless, the important issue is optimal *balance* and a terminological argument that distracted from this point would be unproductive.

The selection pressures pushing both towards and away from inbreeding, are likely to be numerous and varied. Each one may vary in importance from one species to the next. Therefore, the precise balance (or in some cases, balances) will almost certainly vary between animals. Even within a species, the balance is likely to depend on local conditions and on how inbred a population has become. Finally, the sexes may differ, especially when one sex is likely to have more matings than the other. Nonetheless, a general point remains. In choosing a mate an animal may have to pay careful attention to, among other things, similarities between its proposed partner and close kin. When sexual preferences are measured, this possible influence along with many others, must be considered.

Summary

1 Animals may have to strike an optimal balance between inbreeding and outbreeding when choosing a mate. The costs of both inbreeding and outbreeding are likely to be numerous and varied. Not all the costs are genetic in character and even some of the genetic costs could not be readily assessed by laboratory breeding experiments.

2 Two mechanisms for optimal outbreeding are considered. The first involves one sex moving away from the natal area. The second involves recognition of optimally discrepant kin. Both mechanisms may be used in the same species.

3 No firm evidence supports the view that optimal outbreeding depends on an unlearnt recognition of kin. By contrast, a growing body of data suggests that mating preferences are influenced by early experience with particular individuals that are usually close kin. In birds, the learning process is known as 'sexual imprinting'.

4 Experiments with Japanese Quail indicate that sexual preferences are finely tuned by their early experience with members of the

opposite sex. After being reared with siblings, the majority of the quail preferred a novel first cousin. This was true in both males and females.

5 Fine tuning of sexual preferences may be accomplished by a combination of two learning processes. The imprinting process is known to reduce responsiveness to novel animals and an habituation process could reduce responsiveness to familiar animals. The combined effect would be a preference slightly displaced away from the familiar.

6 The optimal outbreeding mechanism slows down the rate at which a population becomes inbred and may eventually act as a safety valve so that one sex moves out of the population in search of an optimally discrepant mate.

I am very grateful to Brian Charlesworth, Tim Clutton-Brock, Nick Davies, Richard Dawkins, Linda Partridge and Michael Reiss for kindly commenting on an earlier version of the chapter.

References

Aberle, D. F., Bronfenbrenner, J., Hess, E. H., Miller, D. R., Schneider, D. M. & Spuhler, J. N. (1963). The incest taboo and the mating patterns of animals. *American Anthropologist*, **65**, 253–65.

Alexander, R. D. (1977). Natural selection and the analysis of human sociality. In *Changing Scenes in Natural Sciences, 1776–1976*, ed. C. E. Goulden, pp. 283–337. Academy of Natural Sciences: Philadelphia.

Andrews, P. W. & Boyse, E. A. (1978). Mapping of an H-2-linked gene that influences mating preference in mice. *Immunogenetics*, **6**, 265–8.

Baker, M. C. & Marler, P. (1980). Behavioral adaptations that constrain the gene pool in vertebrates. In *Evolution of Social Behavior: Hypotheses and Empirical Tests*, Dahlem Konferenzen 1980, ed. H. Markl, pp. 59–80. Verlag Chemie Gmbh.: Weinheim.

Bateson, P. P. G. (1978a). Early experience and sexual preferences. In *Biological Determinants of Sexual Behaviour*, ed. J. B. Hutchison, pp. 29–53. Wiley: Chichester.

Bateson, P. (1978b). Sexual imprinting and optimal outbreeding. *Nature*, **273**, 659–60.

Bateson, P. (1979). How do sensitive periods arise and what are they for? *Animal Behaviour*, **27**, 470–86.

Bateson, P. (1980). Optimal outbreeding and the development of sexual preferences in Japanese Quail. *Zeitschrift für Tierpsychologie*, **53**, 231–44.

Bateson, P. (1982). Preferences for cousins in Japanese quail. *Nature*, **295**, 236–7.

Bateson, P., Lotwick, W. & Scott, D. K. (1980). Similarities between the faces of parents and offspring in Bewick's swan and the differences between mates. *Journal of Zoology, London*, **191**, 61–74.

Bengtsson, B. O. (1978). Avoiding inbreeding: at what cost? *Journal of Theoretical Biology*, **73**, 439–44.

Berlyne, D. E. (1960). *Conflict, Arousal and Curiosity*. McGraw-Hill: New York.

Bischof, N. (1972). The biological foundations of the incest taboo. *Social Sciences Information*, **11**, 7–36.

Buckle, G. R. & Greenberg, L. (1981). Nestmate recognition in sweat bees (*Lasioglossum zephyrum*); does an individual recognise its own odour or only odours of its nestmates. *Animal Behaviour*, **29**, 802–9.

Crow, J. F. & Kimura, M. (1970). *An Introduction to Population Genetics Theory*. Harper & Row: New York.

Cowan, D. P. (1979). Sibling matings in a hunting wasp: adaptive inbreeding. *Science*, **205**, 1403–5.

Dawkins, R. (1979). Twelve misunderstandings of kin selection. *Zeitschrift für Tierpsychologie*, **51**, 184–200.

Dewsbury, D. A. (1982). Avoidance of brother-sister incestuous breeding in two species. *Biology of Behaviour*, **7**, 157–69.

Festing, M. F. W. (1976). Phenotypic variability of inbred and outbred mice. *Nature*, **263**, 230–2.

Greenwood, P. J. (1980). Mating systems, philopatry and dispersal in birds and mammals. *Animal Behaviour*, **28**, 1140–62.

Harvey, P. H. (1980). Mechanisms of kin-correlated behaviour group report. In *Evolution of Social Behavior: Hypotheses and Empirical Tests*, Dahlem Konferenzen 1980, ed. H. Markl, pp. 183–202. Verlag Chemie Gmbh.: Weinheim.

Immelmann, K. (1975). Ecological significance of imprinting and early learning. *Annual Review of Ecology and Systematics*, **6**, 15–37.

Linsenmair, K. E. & Linsenmair, C. (1972). Die Bedeutung familienspezifischer "Abzeichen" fur den Familienzusammenhalt bei der sozialen Wüstenassel *Hemilepistus reaumuri* Audouin u. Savigny (Crustacea, Isopoda, Oniscoidea). *Zeitschrift für Tierpsychologie*, **31**, 131–62.

Lorenz, K. (1935). Der Kumpan in der Umvelt des Vogels. *Journal für Ornithologie*, **83**, 137–213; 289–413.

Maynard Smith, J. (1978). *The Evolution of Sex*. Cambridge University Press: Cambridge.

McClelland, D. C. & Clarke, R. A. (1953). Discrepancy hypothesis. In *The Achievement Motive*, ed. D. C. McClelland, J. W. Atkinson, R. A. Clark & E. L. Lowell, pp. 42–66. Appleton-Century-Crofts: New York.

McGregor, P. K. & Krebs, J. R. (1982). Mating and song types in the great tit. *Nature*, **297**, 60–1.

Miller, D. B. (1979). Long-term recognition of father's song by female zebra finches. *Nature*, **280**, 389–91.

Mourant, A. E., Kopec, A. C. & Domaniewska-Sobczak, K. (1976). *The Distribution of the Human Blood Groups and Other Polymorphisms*. Oxford University Press: London.

Noordwijk, A. J. van & Scharloo, W. (1981). Inbreeding in an island population of the great tit. *Evolution*, **35**, 674–88.

Parker, G. A. (1979). Sexual selection and sexual conflict. In *Sexual Selection and Reproductive Competition in Insects*, ed. M. S. Blum & N. A. Blum, pp. 123–66. Academic Press: New York.

Price, M. V. & Waser, N. M. (1979). Pollen dispersal and optimal out-crossing in *Delphinium nelsoni*. *Nature*, **277**, 294–7.

Pusey, A. E. (1980). Inbreeding avoidance in chimpanzees. *Animal Behaviour*, **28**, 543–52.

Roy, M. A. (1980). *Species Identity and Attachment: A Phylogenetic Evaluation*. Garland: New York.

Salzen, E. A. & Cornell, J. M. (1968). Self-perception and species recognition in birds. *Behaviour*, **30**, 44–65.

Scudo, F. M. (1976). "Imprinting", speciation and avoidance of inbreeding. *Evolutionary Biology*, Prague, pp. 375–92.

Shepher, J. (1971). Mate selection among second generation kibbutz adolescents and adults: Incest avoidance and negative imprinting. *Archives of Sexual Behavior*, **1**, 293–307.

Shields, W. M. (1983). Optimal inbreeding and the evolution of philopatry. In *The Ecology of Animal Movement*, ed. I. R. Swingland & P. J. Greenwood, pp. 132–59. Oxford University Press: Oxford.

Slater, P. J. B. & Clements, F. A. (1981). Incestuous mating in zebra finches. *Zeitschrift für Tierpsychologie*, **57**, 201–8.

Smith, R. H. (1979). On selection for inbreeding in polygynous animals. *Heredity*, **43**, 205–11.

Sonnemann, P. & Sjölander, S. (1977). Effects of cross-fostering on the sexual imprinting of the female zebra finch *Taeniopygia guttata. Zeitschrift für Tierpsychologie*, **45**, 337–48.

Spiro, M. E. (1958). *Children of the Kibbutz*. Harvard University Press: Cambridge, Mass.

Talmon, Y. (1964). Mate selection in collective settlements. *American Sociological Review*, **29**, 491–508.

Thiessen, D. & Gregg, B. (1980). Human assortative mating and genetic equilibrium: an evolutionary perspective. *Ethology & Sociobiology*, **1**, 111–40.

Turkington, R. & Harper, J. L. (1979). The growth, distribution and neighbour relationships of *Trifolium repens* in a permanent pasture. IV. Fine-scale biotic differentiation. *Journal of Ecology*, **67**, 245–54.

Waldman, B. (1981). Sibling recognition in toad tadpoles: the role of experience. *Zeitschrift für Tierpsychologie*, **56**, 341–58.

Westermarck, E. (1891). *The History of Human Marriage*. Macmillan: London.

Williams, G. C. (1975). *Sex and Evolution*. Princeton University Press: Princeton.

Wolf, A. P. (1966). Childhood association, sexual attraction and the incest taboo: a Chinese case. *American Anthropologist*, **68**, 883–98.

Wright, S. (1933). The roles of mutation, inbreeding, crossbreeding and selection in evolution. *Proceedings of the VIth International Congress on Genetics*, vol. **1**, ed. D. F. Jones, pp. 356–66. Brooklyn Botanic Garden: New York.

Wu, H. M. H., Holmes, W. G., Medina, S. R. & Sackett, G. P. (1980). Kin preference in infant *Macaca nemestrina. Nature*, **285**, 225–7.

Yamaguchi, M., Yamazaki, K. & Boyse, E. A. (1978). Mating preference tests with the recombinant congenic strain BALB.HTG. Immunogenetics, **6**, 261–4.

Yamazaki, K., Boyse, A. E., Miké, V., Thaler, H. T., Mathieson, B. J., Abbott, J., Boyse, J., Zayas, Z. A. & Thomas, L. (1976). Control of mating preferences in mice by genes in the major histocompatibility complex. *Journal of Experimental Medicine*, **144**, 1324–35.

Yamazaki, K., Yamaguchi, M., Andrews, P. W., Peake, B. & Boyse, E. A. (1978). Mating preference of F_2 segregants of crosses between MHC-congenic mouse strains. *Immunogenetics*, **6**, 253–9.

12

Assortative mating, mate choice and reproductive fitness in Snow Geese

F. COOKE AND J. C. DAVIES

For biologists interested in the question of mate choice, it is important to ascertain whether choices are in fact being made in the wild (and if so, what the choices are) and whether there is any selective advantage in making a 'correct' choice.

These are difficult objectives to achieve and require both a careful choice of study organism and a willingness to spend many years working on a single population. The work we are going to describe was carried out on a population of 2000–4000 pairs of Lesser Snow Geese breeding in the Canadian Arctic at La Perouse Bay in Northern Manitoba. The work started in 1968 and has continued up to the time of writing. Snow Geese occur in two distinctive colour morphs, white and dark grey (the 'Blue' goose), and as shown by Cooch & Beardmore (1959), there is assortative mating on the basis of colour. These observations suggested that birds may be using plumage colour as a criterion for mate choice.

There has long been confusion regarding the distinctions between sexual selection, assortative mating and mate choice and at least part of this confusion relates to the criteria by which a mate is chosen. In Darwin's (1871) classical definition of the intrasexual component of sexual selection, he imagined that some members of one sex carried a set of phenotypic attributes which made them preferable as mates to all members of the other sex. As such, they would achieve a larger proportion of the copulations and produce more offspring, leading to directional selection favouring those genotypes with the preferred characteristics and, other factors being equal, to a reduction in the genetic variability for the preferred attributes. As Fisher (1930) pointed out, if this led to the fixation of those alleles coding for the preferred attributes, sexual selection could not be effective since selection cannot act without genetic variability. O'Donald (1980)

279

attempted to circumvent this paradoxical conclusion by proposing that while sexual selection in Arctic Skuas favoured the melanic morph, genetic variability was maintained due to countervailing natural selection favouring the pale morph.

In contrast to this classical model of sexual selection, recent authors have drawn attention to mate choices based not on some universally preferred character, but to some quality of the mate's phenotype in relation to the chooser's phenotype. A mate may be chosen on the basis of its perceived phenotypic similarity or dissimilarity to the chooser, rather than to some overall suitability. This is the basis of Bateson's (1978, this volume) Optimal Discrepancy Theory and of the writings of Shields on Inbreeding and Outbreeding Depression (1983). A human example will perhaps clarify the distinction. A man may have a sister who is perceived by the majority of the male population to have attributes which make her an ideal marriage partner. It would nevertheless be unwise for him to marry her because of the potential genetic problems of inbreeding. In animals we assume that mates may be chosen on the basis of either or both of the above criteria, and this could lead to some non-random mating at the population level. Various models of choice and their population consequences are examined in detail by O'Donald (1980, this volume). If choices are being made they do not lead necessarily to non-random mating but it seems reasonable when studying the question of mate choice to examine a population in which non-random mating has been demonstrated.

For researchers attempting to demonstrate mate choice and its evolutionary consequences we suggest that the following five questions be considered.

(1) Is there evidence of non-random mating in relation to some phenotypic character?

(2) Does the non-random mating necessarily imply mate choice?

(3) Is the choice based on the character itself?

(4) Is there genetic variability in the population for the character?

(5) Is there a selective advantage in making the correct choice? Is the choice adaptive?

Most of these questions are difficult to answer, and to our knowledge, no field study on mate choice to date can answer all of these questions. The long-term study by Peter O'Donald on the Arctic Skua (*Stercorarius parasiticus*) population on Fair Isle has provided valuable insights into the question of mate choice but has failed to give unequivocal answers to questions (2) and (3). In our opinion the data for the Snow Goose population at La Perouse Bay come closest to answering the questions, though they provide what superficially may seem to be a surprising answer to question (5).

There are several advantages to working with Snow Geese. Since the Snow Goose nests colonially, it is possible to monitor large numbers of individuals. We collect data on 1500–2500 pairs each season and this large sample allows us to detect even rare events and small differences in reproductive fitness. Moreover, because the Snow Goose is a species of considerable economic importance, much is known about its biology at various stages of its life cycle. It is possible therefore to obtain such basic measurements as clutch size and fledging success and also first year survival, adult survival and age of first breeding. This gives a much more complete picture of the relative fitness of different phenotypes than is possible in most studies. Snow Geese mate for life and thus fitness measures can be obtained not only for known birds for several successive years but also for known pairs. The consequences of mate changes can also be assessed.

Another advantage of working with geese is that they can be readily kept in captivity, thus allowing manipulation under more controlled conditions.

There are a number of disadvantages also. Mate choice occurs very rarely on the breeding grounds. Birds pair in the wintering area of the Gulf coasts of Texas and Louisiana or during the spring migration and so observations on the actual process of pair formation are not possible. Thus, we can observe those birds that did successfully form pairs, but have no knowledge of unsuccessful attempts at pair formation. Problems arise because although the philopatry of female Snow Geese is strong, that of males is not. Most of the female goslings that survive to breeding age return to breed at La Perouse Bay, but very few male goslings do so. This is a consequence of pair formation occurring away from the breeding ground when birds from different breeding colonies associate together in large flocks (Cooke, MacInnes & Prevett, 1975).

We will now review the evidence for mate choice in Snow Geese. This will be related primarily to choice based on plumage colour, but later in the chapter we consider briefly the effect of body size on mate choice. The evidence from the La Perouse Bay colony will be reviewed in relation to the five questions listed above.

Plumage colour

(1) *Is there evidence of non-random mating?*

Cooch & Beardmore (1959) showed that at Boas River, Southampton Island in the North West Territories, Canada, far fewer mixed pairs occurred than would be expected on the basis of random mate choice in terms of plumage colour. Table 12.1 shows a similar situation at the La Perouse Bay colony for 13 years. With random mating, one would expect approximately 39% rather than 15–19%, of all pairs to be mixed. The discrepancy is strong evidence of non-random mating with respect to plumage colour. In addition, we see that the two types of mixed pairs, blue female × white male and blue male × white female are not equally frequent. When mixed pairs occur, it is more likely that the male will be blue. The significance of this will be discussed later when we consider possible sexual differences in mate choice.

(2) Does the non-random mating necessarily imply mate choice?

Just because we observe non-random mating in terms of plumage colour, we cannot automatically assume that the birds are necessarily making a choice. If, for example, the blue morphs wintered predominantly in one area and the white morphs in another and mating occurred at random in the different wintering areas, then this would lead to paucity of mixed pairs on the colony. Birds would be choosing at random, but birds

Table 12.1. *Pair bond frequencies and phase ratio of blue and white Lesser Snow Geese at La Perouse Bay, Manitoba 1968–1980*

Year	W × W No.	W × W %	B♀ × W♂ No.	B♀ × W♂ %	W♀ × B♂ No.	W♀ × B♂ %	B × B No.	B × B %	% Blue phase
1968	242	63	20	5	53	14	70	18	28
1969	439	70	36	6	55	9	98	16	23
1970	619	67	55	6	92	10	162	17	25
1971	411	68	28	5	63	10	102	17	24
1972	850	66	80	7	125	10	231	18	26
1973	929	65	91	6	144	10	272	19	27
1974	900	64	85	6	137	10	279	20	28
1975	947	64	99	7	146	9	286	20	28
1976	893	63	113	8	134	10	271	19	28
1977	984	62	129	8	165	10	310	20	29
1978	1039	64	133	8	150	9	292	18	27
1979	950	65	113	9	143	10	261	18	27
1980	1089	65	143	9	150	9	290	17	26

Updated from Cooke, 1978.

of a similar colour would be available where the choices were being made. There is some evidence (Lemieux & Heyland 1967; Cooke *et al.*, 1975) that blue phase birds have a more easterly wintering distribution on the whole than the white phase birds, although there is considerable overlap, and both colour phases can be found along the entire Gulf coast wintering area. Cooke, Finney & Rockwell (1976) drew attention to this alternative explanation for the non-random mating pattern and referred to the alternative hypotheses as 'preference' where a choice is postulated and 'prevalence' where differential availability of mates is sufficient to explain the pattern. This has also been referred to as 'active' or 'passive' mate choice. 'Passive' choice seems to be a contradiction in terms. Other workers such as Coulson & Thomas (this volume) studying Kittiwakes (*Rissa tridactyla*) explained non-random mating as a function of differential availability of birds of a suitable age. Birkhead & Clarkson (1980) explain the non-random mating of *Gammarus pulex* in terms of body size by suggesting that animals of a certain size choose a particular type of substrate and mate randomly within that substrate type.

To show that Snow Geese were actively choosing on the basis of colour, we conducted studies on mated pairs under both field and experimental conditions. These studies have been reported elsewhere (Cooke, Mirsky & Seiger, 1972; Cooke & McNally, 1975; Cooke *et al.*, 1976; Cooke, 1978), and we will give only a brief summary here.

The studies arose from the hypothesis that Snow Geese choose their mates not on the basis of their own colour, but rather according to the plumage colour of their parents. It was assumed that during the pre-pairing period, juveniles learned the plumage of their parents and subsequently paired with a mate of a similar colour. Thus birds with white parents would choose a white mate, those with blue parents would prefer a blue mate and those that had one parent of each colour would choose a mate of either colour. This hypothesis was originally developed by Cooke & Cooch (1968) because of anomalies in the genetic segregation ratios of various Snow Goose crosses. If the geese do indeed show such colour preference as a result of some learned experience prior to mate choice, it should be possible to demonstrate this in both field and laboratory situations.

In the field, this involved: (1) finding a large number of nests (approximately 2000 per year) and recording the colour phase of the parents; (2) individually marking the goslings, such that we would have a record of the colour of their parents; and (3) waiting at least two years until some of the birds returned with a mate and recording the colour phase of the mate. This natural experiment took a considerable time and large numbers of goslings had to be marked in order to have an adequate sample size. Fig. 12.1 shows the mate choice of geese in relation to the plumage colour of their parents. Birds of white parentage usually returned with white mates, those of blue parentage with blue mates, and birds of mixed parentage with mates of either colour with approximately 60% having white mates and 40% blue mates. This 6:4 ratio is approximately the ratio of the two colour phases in that part of the Gulf Coast wintering area frequented by birds from La Perouse Bay.

The data in Fig. 12.1 suggest strongly that parental colour influences subsequent mate choice but other explanations are possible. Because of the genetic basis of colour, the offspring of white parents are themselves usually white coloured and so one might get similar results if the birds were to choose mates similar to their own colour. However, this is not the case, since offspring from mixed parents often choose mates of a colour opposite to their own.

Field observations, while suggestive, could not completely rule out choice based on prevalence. A laboratory experiment which consisted of raising incubator-hatched snow goslings with various combinations of parental and sibling colouration was described by Cooke *et al.* (1976). The results showed choice patterns very similar to those obtained in the wild and thus indicated that there was colour preference. They also showed that sibling colour influenced subsequent mate choice, a finding which would

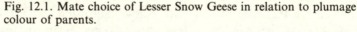

Fig. 12.1. Mate choice of Lesser Snow Geese in relation to plumage colour of parents.

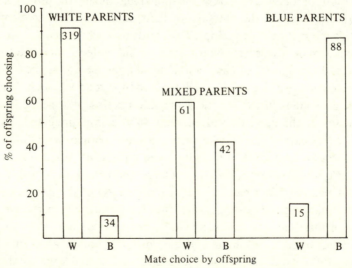

have been difficult to detect in the field. This necessitated a revision of the original hypothesis to state that family colour (parents and/or siblings) influences subsequent mate choice.

As further proof that the assortative mating pattern really does indicate mate choice, a large group of incubator-hatched goslings of both colours were raised in a mixed flock and allowed to choose their mates. There was no evidence of assortative mating in this population. Thus, we concluded that the assortative mating pattern found in Snow Geese does indeed indicate that the birds are making choices.

Are there differences in mate choice among the two sexes? It has been shown that among goslings of mixed parentage, neither parent was more important than the other in influencing the mate choice of its offspring (Cooke, 1978). We have also investigated the influence of sex on mate choice. In Snow Geese, both parents play an active role in parental care. Although only the female incubates, the male stands guard throughout the incubation period and both sexes defend the young. The pair bond is maintained throughout the year and juveniles remain with their parents throughout the first year of life (Prevett, 1972). Snow Geese mate for life and 'divorce' is apparently rare (Cooke, Bousfield & Sadura, 1981). From these facts one would deduce that the investment of each parent is considerable and that for each sex it would be adaptive to choose correctly. One would expect that choices would be made by both sexes during the pairing process. Copulations outside the pair bond do occur occasionally with males occasionally copulating with females from nearby nests (Mineau & Cooke, 1979). Since these are initiated by males, one might expect them to be slightly less choosy than females.

Males return to their natal colony much less frequently than females, and thus it has been difficult to obtain an adequate male sample size to test the relative choosiness of the two sexes. It will be noted from Fig. 12.1 that a small proportion of birds choose a mate of the opposite colour to that of their parents. Thirty-four offspring of white parents chose a blue mate and 15 offspring of blue parents chose a white mate. If one classifies these choices as 'incorrect' (according to the mating scheme) then one can compare the frequency of 'incorrect' choices among the two sexes. Ten per cent of 435 females and 24% of 21 males of known parentage chose 'incorrectly'. While differences between the sexes are significant ($P < 0.05$), they are based on too small a male sample to draw firm conclusions. We can, however, say that at least one of the sexes is choosing on the basis of colour, and if only one sex is choosy, it is likely to be the female.

Another difference between the sexes has been mentioned previously. Among mixed pairs in the colony, blue ♂ × white ♀ pairs are significantly more frequent than the reciprocal (Table 12.1). Does this tell us anything about mate choice? O'Donald (1980) has explained the non-random mating pattern in Arctic Skuas by postulating sexual preferences by female skuas for dark phase male skuas. Assuming that this preference leads to some light phase males obtaining no mate at all, one might expect an asymmetry with an excess of dark males among mixed pairs. An alternative hypothesis to explain our findings involves not sexual selection, but gene flow. Pair bonds form away from the breeding colonies, at a time when birds from different breeding colonies are intermingled. If birds from two different breeding colonies pair, one of the birds must go to a non-natal colony. In Snow Geese, the pair usually returns to the natal colony of the female. Thus most immigrants to the La Perouse Bay colony are males and because La Perouse Bay is a small community relative to the total wintering population, most males are immigrants. If the phase ratio of immigrants is different from that of non-immigrants, this would result in a different phase ratio among the two sexes and thus asymmetry between the two types of mixed pairs. Snow Goose colonies differ considerably in phase ratio (Dzubin, Boyd & Stephen, 1973) with westerly colonies (such as La Perouse Bay) having an excess of white birds, and easterly colonies (such as Cape Henrietta Maria) having more blues (Table 12.2). In the Gulf coast wintering grounds there is probably a slight excess of whites. Thus immigrants (which are males) into the La Perouse Bay colony would in general have a higher frequency of blue phase birds than the non-immigrants (which are female). This would result in an excess of blue ♂ × white ♀ crosses among the mixed pairs.

To discriminate between these alternative hypotheses one needs only to look at the types of mixed pairs at other colonies. If sexual selection is

Table 12.2. *Mixed pair ratios in relation to phase ratios in different Lesser Snow goose colonies*

Colony	% white phase	Ratio W♀B♂/B♀W♂
Baffin Island	15.0	0.10
Cape Henrietta Maria	31.0	0.40
Southampton Island	63.5	1.14
La Perouse Bay	73.4	1.45

operating throughout the breeding range of the Snow Goose then all colonies should show an excess of blue males among the mixed pairs. If the gene flow hypothesis is correct, then at the predominantly blue phase colonies of the Eastern Arctic white♂ × blue ♀ crosses should predominate among the mixed pairs. Data from the predominantly blue phase Snow Goose colony at Cape Henrietta Maria in Northern Ontario, generously donated by Dr. J. P. Prevett, are shown in Table 12.3. One can readily see that the pattern of mixed pairs is the opposite to that observed at La Perouse Bay. White ♂ × blue ♀ crosses greatly outnumber the reciprocal crosses. Fig. 12.2 summarises the data from other Snow Goose colonies, and shows a reasonably straightforward relationship between the phase

Table 12.3. *Pair bond types at Cape Henrietta Maria, Ontario 1979, 1980*

Year	W × W	W♂ × B♀	B♂ × W♀	B × B	W × B sex unknown	% blue
1979	213	79	33	526	25	68
1980	257	107	40	722	32	70

Data by courtesy of J. P. Prevett.

Fig. 12.2. Mixed pair ratios in relation to phase ratios in different Lesser Snow Goose colonies.

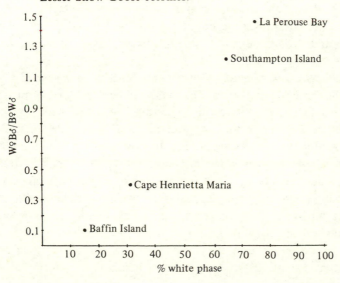

ratio of the colony and the relative frequency of the two types of mixed pairs. This is consistent with the gene flow hypothesis and provides no support for the sexual selection hypothesis.

It appears then that in Snow Geese there is no evidence of a global preference for a particular plumage colour as postulated by O'Donald for Arctic Skuas, but the non-random mating pattern among mixed pairs reflects immigration by males, whose phase ratio differs from that of the non-immigrant females.

To summarise, the second question – does the non-random mating in Snow Geese imply mate choice – can be answered affirmatively and we have provided indications that female choice is stronger than male choice. There is no evidence of an overall preference for a particular plumage colour.

(3) *Is mate choice based on the character itself?*

If sexual selection were operating, a gene would increase in frequency if the character, or pleiotropically related characters, were being chosen preferentially. To determine whether plumage colour was the relevant character in mate choice, we dyed several white phase birds pink and monitored the approach response of goslings to unknown geese of either blue, white or pink plumage in relation to the plumage of the goslings' parents. In all these experiments, goslings including those with pink-dyed parents preferentially approached geese of similar plumage colour to their parents, thus indicating preference for the colour itself. These results, described in more detail by Cooke & McNally (1975), showed that approach response choices are indeed based on plumage colour *per se* and strongly suggest that this is true for mate choice as well.

(4) *Is there genetic variability for the character in question?*

If the variability of a trait on which choice is based is purely environmental, then selection cannot operate. Selection acts on the additive genetic component of phenotypic variance. If one can demonstrate genetic variability it becomes legitimate to consider the evolutionary consequences of potential changes in the frequency of particular characters. Many of the studies involving assortative mating by size are in organisms with indeterminate growth patterns, such that size is age-dependent (e.g. fish and amphibians). Thus the additive genetic component of size variation may be small, and although the experiments may tell us something of mate choice, they tell us little about sexual selection *per se*. It is important for those studying mate choice in organisms with indeterminate growth to try to differentiate between the genetical and non-genetical causes of size variation.

Fortunately the genetic basis of plumage colouration in geese is well known (Cooke & Cooch, 1968; Cooke, Mirsky & Seiger, 1972), The blue plumage colour is a consequence of a semidominant allele B; such that homozygotes BB and heterozygotes Bb have blue plumage, homozygous recessives are white. A recent analysis by Rattray (1981) has confirmed this interpretation using the large data base from La Perouse Bay. Since the phenotypic variation reflects underlying genetic variability, there could indeed be evolutionary consequences of mate choice processes in Snow Geese.

(5) *Is there any selective advantage in making the correct choice?*

From an evolutionary perspective, it would be satisfying if we could demonstrate that mate choice affected an individual's fitness. However, even if no selective advantages were detected, it could be argued that an advantage to correct choice had occurred in the past, or that some component of fitness had not been measured.

With Snow Geese, we have shown that there is not an overall preference for a particular colour (as would be expected in sexual selection), but a preference determined by the pre-pairing experience of the geese. Some geese prefer a white mate, others a blue mate. Nevertheless, some birds, despite being raised in a family of a particular plumage colour, have chosen (and/or been chosen by) a bird of the opposite colour. Geramita, Cooke & Rockwell (in press) have shown, using a modelling approach, that a large proportion of mixed pairs on the colony arise as a result of choosing a mate not of the family colour. If there is any selective disadvantage in making an incorrect choice, this should show up in lowered reproductive fitness amongst the mixed pairs when compared with pure pairs. Smith (1979) investigated reproductive fitness measures between the two colour phases and between the four pair types by comparing clutch size, egg loss, nest loss, fledging success, first year and adult survival for all years where adequate data were available. While white phase females produced a larger average clutch than blue phase females, they also suffered increased post-hatch gosling mortality. As a result, the average brood size at fledging of families of all four pair types did not differ. There were no differences detected in the post fledging or adult mortality of offspring of mixed pairs compared to pure pairs. Offspring from mixed pairs entered the breeding population as frequently as those of pure pairs. Large sample sizes were available throughout the study and yet there was no evidence of reduced reproductive fitness of mixed pairs, and thus no evidence that incorrect choice results in any reproductive penalty.

Evolutionarily, these results are rather surprising. There are, however, several possible explanations. When studying mate choice, it is important to be aware of the distinction between intra- and interspecific mechanisms for choice. The penalties for an animal that chooses a mate of the wrong species is usually genetical death. An animal that chooses a less suitable member of its own species may incur only a slight penalty. It might be imagined, therefore, that mate choice mechanisms have evolved largely as a result of selection against interspecific matings (Lorenz, 1935) and the actual choice of a mate within a species is a relatively unimportant extension of the species recognition mechanism. Lorenz also proposed that the most important function of sexual imprinting was to enable the animal to recognise members of its own species. The young animal must be able to generalise from the particular appearance of its own parents to species-specific characters. Such a mechanism more finely tuned might assist the animal to discriminate intraspecifically.

The geographical co-occurrence of the two Snow Goose colour phases may be a recent event. As mentioned earlier, the blue phase birds predominate in the eastern Arctic breeding areas and in the Louisiana wintering grounds; the white phase birds are more prevalent in the western Arctic and in Texas. This difference was much more pronounced in the eighteenth century when Graham (1768) reported

> 'At Prince of Wales, York and Severn Settlements [Western Hudson Bay] are killed yearly above ten thousand of these [white] geese only. The blue geese are the size, shape and make of the white geese and are as numerous at Albany, Moose and East-main settlements [more easterly locations] as the white geese are at Prince of Wales, York and Severn; but they have very few white geese at the Southern Settlements, and as few blue at the northern there not being above 20 or 30 blue geese killed at Prince of Wales Fort etc'.

This observation shows less than 0.3% blue phase in Western Hudson Bay in the eighteenth century in contrast to the 30% blue phase there at the present time, and suggests the sympatry of the two colour phases has been re-established recently.

A perfectly reasonable explanation of the assortative mating is that it represents an outgrowth of the species-recognition mechanism. Conceivably, the wrong colour phase normally is not recognised as a member of the same species by birds from a pure family. Perhaps the birds have simply not learned that there are no disadvantages in choosing the opposite colour phase. It may be difficult to generalise to the species as a whole, when morph plumage differences are so great.

Even if this is the explanation for the non-random mating, there is still the potential for intra-specific discrimination of mates. In our study approximately ten percent of birds from pure families chose a mate of the non-family colour, and it would be interesting if we could show that these birds differed in some way from those who chose the family colour. Cooke (1978) speculated that some birds may be tradition breakers and may show more tradition breaking behaviour than the others. This is an extremely difficult hypothesis to test and must therefore remain speculative. Another approach offers more promise and may give us additional insight into the mate choice process. We will refer to this second theory as the 'buxom redhead' hypothesis. The idea simply is that individuals are unlikely to choose a mate solely on the basis of a single character. Indeed Burley (1981) has shown that several different characters are used by domestic pigeons. Individuals perhaps have a list of independent attributes which are perceived as desirable in their mate but may have to settle for a partner who does not match up in all details with the list. For example, if a group of men had a preference for buxom redheads it is unlikely that they would all be successful, since redheads are relatively rare, and buxom redheads rarer still. Some would have to settle for non-buxom redheads, others buxom non-redheads. At the population level, assuming that some females remain mateless, this would result in the non-redhead mates being on average more buxom than the redheaded mates. In terms of the Snow Goose, perhaps those geese that did not choose a mate of their family colour, chose on the basis of some other desirable attribute. In this way, any possible disadvantage associated with choosing the wrong colour is counterbalanced by the advantage accrued by the acquisition of a mate with the other attribute(s).

This provides a possible method for seeking other characters used in mate choice, since such characters may be over-represented among mates of birds who have chosen 'incorrectly' in terms of family colour. One character of potential importance is body size. Fortunately, geese reach adult body size before pair formation occurs. We can ask the same questions in relation to body size that we did for plumage colour.

Body size

Non-random mating in terms of body size was first shown by Ankney (1977). Using culmen length as a measure of body size, he showed that female Snow Geese paired with males with a culmen larger than themselves more frequently than would be expected by chance. He interpreted this to mean that females were choosing males larger than themselves, but several other interpretations are possible. Davies (unpublished), using both culmen length and body weight as a measure of size, did not find the phenomenon described by Ankney but did find a small but highly significant positive correlation between the sizes of each member of the pair. These data indicate positive assortative mating on the basis of body size, and suggest that size is another potential character by which individuals choose their mates.

Although there is non-random mating in terms of body size there is no evidence that birds are actually choosing on the basis of size. It would be extremely difficult to obtain direct evidence of this given the difficulty of observing the pair formation process in the field.

We also do not know with certainty that size is actually the character used in mate choice. If mate choice were based on size it would be difficult to isolate which cues were actually involved.

We do know that size has a high heritable component. Both culmen length and body weight show high heritability based on mother-daughter regressions. Unless the similarity arises from correlated environments, there appears to be a genetic component to structural size variation.

There does appear to be some selective advantage associated with larger-sized pairs, at least in terms of number of eggs laid and number of eggs hatched (Tables 12.4 and 12.5). The large × large pairs also have a larger average brood size at fledging but differences are not significant, probably because of small sample size. It is interesting that the greater clutch size is associated not with large $\male$ size alone, or large $\female$ size alone but with large × large pairs, suggesting that a large bird will attain a higher

Table 12.4. *Clutch size in relation to size of parents: Snow Geese data, La Perouse Bay, Manitoba, 1977–1979*

Male size	Female size		
	Small	Medium	Large
Small	4.6 ± 1.4^a (35)	4.5 ± 1.7 (30)	4.2 ± 0.4 (10)
Medium	4.5 ± 1.6 (37)	4.6 ± 0.7 (24)	4.6 ± 1.6 (24)
Large	4.4 ± 0.6 (8)	4.7 ± 0.8 (30)	5.4 ± 1.7 (20)

Sample size is indicated in parentheses.
^{a} S.D.

clutch size only if he or she can choose a large mate. Clutch size and body size are thus correlated characters and a function of both male and female genotype.

If large size does confer some sort of a selective advantage, then one might expect it to be used as a cue for intraspecific mate choice in Snow Geese. We still do not know whether birds that have chosen a mate of the 'wrong' colour have done so because those birds were preferred because of their larger size. We have to wait until we have an adequate sample size to test the 'buxom redhead' hypothesis. What we have however is one of the few cases in which we can look at two distinct phenotypic characters both of which lead to assortative mating. Thus we should in time be able to assess the relative importance of colour *versus* size in mate choice in Snow Geese.

Summary

We have shown in Snow Geese that there is non-random mating in terms of both plumage colour and body size but that only in the former case are we satisfied that the birds are using the character in making their choice. We have shown that *variation* in both plumage colour and body size have an underlying genetic basis, the former due to a single major gene, the latter presumably polygenically determined.

There appears to be no obvious selective advantage in making a correct choice in terms of plumage colour, but there may be an advantage in choosing a large mate. It seems reasonable that mate choice on the basis of plumage colour may simply be a misapplication of a species recognition mechanism at a colour morph level. However, it seems likely that such a mechanism could also be used to choose more suitable mates intra-

Table 12.5. *Number of eggs hatched in relation to size of parents: Snow Geese data, La Perouse Bay, Manitoba, 1977–1979*

Male size	Female size		
	Small	Medium	Large
Small	4.2 ± 1.4^a (34)	4.1 ± 1.2 (30)	3.8 ± 1.1 (10)
Medium	4.1 ± 1.7 (37)	4.0 ± 1.2 (24)	4.1 ± 1.5 (24)
Large	3.4 ± 0.8 (8)	4.2 ± 0.9 (30)	5.2 ± 1.7 (20)

Sample size is indicated in parentheses.
[a] S.D.

specifically and to allow an animal to choose a partner that would enhance its reproductive fitness.

References

Ankney, C. D. (1977). Male size and mate selection in Lesser Snow Geese. *Evolutionary Theory*, **3**, 143–8.

Bateson, P. P. G. (1978). Sexual imprinting and optimal outbreeding. *Nature*, **273**, 659–60.

Birkhead, T. R. & Clarkson, K. (1980). Mate selection and precopulatory guarding in *Gammarus pulex*. *Zeitschrift für Tierpsychologie*, **52**, 365–80.

Burley, N. (1981). Mate choice by multiple criteria in a monogamous species. *American Naturalist*, **117**, 515–28.

Cooch, F. G. & Beardmore, J. A. (1959). Assortative mating and reciprocal differences in the blue-snow complex. *Nature*, **183**, 1833–4.

Cooke, F. (1978). Early learning and its effect on population structure. Studies of a wild population of snow geese. *Zeitschrift für Tierpsychologie*, **46**, 344–58.

Cooke, F., Bousfield, M. A. & Sadura, A. (1981). Mate change and reproductive success in the Lesser Snow Goose. *Condor*, **83**, 322–7.

Cooke, F. & Cooch, F. G. (1968). The genetics of polymorphism in the Snow Goose, *Anser caerulescens*. *Evolution*, **22**, 289–300.

Cooke, F., Finney, G. H. & Rockwell, R. F. (1976). Assortative mating in Lesser Snow Geese. *Behavior Genetics*, **6**, 127–40.

Cooke, F., MacInnes, C. D. & Prevett, J. P. (1975). Gene flow between breeding populations of Lesser Snow Geese. *Auk*, **92**, 493–510.

Cooke, F. & McNally, C. M. (1975). Mate selection and colour preferences in Lesser Snow Geese. *Behaviour*, **53**, 151–70.

Cooke, F., Mirsky, P. J. & Seiger, M. B. (1972). Colour preferences in the Lesser Snow Goose and their possible role in mate selection. *Canadian Journal of Zoology*, **50**, 529–36.

Darwin, C. (1871). *The Descent of Man and Selection in Relation to Sex*. Murray: London.

Dzubin, A., Boyd, H. & Stephen, W. J. D. (1973). Blue and Snow Goose distributions in the Mississippi and Central Flyways: a preliminary report. *Progress Notes. CWS*.

Fisher, R. A. (1930). *The Genetical Theory of Natural Selection*. Clarendon Press: Oxford.

Geramita, J. M., Cooke, F. & Rockwell, R. F. Assortative mating and gene flow in the Lesser Snow Goose: a modelling approach. *Theoretical Population Biology* (in press).

Graham, A. *Diary written between 1768 and 1769. Observations on Hudson's Bay, Book 2.* Located at Hudson's Bay Company Archives, Winnipeg, Manitoba.

Lemieux, L. & Heyland, J. (1967). Fall migration of the Blue Geese and Lesser Snow Geese from the Koukdjuak River, Baffin Island, Northwest Territories. *Naturaliste Canadien*, **94**, 677–94.

Lorenz, K. (1935). Der Kumpan in der Umwelt des Vogels. *Journal für Ornithologie*, **83**, 137–213: 289–413.

Mineau, P. & Cooke, F. (1979). Rape in the Lesser Snow Goose. *Behaviour*, **70**, 280–91.

O'Donald, P. (1980). Sexual selection by female choice in a monogamous bird: Darwin's theory corroborated. *Heredity*, **45**, 201–17.

Prevett, J. P. (1972). *Family Behavior and Age-Dependent Breeding Biology of the Blue Goose* (Anser caerulescens). Unpublished Ph.D. Thesis, University of Western Ontario, London, Ontario.

Rattray, A. B. (1981). *Genetics of the Colour Polymorphism of the Lesser Snow Goose: Revisited*. Unpublished B.Sc. Thesis, Queen's University, Kingston, Ontario.

Shields, W. M. (1983). Optimal inbreeding and the evolution of philopatry. In *The Ecology of Animal Movement*, ed. I. R. Swingland & P. J. Greenwood, pp. 132–59. Oxford University Press: Oxford.

Smith, J. A. (1979). *Fitness Differences Between the Blue and White Phenotypes of the Lesser Snow Goose* (Anser caerulescens caerulescens). Unpublished M. Sc. Thesis, Queen's University, Kingston, Ontario.

13

Mate choice in the Mallard

DIANE M. WILLIAMS

Courting parties of Mallard drakes are a familiar sight throughout most of the Northern Hemisphere. They provide an eye-catching spectacle as their striking plumage is accentuated by the performance of special movements and vocalisations in social display groups. Yet Mallard form monogamous pairs which may endure for several months before breeding commences. Many of the displaying males may already be paired. This prompts enquiry into the questions: are plumage and display important for mate choice and pair formation? Are other factors also important?

This chapter will not discuss the constraints which have shaped anatid signalling systems other than to mention excellent papers by Kear (1970), McKinney (1975) and Milstein (1979). The chapter contains a brief description of the annual cycle of social behaviour in the Mallard and a description of the behaviour of the birds in the social display groups. The evidence concerning the involvement of plumage, displays and other cues in mate choice in the Mallard will be summarised in an attempt to answer the above questions. The sources of information about mate choice in Mallard are from studies of the behavioural and morphological similarities and differences between duck species, investigations of interspecific hybridisation and direct experiments.

Annual cycle of social behaviour

Mallard flocks assemble in autumn after moult and migration. Courtship, mating and social display begin immediately. In some resident populations the majority of birds are paired by the end of October (Bezzel, 1959; Lebret, 1961) and in migratory populations most birds are paired by February (Johnsgard, 1960a; Raitasuo, 1964). Thus pairs may be formed up to six months before the birds are fertile although some of the early pairs observed may be temporary 'trial liaisons' (Weidmann, 1956). Mallard usually form monogamous pairs but occasional trios are usually composed of two males and one female (Weidmann, 1956; Lebret, 1961; Raitasuo, 1964). In most populations the sex ratio is skewed, with more males than females (documented for Western Palearctic populations in Cramp & Simmons, 1977, and for North American populations in Bellrose, Scott, Hawkins & Low, 1961) and some males will be unable to form a monogamous pair. Some females may also remain unpaired (Raitasuo, 1964). Social display sessions continue throughout the winter. Males' participation in display sessions is irrespective of their pair status. Weidmann (1956) and Lebret (1961) both reported males leaving their mates asleep on the bank to join a displaying group of males.

Residential flocks remain integrated until February or March when pairs disperse to seek nest sites. Migrant populations usually disperse soon after arrival on the breeding grounds. The pair prospect for a nest site together and then remain on a home range which includes the nest site. When members of a pair forage together males spend more time alert and less time feeding than their mates (Kaminski & Prince, 1981). Females need protein-rich foods to lay eggs although they also draw heavily on lipid reserves during the laying and incubation of the first clutch (Krapu, 1981). At this time the male is intolerant of other Mallard. He will defend his female from forced copulation attempts by other males (Goodwin, 1956; Barrett, 1973; Barash, 1977). He will also behave aggressively toward or attempt forced copulation on other females (review in McKinney, 1969). This has the effect of spacing out nesting females (McKinney, 1965; Dzubin, 1969) which affects brood survival (Dzubin, 1969) and probably conserves females' food supply and reduces predation on the nests.

Females construct the nest, incubate the eggs and care for the precocial young. Pair bonds usually break during the first week of incubation as the male associates to an increasing extent with other males. Males make many flights after females and as many as 20 males may pursue a female over long distances in forced copulation attempts (Cramp & Simmons, 1977). Forced copulations have been shown to fertilise eggs in groups of captive Mallards (Burns, Cheng & McKinney, 1980) and probably do so in the wild. It is quite common for Mallard females to re-nest if their first clutch is destroyed and, exceptionally, even if they lose the ducklings from their first brood (Cramp & Simmons, 1977). The second clutch will normally be fertilized by forced copulation unless the female establishes a temporary pair bond with a new male or re-establishes the bond with her old mate (Sowls, 1955; Weidmann, 1956; Lebret, 1961).

An average male will therefore fertilise most of his mate's first clutch and a variable number of other females' eggs. He will have made a considerable investment in his pair bond and in mate guarding and a small investment in displaying to, chasing and performing forced copulation attempts on other females. The number of eggs in a female's first clutch which are fertilised by her mate will depend on his success in protecting her. If her first clutch fails and she re-nests her eggs will usually be fertilised by several males. In choosing a partner a Mallard needs to establish that the prospective mate is of the correct species and sex, is sexually competent and has genes which will contribute to the survival and reproductive ability of the offspring. In addition a female should prefer a male who will remain attentive to her, warn her of predators and fight off males who are attempting forced copulations, and keep other nesting females away from her nest area. A male should prefer a female who would successfully rear many ducklings from her first clutch.

Dabbling ducks: behavioural and morphological comparisons

Ducks have two separate body moults per year and may assume a different plumage colouration after each moult. For most of the year male Mallard are in the familiar, brightly coloured, 'nuptial' plumage but during wing moult they assume a dull 'eclipse' plumage. This eclipse plumage is very similar to the female and juvenile plumage. (A full description of Mallard plumage is given in Cramp & Simmons, 1977.) This dimorphic plumage pattern, with brightly coloured males and dull females, is common to most Northern Hemisphere dabbling ducks. Despite the close taxonomic affinities between many members of the genus *Anas* male nuptial plumages of different species are often strikingly different whereas female and male eclipse plumages are often alike.

Closely related *Anas* species often share many of the homologous social displays; for instance Mallard share the head-up-tail-up display with at least 14 other species (Johnsgard, 1962). However, differences in the temporal sequences of these displays, performed by males of different species, may produce a very different overall effect (Johnsgard, 1963). Potentially, therefore, females could use male plumage and social displays for species recognition as both these characters differ greatly from species to species. This is in striking contrast with the pair displays of leading and inciting (Weidmann, 1956), and pre-copulatory behaviour which are remarkably uniform across the genus (Lorenz, 1941; Johnsgard, 1960*b*, 1963). For most ducks, therefore, the behavioural and morphological characteristics which differ most between species are those that are evident early in the pair formation process while the behaviour patterns that consolidate the pair bond differ little.

Hybridisation

Although drakes appear to exhibit clear species identifying signals an embarrassing wealth of anatid hybrids have been reported. One hundred and fifteen intrageneric combinations have been recorded among 32 species (Johnsgard, 1960*c*). Of these at least 39 combinations have produced fertile offspring and 38 combinations have occurred in the wild (Phillips, 1915; Johnsgard, 1960*c*, 1963). Mallard have hybridised with approximately 40 other species (Johnsgard, 1968). This suggests that the signal characters that function in species recognition are not particularly effective. However, recent evidence (Milstein, 1979) suggests that hybrids are even more common among Southern Hemisphere ducks in the wild than among Northern Hemisphere ducks. Many Southern Hemisphere ducks are monomorphic and the males do not have an elaborate nuptial plumage. Although males of monomorphic species do perform social displays the movements are not enhanced by complementary plumage features and they may have a less distinctive overall effect. So even though fewer Southern Hemisphere ducks are sympatric, their inefficient isolating mechanisms predispose them to produce relatively more hybrids than Northern Hemisphere ducks, many of which are sympatric. Early hypotheses about the significance of male plumage and displays (Sibley, 1957) had been based on the erroneous information that there were few hybrids among Southern Hemisphere monomorphic ducks.

The greatest incidence of hybridisation between two duck species in the wild occurs between Mallards and American Black Ducks. Hybrids are numerous, comprising up to 12% of the total Mallard/Black Duck population in some areas (Johnsgard, 1967; Heusman, 1974; Alison & Prevett, 1976). Hybrids bred in captivity are fertile (Phillips, 1915) and there is no reason to suppose that wild hybrids are different. The males of the two species perform identical social displays with only slight differences in the frequency of occurrence of the various displays (Johnsgard, 1960*a*). The plumage of the two species differs; Black Ducks are monomorphic, both sexes having dark brown plumage. Despite the high incidence of hybridisation most matings in the wild are assortative, even in areas of considerable sympatry, and the plumage difference may play a part in this. Different habitat preferences may also separate the species during pair formation. Indeed it has been suggested that the high incidence of hybridisation has been brought about by the large-scale artificial rearing and releasing of Black Ducks and Mallards and would not have occurred without this (Milstein, 1979).

Experimental findings
Sexual imprinting

Female Mallards have no early opportunity to learn the characteristics of male nuptial plumage as duckling broods are cared for by the mother only and split up while the males are still in juvenile plumage. However, male Mallards will have had several weeks to learn the plumage characteristics of their mother and sisters. The consequences of these differing opportunities are demonstrated by studies of sexual imprinting in Mallards – work pioneered by Schutz (1965). After experiments involving 232 birds from 10 different species he concluded that the females of dimorphic duck species 'are almost incapable of becoming imprinted as they react innately to the releasers of the male courtship dress'. In contrast about two-thirds of Mallard drakes reared by a foster mother or with a foster sibling of a different species later attempted to pair with an individual of that species. Schutz (1965) argued that innate factors were also important in determining males' mate preferences. The remaining third of the males preferred female Mallards even though they had been reared with individuals of a different species and many of the males who paired with individuals of the foster species only did so after bonds with female Mallards had been broken. Further work on imprinting in female Mallards has shown that females do learn about the characteristics of their foster mother or foster siblings but that this information is normally overridden by the strong preference for male Mallards (Schutz, 1975). Females may also spontaneously revert to preferring male Mallards after an initial period of preferring an individual of the foster species (Schutz, 1975; Klint, 1975, 1978). Male Mallard appear to use information gained during the brood period to specify their eventual sexual preferences (Schutz, 1971; Klint, 1978) but have a predisposition to learn 'female Mallard' characteristics (Schutz, 1965, 1971). On the other hand early experience plays little part in determining females' sexual preferences.

Kaspar Hauser females

The precision of the females' unlearnt 'model' of a male Mallard has been examined using Kaspar Hauser females (i.e. females reared in isolation) and females reared in female-only groups. Schutz (1965) reared three females in optical and auditory isolation for nine weeks and found that they later formed pairs with male Mallards. Incidentally, three males reared under the same conditions also paired normally with Mallard females. A criticism of Schutz's experiments is that the birds were tested in a free choice situation among many anatids and it is impossible to determine which elements of behaviour or morphology contributed to the establishment of each pair bond. More experiments were performed by Klint (1973, 1978, 1980) using both normally coloured and white Kaspar Hauser females. In these experiments the females were isolated from hatching for 19 weeks. All of the test males used had been imprinted with the type of the female being tested. Klint (1973, 1978, 1980) found that 19 out of 21 white Kaspar Hauser females preferred males in normal nuptial plumage when given a choice between these and white males. His investigations with normally coloured Kaspar Hauser females were more detailed (Klint, 1980) and included females reared in female-only groups or reared in mixed-sex groups with experience of males in nuptial plumage. Females from all categories preferred males in normal nuptial plumage to white males or to males with the green head colour removed. When given a choice between males in normal nuptial plumage and males with the brown chest colouration removed the females who had been reared in groups again preferred the normally coloured males. However, the Kaspar Hauser females either showed no preference or preferred the male with abnormal plumage. Interestingly an earlier experiment (Klint, 1973) had shown that even females with experience of males in normal nuptial plumage could prefer (three out of five) a 'mutant' male with a grey instead of a brown chest rather than a male in full nuptial plumage. These experiments demonstrate that females do not need prior experience with Mallard males in full nuptial plumage to prefer them to males with non-Mallard-like or incomplete plumage. Klint's (1980) experimental removal of the blue secondary feathers from males' plumage had no apparent effect on female choice but the males in the experiment did not perform the displays which emphasise these feathers. Looking at the problem from a different viewpoint: perhaps sympatric male dabbling ducks have to have such distinctive and different plumages simply because females have only a very basic innate model of the conspecific male which cannot be greatly improved by learning during the brood period.

Behavioural cues

Many practical difficulties arise in investigations of the importance of Mallard social displays in mate choice. It is a complex activity. A Mallard social display session involves a number of birds, both male and female, swimming together in a fairly close group, constantly adjusting their positions and intermittently performing characteristic display movements and vocalisations. Females may nod-swim, and this facilitates male performance of social displays (Weidmann & Darley, 1971*a*), but the organisation of the 'bursts' of the major displays depends on interactions between the participating males (Weidmann & Darley, 1971*b*). There are three major displays – the grunt-whistle or water-flick, the down-up and the head-up-tail-up complex which includes the head-up-tail-up proper, male nodswimming and turn-the-back-of-the-head. A full description of the displays is given in Cramp & Simmons (1977). Performance of the major displays may be highly synchronised. There are also a variety of Introductory Shakes (Simmons & Weidmann 1973). When several males display to a single female, Weidmann & Darley (1971*a*) found that the males take up positions in a circle around the female with their bodies oriented at right angles to her before performing grunt-whistles and head-up-tail-ups. Dominant males appeared to take favoured positions; for instance a dominant male would usually perform a head-up-tail-up when he was straight in front of the female while lower-ranking males would display from more variable positions (illustrated in Halliday, in press). The display movements involved in grunt-whistle and head-up-tail-up also include components which have a special orientation with respect to a preferred female and the introductory shakes given by the males usually start with a turn of the head towards the preferred female (Simmons & Weidmann, 1973). A female indicates her preference for a particular male by swimming beside him inciting from him, often when he turns-the-back-of-the-head and leads her (Lorenz, 1941; Weidmann, 1956).

Observations on geese and ducks led Schutz (1971) to suggest that females may respond innately to male displays and their plumage may not be as important, although in his free choice tests these properties will have been confounded. The problem therefore, has been to separate the effects of performance of male social displays and possession of male nuptial plumage. This problem was partially solved by Kruijt & Bossema (1975) when they demonstrated that Mallard females (both wild type and domesticated white) preferred males who were imprinted with their type and therefore displayed interest in them. This was irrespective of the colour of the males used (white or wild type) and of the females' early experience. A drawback of the experimental method was that the males did not perform social displays but showed interest in a female by approaching her. It should be noted that directly contradictory results had been obtained by Klint (1973). He found that white females, reared with a white mother and siblings, did not show any sexual response to normally coloured males who had been imprinted with white females. However, these results were obtained from only five females and are outweighed by the results obtained by Cheng, Shoffner, Phillips & Lee (1978, 1979).

Cheng *et al.* (1978, 1979) used two strains of Mallard – wild type and game farm. The two strains have similar plumages but game-farm Mallards have a heavier adult body weight. They perform identical displays. The birds (48 of each sex) were reared, and lived, in pure-strain or mixed-strain groups. In any group all birds of the same sex were the same strain. Initial preference tests (Cheng *et al.*, 1978) were carried out when the birds were about 150 days old. Each bird was tested separately by introducing it into a room with six, penned, unfamiliar birds of the opposite sex. These were arranged so that three game-farm birds were on one side of the room while three wild-type birds were on the other side of the room. In these tests females from all rearing groups did not show a significant preference for males of either strain although, with one exception, all females did make a choice. Males who had been reared in pure-strain groups showed a significant preference for females of their own strain. Males reared in mixed-strain groups showed no significant preference. Cheng *et al.* (1979) carried on to test the birds' pairing preferences when they were 36 weeks old. For each test four males and four females, all initially strangers, were released into a pen. Each group of eight birds was composed of a wild-type male and female and a game-farm male and female reared in pure-strain groups, and a wild-type male and female and a game-farm male and female reared in mixed-strain groups. They found that males reared in pure-strain groups courted and were successful in pairing only with females of their own strain while males reared in mixed-strain groups courted and were successful in pairing with females of either strain. Females paired with males who were imprinted with their own strain, regardless of the strain of the male and of the early experience of the female. In this experiment males did occasionally perform two of the major social displays, grunt-whistles and head-up-tail-ups. No males were observed to perform down-ups. The males mainly showed interest in particular females by approaching them and by turning-the-back-of-the-head. While this experiment did not demonstrate that females pay attention to male social displays it did show that they are sensitive to cues indicating whether or not a male is interested in them. The females may have been able to distinguish between the males of the two strains but they did not use this information in mate choice. On the other hand the males did discriminate between the two strains of female, even though their plumage was very similar.

In this experiment the males and females were solving two different problems. Males were choosing a mate of the correct species and were making very fine discriminations between females of the two strains in order to do so. Females were attempting to choose the best males and regarded all of the males as Mallard males. An important cue for the females appeared to be male interest in them, an individual, not a species, characteristic. However, some females attempted to pair with males that had shown no interest in them, indicating that other cues may also have been important.

Sexual selection

Published work to date has concentrated on the importance of species recognition in mate choice in Mallards. While male plumage undoubtedly serves to prevent interspecific hybridisation and social displays may also do so, they may also reflect male/male competition for mates and female choice between males. Females may use plumage differences to discriminate between mallard males. After observing wild birds in Finland, Raitasuo (1964) wrote 'exaggerated colour shades of the species-specific masculine characteristics such as unusually yellow colouration of the bill or unusual breadth of the white collar seem to evoke the sympathy of the females more effectively than normal colouration'. Titman & Lowther (1975) reported that males with undamaged plumage won more fights than males with damaged plumage. A female could potentially judge a male's 'fighting ability' by the condition of his plumage. Females could also potentially judge a male's skill, strength, stamina, aggression and interest in her from his performance in a social display session. There is a great deal of competition between males as they jockey for position in a display group and outbreaks of overtly aggressive behaviour are quite common (Weidmann & Darley, 1971a). Both males and females may initially direct displays towards several individuals of the opposite sex before establishing a firm pair bond. In these trial liaisons they could test the fidelity of the mate and their efficiency at copulation. The long pair bond would make it very difficult for a bird to fake some quality which he or she did not possess.

Finally a brief mention must be made of the effects of familiarity on pair formation. Mallards may re-pair with their old mates in sedentary populations (Weidmann, 1956; Lebret, 1961; Raitasuo, 1964) and even in migratory populations (Dwyer, Derrickson & Gilmer, 1973). However, the mortality rate amongst adult Mallards is approximately 50% (Cramp & Simmons, 1977) so re-pairing will only be possible for a minority of adult birds. The information about pairings between close relations in captive mallards is contradictory. Kaltenhaüser (1971) stated that birds formed sibling pairs when quite young and that the males' first displays were always directed towards their mother. Klint (1978) found that 35% of the pairs formed during an experiment were sibling pairs. However, Schutz (1965) stated that it was rare for pairing to involve the same individuals that had been reared together. In migratory Mallards there is evidence to show that siblings do not migrate together and may end up on different wintering grounds (Martinson & Hawkins, 1968). Most pairing in Mallards will therefore usually involve unfamiliar birds.

Concluding remarks

Returning to the courting party of Mallard drakes; there is strong evidence to suggest that a normal Mallard drake will have learnt the characteristics of his mother and siblings and will address his courtship selectively towards Mallard females and specifically towards one, or a few, preferred potential mates. No investigations have been carried out into male choice between individual females. A male will have little, if anything, to lose by being extremely unselective when performing forced copulation attempts.

There is little published evidence to suggest that females pay any attention to the performance of social displays by the males. They may indicate preferences for particular males in the absence of any social display (Kruijt & Bossema, 1975; Cheng *et al.*, 1978) and the importance of this complex activity remains unexplained. There is rather more evidence to suggest that they do pay some attention to male plumage but I would hypothesise that females pay most attention to cues which signal males' interest in them and male ability to protect and defend them.

Summary

The annual cycle of social behaviour in the Mallard is briefly described. A comparison between anatid species reveals that male nuptial plumages and social display patterns are very different in closely related sympatric species. These characters probably function as an isolating mechanism preventing interspecific hybridisation. Mallard drakes learn the characteristics of their mother and siblings in sexual imprinting. Mallard females have a simple unlearnt model of a Mallard drake, specifying that he should have a green head and a brown breast. Females also use behavioural characteristics of males in mate choice but the involvement of social displays in pair formation has not been convincingly demonstrated.

References

Alison, R. M. & Prevett, J. P. (1976). Occurrences of duck hybrids at James Bay. *Auk*, **93**, 643–4.

Barash, D. P. (1977). Sociobiology of rape in Mallards (*Anas platyrhynchos*): responses of the mated male. *Science*, **197**, 788–9.

Barrett, J. (1973). *Breeding Behaviour of Captive Mallards*. MS Thesis, University of Minnesota.

Bellrose, F. C., Scott, T. G., Hawkins, A. S. & Low, J. B. (1961). Sex ratios and age ratios in North American ducks. *Illinois Natural History Survey Bulletin*, **27**, 391–474.

Bezzel, E. (1959). Beiträge zur Biologie der Geschlechter bei Entenvögeln. *Anzeiger der Ornithologische Gesellschaft in Bayern*, **5**, 269–355.

Burns, J. T., Cheng, K. M. & McKinney, F. (1980). Forced copulation in captive Mallards. 1. Fertilization of eggs. *Auk*, **97**, 875–9.

Cheng, K. M., Shoffner, R. N., Phillips, R. E. & Lee, F. B. (1978). Mate preference in wild and domesticated (game farm) mallards (*Anas platyrhynchos*): I. Initial preference. *Animal Behaviour*, **26**, 996–1003.

Cheng, K. M., Shoffner, R. N., Phillips, R. E. & Lee, F. B. (1979). Mate preference in wild and domesticated (game farm) mallards: II. Pairing success. *Animal Behaviour*, **27**, 417–25.

Cramp, S. & Simmons, K. E. L. eds. (1977). *The Birds of the Western Palearctic*, vol. 1, pp. 505–19. Oxford University Press: London.

Dwyer, T. J., Derrickson, S. R. & Gilmer, D. S. (1973). Migrational homing by a pair of mallards. *Auk*, **90**, 687.

Dzubin, A. (1969). Comments on carrying capacity of small ponds for ducks and possible effects of density on mallard production. *Canadian Wildlife Service Reports Series No. 6. Saskatoon Wetlands Seminar*, pp. 138–60.

Goodwin, D. (1956). Displacement coition in the Mallard. *British Birds*, **49**, 238–40.

Halliday, T. (in press). *Courtship in Animals*. Edward Arnold: London.

Heusman, H. W. (1974). Mallard – Black Duck relationships in the Northeast. *Wildlife Society Bulletin*, **2**, 171–7.

Johnsgard, P. A. (1960a). A quantitative study of the sexual behaviour of mallard and black ducks. *Wilson Bulletin*, **72**, 133–55.

Johnsgard, P. A. (1960b). Pair-formation mechanisms in *Anas* (Anatidae) and related genera. *Ibis*, **102**, 616–18.

Johnsgard, P. A. (1960c). Hybridization in the Anatidae and its taxonomic implications. *Condor*, **62**, 25–33.

Johnsgard, P. A. (1962). Evolutionary trends in the behaviour and morphology of the Anatidae. *Wildfowl Trust Annual Report*, **13**, 130–48.

Johnsgard, P. A. (1963). Behavioural isolating mechanisms in the family Anatidae. *Proceedings of the XIIIth International Ornithological Congress*, 531–43.

Johnsgard, P. A. (1967). Sympatry changes and hybridization incidence in Mallards and Black Ducks. *American Midland Naturalist*, **77**, 51–63.

Johnsgard, P. A. (1968). *Waterfowl: Their Biology and Natural History*. University of Nebraska Press: Lincoln, USA.

Kaltenhaüser, D. (1971). Über Evolutionsvorgänge in der Schwimmentenbalz. *Zeitschrift für Tierpsychologie*, **29**, 481–540.

Kaminski, R. M. & Prince, H. H. (1981). Dabbling duck activity and foraging responses to aquatic invertebrates. *Auk*, **98**, 115–26.

Kear, J. (1970). The adaptive radiation of parental care in waterfowl. In *Social Behaviour in Birds and Mammals*, ed. J. H. Crook, pp. 357–92. Academic Press: London & New York.

Klint, T. (1973). Praktdräkten som 'sexuell utlösare' hos grasänd. *Zoologisk Revy*, **35**, 11–21.

Klint, T. (1975). Sexual imprinting in the context of species recognition in female mallards. *Zeitschrift für Tierpsychologie*, **38**, 385–92.

Klint, T. (1978). Significance of mother and sibling experience for mating preferences in the Mallard (*Anas platyrhynchos*). *Zeitschrift für Tierpsychologie*, **47**, 50–60.

Klint, T. (1980). Influence of male nuptial plumage on mate selection in the female mallard (*Anas platyrhynchos*). *Animal Behaviour*, **28**, 1230–8.

Krapu, G. L. (1981). The role of nutrient reserves in mallard reproduction. *Auk*, **98**, 29–38.

Kruijt, J. P. & Bossema, I. (1975). Partner choice in the female mallard (*Anas platyrhynchos*). *Paper presented at the XVth International Ethological Conference, Parma*.

Lebret, T. (1961). The pair formation in the annual cycle of the Mallard, *Anas platyrhynchos* L. *Ardea*, **49**, 97–158.

Lorenz, K. (1941). Vergleichende Bewegungsstudien an Anatiden. *Journal für Ornithologie*, **89**, 194–294. Translated in K. Lorenz (1971) *Studies in Animal and Human Behaviour*, vol. II, pp. 14–114. Methuen & Co. Ltd: London.

Martinson, R. K. & Hawkins, A. S. (1968). Lack of association among duck broodmates during migration and wintering. *Auk*, **85**, 684–6.

McKinney, F. (1965). Spacing and chasing in breeding ducks. *Wildfowl Trust Annual Report*, **16**, 92–106.

McKinney, F. (1969). The behaviour of ducks. In *The Behaviour of Domestic Animals*, ed. E. S. E. Hafez (2nd edn), pp. 593–626. Baillière, Tindall & Cassell: London.

McKinney, F. (1975). The evolution of duck displays. In *Function and Evolution in Behaviour: Essays in Honour of Professor Niko Tinbergen, F.R.S.*, ed. G. P. Baerends, C. Beer & A. Manning, pp. 331–57. Clarendon Press: Oxford.

Milstein, P. Le S. (1979). The evolutionary significance of wild hybridization in South African high veld ducks. *Ostrich*, Supplement **13**, p. 48.

Phillips, J. C. (1915). Experimental studies of hybridization among ducks and pheasants. *Journal of Experimental Zoology*, **18**, 69–144.

Raitasuo, K. (1964). Social behaviour of the Mallard (*Anas platyrhynchos*) in the course of the annual cycle. *Papers on Game Research*, **24**, p. 72. Helsinki.

Schutz, F. (1965). Sexuelle Prägung bei Anatiden. *Zeitschrift für Tierpsychologie*, **22**, 50–103.

Schutz, F. (1971). Prägung des Sexualverhaltens von Enten und Gänsen durch Sozialeindrücke während der Jugendphase. *Journal of Neuro-Visceral Relations*, Supplement **10**, 339–57.

Schutz, F. (1975). Der Einfluss von Testosteron auf die Partnerwahl bei geprägt aufgezogenen Stockenten weibchen: Nachweis latenter Sexualprägung. *Verhandlungen der Deutschen zoologischen Gessellschaft*, **67**, 339–44.

Sibley, C. G. (1957). The evolutionary and taxonomic significance of sexual dimorphism and hybridization in birds. *Condor*, **59**, 166–87.

Simmons, K. E. L. & Weidmann, U. (1973). Directional bias as a component of social behaviour with special reference to the mallard, *Anas platyrhynchos*. *Journal of Zoology, London*, **170**, 49–62.

Sowls, L. K. (1955). *Prairie Ducks*. Stackpole Co.: Harrisburg, Pennsylvania.

Titman, R. D. & Lowther, J. K. (1975). The breeding behaviour of a crowded population of Mallards. *Canadian Journal of Zoology*, **53**, 1270–83.

Weidmann, U. (1956). Verhaltensstudien an der Stockente (*Anas platyrhynchos* L.). I. Das Aktionssystem. *Zeitschrift für Tierpsychologie*, **13**, 208–71.

Weidmann, U. & Darley, J. (1971*a*). The role of the female in the social display of mallards. *Animal Behaviour*, **19**, 287–98.

Weidmann, U. & Darley, J. (1971*b*). The synchronisation of signals in the 'social display' of mallards. *Revue Comparative Animal*, **5**, 131–5.

14

Early experience and sexual preferences in rodents

BRUNO D'UDINE AND ENRICO ALLEVA

In order to maintain reproductive barriers between species, rodents have evolved a variety of genetic isolating mechanisms, most of which involve behaviour.

On the other hand, within a species behavioural mechanisms leading to genetic recombination have been suggested. Assortative mating (i.e. the tendency to depart from random mating preferences) has been considered an important mechanism in the determination of the genetic composition of natural populations of rodents and other species. Negative assortative mating occurs when there is a tendency to prefer a novel mate to a familiar one. Positive assortative mating is the opposite tendency (see Bateson, this volume). Assortative mating is one of the sources of deviation from the Hardy-Weinberg equilibrium (Yanai & McClearn, 1972a). Assortative mating, either negative or positive, has been thought to influence the degree of homozygosity, the total variance of any character and the similarity between relatives in the population. Crow & Felsenstein (1968) summarised and reviewed these effects.

Interspecific cross-fostering

The aim of the first part of our chapter is to summarise briefly work on rodents where an early experience, mainly cross-fostering, affects sexual preferences and, in some cases, breaks the behavioural reproductive barriers between species. Interspecific cross-fostering is a common experimental procedure used to study the effects of an early adoption of the pups by different species on subsequent patterns of behaviour.

In the papers we examined, there has been a fairly confusing use of the terms sexual or social preferences and sometimes no definite measures of proper sexual behaviour were recorded. Reluctantly we shall use the term 'sexual' even in cases where we feel it was used inappropriately by the authors, since animals only approached or spent some time close to the possible mate, without any more substantial observation of copulatory pattern.

In Table 14.1 we have listed studies in which an experimental manipulation at an early stage of life was carried out on precocial species. Pups were exposed to a variety of stimuli or surrogates and the influence of early exposure was subsequently tested. Table 14.2 lists studies in which young of several altricial species were cross-fostered to a different altricial species in order to test the effects of early exposure on later social preference. Early exposure resulted mainly in a reduced preference for conspecifics and in an enhanced preference for the cross-fostering species.

From all these data the following points may be made:

(i) Manipulation of early experience, instead of redirecting the 'species awareness' towards a different species (Lorenz, 1937), results in broadening of the species identity in order to include the foster species or surrogate. Huck & Banks (1980*a*, *b*) working on Lemmings suggested that in some cases there is evidence of a decreased frequency in social and sexual contacts with conspecifics so there is not a complete reorientation of species identity. Lagerspetz & Heino (1970) found that mice raised by rat mothers engaged in more sexual behaviour with a small rat in premature oestrus than did mouse-reared animals. Sexual behaviour directed toward mice was lower in the rat-reared animals. Similarly, male *Mus musculus* previously cross-fostered to *Baiomys taylori* dams subsequently mounted *Baiomys* (Quadagno & Banks, 1970). McCarty & Southwich (1977) reported that cross-fostered male and female Southern Grasshopper Mice (*Onychomys torridus*) and female White-footed Mice (*Peromyscus leucopus*) showed a reduction or elimination of preference for conspecifics. Similar results were obtained by Murphy (1980) in hamsters.

Only in one precocial species, the Guinea Pig, has it been reported that some hand-reared males directed precopulatory responses to the experimenter's hand. In the same study comparisons between different stimuli to which animals had been exposed suggested that some of them were more 'adequate' than others (Beauchamp & Hess, 1973). In summary, early social experience with an appropriate conspecific seems to affect the pup differently from experience with other stimuli.

(ii) Some behaviour patterns such as allogrooming and other social interactions are labile and easily changeable, while others, such as copulation, are more fixed and less subject to modification. Frank Beach (1976) proposed that the various aspects of reproductive behaviour,

Table 14.1. *Effects of early exposure in precocial rodents*

Author(s)	Exposed species	Exposure duration (days)	Stimulus	Age at test (days)	Effect of early exposure
Kunkel & Kunkel, 1964; Harper, 1970	♂ *Cavia porcellus*	1–21	Hand	40–60	Attempt to copulate with hands[a]
Beauchamp & Hess, 1971	♂ *Cavia porcellus*	1–90	Chicks	1–21	Preference for chicks instead of conspecifics[a]
Beauchamp & Hess, 1971	♀ *Cavia porcellus*	1–90	Chicks	1–49	Preference for chicks instead of conspecifics
Carter, 1972	♂ *Cavia porcellus*	1–21	Acetophenone or ethyl benzoate	75	Enhanced attractiveness of the female in presence of the stimulus
Beauchamp & Hess, 1973	♂ *Cavia porcellus*	1–42	Rat	70	Strong interest for the rat[a]
Porter & Etscorn, 1974, 1975, 1977	♂ + ♀ *Acomys cahirinus*	1–2	Cinnamon or cumin	2	Strong preference for the stimulus
Porter et al., 1977	♂ + ♀ *Acomys cahirinus*	1–3	Mouse	3	Strong preference for mouse odour

[a] Sexual activity (attempts to mount, etc.).

Table 14.2. *Effects of cross-fostering in altricial rodents*

Author(s)	Species Fostered	Species Fostering	Fostering period (days)	Age at preference test (days)	Preference for Natural species	Cross-fostering species
Denenberg, Hudgens & Zarrow, 1964	*Mus musculus* ♂	*Rattus norvegicus* ♂	3–63	64–68	Almost absent	Greatly enhanced
Lagerspetz & Heino, 1970	*Mus musculus* ♂	*Rattus norvegicus* ♂	2–21	40	Greatly reduced	Greatly enhanced
Quadagno & Banks, 1970	*Baiomys taylori* ♂	*Mus musculus*	1–21	80–115	—	Enhanced
	Baiomys taylori ♀	*Mus musculus*	1–21	80–115	Greatly reduced	Enhanced
	Mus musculus♂	*Baiomys taylori*	1–21	80–115	Greatly reduced	Enhanced[a]
	Mus musculus♀	*Baiomys taylori*	1–21	80–115	Greatly reduced	Greatly enhanced
McCarty & Southwich 1978	*Onychomys torridus* ♂	*Peromyscus leucopus*	2–25	30–110	Reduced	Enhanced
	Onychomys torridus ♀	*Peromyscus leucopus*	2–25	30–110	Reduced	Enhanced
	Peromyscus leucopus ♂	*Onychomis torridus*	2–25	30–110	Reduced	Greatly enhanced
	Peromyscus leucopus ♀	*Onychomis torridus*	2–25	30–110	Reduced	Greatly enhanced
McDonald & Forslund 1978	*Microtus montanus*♂	*Microtus canicaudus*	1–28	80	Reduced	Greatly enhanced
	Microtus montanus ♀	*Microtus canicaudus*	1–28	80	Reduced	Enhanced
	Microtus canicaudus ♂	*Microtus montanus*	1–28	80	—	Almost unaffected
	Microtus canicaudus ♀	*Microtus montanus*	1–28	80	Reduced	—
Kirchhof-Glazier, 1979	*Mus musculus* ♀	*Peromyscus maniculatus*	1–18	44	Enhanced	Reduced
Murphy, 1980	*Mesocricetus auratus* ♂	*Mesocricetus brandti*	2–31	210	Greatly reduced	—
	Mesocricetus brandti ♂	*Mesocricetus auratus*	2–31	210	Reduced	—
Huck & Banks, 1980*a, b*	*Dicrostonyx groenland* ♀♂	*Lemmus trimucronatus*	1–18	60	Reduced	Greatly enhanced[a]
	Dicrostonyx groenland ♀	*Lemmus trimucronatus*	1–18	60	Greatly reduced	Enhanced
	Lemmus trimucronatus ♂	*Dicrostonyx groenland*	1–18	60	Reduced	Enhanced
	Lemmus trimucronatus ♀	*Dicrostonyx groenland*	1–18	60	Greatly reduced	Enhanced[a]

Starting from the left of the table, parental species are listed, followed by the cross-fostering species, the age at which cross-fostering was initiated and terminated, and age at later tests.

[a] Sexual activity (attempts to mount, lordosis, etc.).

including preference and copulation, may be controlled by different neural, hormonal, experiential, and situational factors. The same possibility had been considered by Quadagno & Banks (1970) when arguing that such 'social' behaviour, e.g. allogrooming and approach, are labile, but that sexual behaviour is more fixed and less subject to early experimental modifications. Indeed, cross-fostering of *Mus musculus* pups to *Baiomys taylori* affected allogrooming, aggressive behaviour and approach-avoidance behaviour, but did not affect their ability to mate with a conspecific. Murphy (1980) also reported that the total amounts of social interest and attempted copulation shown by hamsters were unaffected by fostering by another species. Huck & Banks (1980*a*, *b*) in a complex set of experiments reported that only cross-fostered male *Dicrostonyx* engaged in sexual behaviour with *Lemmus* females clearly demonstrated the profound effect of cross-species rearing on the subsequent behaviour of males of this species. The absence of ejaculation suggested that the non-conspecific females failed to provide adequate positive feedback in their behavioural response to male attempts to mate.

(iii) Differences between sexes. Males are generally said to display weaker sexual preferences than females of the same species (Doty, 1974). Observations of rodent sexual behaviour suggest that males do not show very much discrimination when attempting to mount. Males will mount other males of the same and different species and they will also mount conspecific as well as heterospecific females. This observation is in agreement with theoretical studies to the effect that, in the general case, selection for responses important for maintaining sexual isolation, and thereby minimising hybridisation, would be expected to act more strongly on females than on males.

In some cases, the preference may represent a premating, behavioural, sexual isolating mechanism. Thus, preference tests performed with allopatric species may give different results from studies in which sympatric species are used (Godfrey, 1958; Smith, 1965). Sensitivity to early olfactory cues may, in fact, be a significant factor in the maintenance of species isolation in areas where closely related species are sympatric. This argument has been used to explain results of preference tests in two species of hamsters (Murphy, 1980).

Effects of early experience on mating preferences in house mice

It is particularly important to have information on mating preferences in house mice because this species has been the principal laboratory mammal used in behavioural genetics. Nevertheless, research on preferential mating in mice has been comparatively neglected, and work on wild populations, even more so.

The early work in this field was done by Mainardi and co-workers (1963*a*, *b*, 1964, 1965*a*, *b*). In one study, females of *Mus musculus domesticus* had oestrus induced by injection of oestrogen. During a 25-h observation period these females preferred to associate more with males of their own subspecies than with those of another subspecies, *Mus musculus bactrianus* (Mainardi, 1963*a*). This preference was argued to be due to imprinting or some related process since it only appeared if the father had been present during rearing (Mainardi, 1963*b*). Females reared in presence of the mother only did not display any clear sexual preference. Females of the Swiss and C57BL strains associated more often with males of the opposite strain (Mainardi, 1964). As in the previous case, presence of the father during rearing was necessary for the preference to appear (Mainardi, 1964). Male mice did not show any sexual preference (Mainardi *et al.*, 1965*a*). In an initial effort to characterise the behavioural mechanism of preference in females, Mainardi and co-workers (1965*b*) established the importance of olfactory stimuli.

Yanai & McClearn's (1972*a*) experiments using C57BL/Ibg and DBA/Ibg inbred strains of mice whose sexual behaviour was known to be consistently different, confirmed Mainardi's results (1964), since females from the two strains preferred to associate more with the male of the different strain while in a state of induced oestrus. Subsequently Yanai & McClearn (1972*b*) used a different strain, HS/Ibg. In this experiment daughters were reared with their fathers until testing (long exposure), or until weaning (short exposure). Females that stayed with their fathers until the day before testing preferred to associate and mate more with an unfamiliar male. However, the females that had been reared with their fathers until weaning only did not show any preference. These results clash with those of females of some inbred strains and F_1s that had also been reared by their parents until weaning only and that did show a mating preference (Mainardi *et al.*, 1965*b*; Yanai & McClearn, 1972*a*, *b*). A possible explanation is that members of the same inbred strain in the earlier experiments were reared until 56 days of age in the same breeding shelf, and thus in range of possible olfactory or auditory stimuli peculiar to the strain.

In a further experiment Yanai & McClearn (1973*a*) tested five inbred strains, DBA/Ibg, C57BL/Ibg, C57BL/J, BALB/Ibg, and C3H/J. The choice was between males from their own strain and males from another strain. A general consistency with previously reported results was found, in that the females preferred to associate and mate with males of the opposite strain. However, no preference was found in the case of the strains BALB/Ibg and C3H/J. This study suggested the existence of strain-dependent differences in female mating preferences.

In order to prove this, females BALB/Ibg and DBA/Ibg and females from the reciprocal crosses between the strains, that had been fostered by BALB and DBA males, were tested for mating preference between BALB and DBA males. In these strains it was found that the main influence of females' mating preference is for the genotype of the foster-father. The route of the genetic influence on female mating preferences is therefore indirect. It is suggested that owing to their genotype, DBA males provide social stimuli inducing a tendency for mating preference for the less-preferred male in their daughters, whereas BALB males do not induce any tendency for mating preference in their daughters. Yanai & McClearn (1973b) conclude that DBA males provide adequate negative 'imprinting' stimuli and BALB males do not.

Recently Alleva, D'Udine & Oliverio (1980), using two inbred strains, C57 and SEC, characterised by several contrasting biochemical, physiological and behavioural patterns, investigated the effects of early olfactory experience on the sexual preferences of the two strains. According to Mainardi, female mice raised by parents scented with Parma Violet perfume, on reaching adulthood, preferred a scented male to a non-scented one. In Alleva's experiment, during a 24-h test, each female was allowed to choose between a scented male and a non-scented one, both confined by a yoke at the two ends of a cage divided in three equal compartments. An automatic device recorded the female's presence in each compartment.

Experimental females of both strains (E in Fig. 14.1) were raised by parents that had been artificially scented through the weaning time of pups. Control females (C in Fig. 14.1) were raised by non-scented parents. The mean percentage of female choices is shown; the cross-hatched area indicates preference for the scented male, while the white area indicates preferences for the non-scented males. It is evident that experimental C57 females strongly preferred males characterised by the same familiar odour as the father, in this case artificially altered by the Parma Violet. In contrast, experimental SEC females showed no difference *vis-à-vis* the control group. Our experiment establishes that at least for the C57 strain, an early olfactory experience can strongly redirect the adult preferences of the female.

Frank Oedberg (1976) specifically criticised this type of experiment. His paper 'Failure to demonstrate imprinting on an artificial odour in two strains of mice' suggested that the general tendency is an avoidance of the stimulus animal when it is scented with an artificial odour (geraniol) and concluded that no positive effect of early experience was found in his studies. Oedberg's results do not disprove Mainardi's or our work, as several conditions were different: (i) other strains of mice were used; (ii) the durations of the exposure to odour and the test itself were shorter; (iii) the father was not present during rearing and, according to Mainardi, female mice reared without an adult male show no sexual preference between different strains. Oedberg's conclusions stress the need for studies that closely control such variables as the odours used. Also, the result of our experiment on mate choice could depend greatly on where the 'novel' partner lay in relation to optimal discrepancy between a novel and a familiar member of the opposite sex (see Bateson, this volume).

Summarising, the experiments on inbred strains seem to produce a confusing picture because of unstandardised experimental conditions. Inbred mice might show very different behaviour either within strains or in comparison with wild mice for a number of different reasons.

A better approach to a study of normal olfactory and mating preferences

Fig. 14.1. Percentage of female mice choice for the two compartments during the 24 h of the test (Alleva *et al.*, 1981). A χ^2 test demonstrates that there are differences between strains ($P < 0.001$) when one considers the choices at a higher level than 75% in the mice tested ($\chi^2 = 30.40$). Differences between the control group mice of the two strains are not significant ($\chi^2 = 0.415$, $P > 0.05$). Cross-hatched, test males; white, control males.

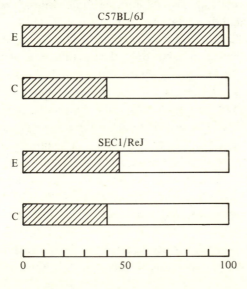

would be to use wild House Mice. In fact, little work has been done on the relevance of mating preferences of females to wild-living populations. Mice are known to live in small demes where the dominant male is assumed to be the sire of most of the offspring (Anderson, 1964; Crowcroft & Rowe, 1963; Reimer & Petras, 1967). Under such stable conditions, especially when migration is rare, female preference may not be very significant. However, there is also evidence of large deviations from these stable conditions (Bronson, 1979). It is known that migration of the young may take place when the population becomes overcrowded and migration of mice of all ages may occur with seasonal changes in food or temperature. This may also happen when the mice are too inbred. Mice migrate either to unoccupied areas in order to establish new populations or possibly into established populations (Delong, 1967; Rowe, Taylor & Chudly, 1963). The latter is possible since mice tend to accept intruders if they invade in large numbers (Reimer & Petras, 1967). If female preference exists in the wild it is more likely to be important under such circumstances.

Up to recent times male mice have been considered not to show any significant preference for females of their own or other strains (Mainardi *et al.*, 1965*a*; Yanai & McClearn, 1973*a, b*). However, Yamazaki *et al.* (1976, 1978) pointed out that mating preferences of male mice exist and are affected by genes in the major histocompatibility complex. Sometimes this results in a preference for a female with the same genotype as the male being tested, sometimes for the other genotype, depending upon the particular male and female genotype used. Yamazaki suggests that males of a particular H-2 type may prefer females of similar or dissimilar H-2 type, depending on which particular H-2 type is offered as the alternative. This suggests a scale of preferences in which the similar H-2 type of the female may rank lower or higher than other H-2 types.

Of the several purposes mating preference might serve in nature, the most easily comprehensible is maintenance of heterozygosity of genes in the proximity of H-2. One obvious advantage of H-2 heterozygosity arises because this region includes Ir (immune response) genes with dominant alleles conferring strong responsiveness to particular antigens. Where infections are a prominent environmental hazard, hybrids would enjoy the advantage of a wider range of immune defences. Genes in the major histocompatibility complex may then be involved in male mouse preferences and further experiments are needed to test the possibility of a tendency of a male to mate with a 'self' or a 'non-self' as guided by the recognition of the species, the subspecies, the strain or the H-2 complex. Bateson (1979) explained the seemingly contradictory evidence obtained from mate choice in mice in terms of the optimal discrepancy hypothesis. Sexual preferences for both familiar and novel stimuli have been demonstrated depending, it seems, on the choices offered to the mice (e.g. Mainardi *et al.*, 1965a, b; Oedberg, 1976; Gilder & Slater, 1978). A similar interpretation may apply to the results of Yamazaki *et al.* (1976) who found that in four sets of crosses out of six, male mice mated significantly more with females differing from themselves in genes determining histocompatibility than with females that were genetically the same. In one set of crosses the males mated to a significantly greater extent with females with identical genes determining histocompatibility. Yamazaki *et al.* argued that the genes in the major histocompatibility complex determine both the female smell and the male recognition system. However, the males may be influenced by their own smell and prefer to mate with a female whose odour is 'optimally' different.

An explanation of the biological functions of early experience has been proposed by Bateson as the requirement for recognition of close kin so that, by choosing males that are slightly different, the animal is able to strike an optimal balance between inbreeding and outbreeding (Bateson, 1978, 1979). According to this model, Gilder & Slater (1978) have suggested that female mice may prefer a male that is slightly unfamiliar to one which is very familiar or very unfamiliar. This is consistent with their finding that females of two inbred mouse strains reared in the presence of their fathers prefer the smell of a non-sibling male of the same strain to that of either a brother or a male of the other strain, thus establishing that in mice olfactory early experience provides the yardstick by which unfamiliarity is judged. Hayashi & Kimura (1978) demonstrated that proximity of males during early postnatal life has a definite effect on female preference for males in later life.

Recently D'Udine & Partridge (1982) attempted to establish whether (i) Gilder and Slater's suggestions apply to two different mouse strains; (ii) male mice show consistent patterns of choice; and whether (iii) cross-fostering between the strains has any effect on the pattern of choice by either sex. Two inbred strains, C57 and SEC, were used.

All the litters were fostered before day two and reared by both sexes of foster parents. Mice of both sexes were tested when they were 80 days old, females being put on artificial oestrus. Every mouse was given two olfactory choice tests using soiled bedding (sugar beet shavings) from home cages as the source of smell. In every test the bedding came from the cages of two mice of the opposite sex to the animal being tested. The two choice tests were (i) between bedding from C57 and from SEC, never using bedding from a sibling of the animal being tested, and (ii) bedding from a sibling and a non-sibling of the same strain as the test animal.

The cages used for testing were divided into three equal-sized compartments by two Perspex partitions each with a hole 25 mm in diameter at floor level. This hole could be opened and closed by means of a sliding door and when the door was open the mouse could move between the compartments. The partitions between the three compartments were also perforated at floor level by 16 holes through which the mouse could sniff the adjacent compartments.

Four days before a test the stimulus animals were given clean bedding. For the test, the four-day-old bedding from the two stimulus animals was transferred to the testing cage, bedding from one stimulus animal being put in each compartment. The centre compartment contained clean bedding. The test animal was then placed in the central compartment of the testing cage for 15 min with the sliding doors to the end compartments closed. During this period the mouse sniffed the end compartments through the smell holes in the partitions. The sliding doors were then opened, and the test mouse was able to enter the two end compartments. The position of the mouse (which compartment it was in) was then noted every 20 s for the next half hour. During this period most of the mice moved between the two end compartments fairly frequently. The data listed in Table 14.3 are now discussed.

(1) Preference for familiarity

It is not easy to explain the results of Table 14.3 merely in terms of preference for slight unfamiliarity (Gilder & Slater, 1978). C57 females, fostered on their own strain, showed a relatively conservative pattern of choice, preferring siblings to non-siblings and showing no significant strain preference. It may be that these females treat the smells of all non-sibling male mice as equal and very unfamiliar. SEC females fostered on their own strain showed a less conservative pattern of choice, preferring the smell of their own strain but showing no significant sibling preference. They may therefore treat other strains as unfamiliar, and all members of the same strain as equally familiar. These results are therefore consistent with the notion that females choose the smells of males on the basis of their degree of familiarity, although if they do so then in these experiments, what was judged as familiar–unfamiliar differed for the two strains used.

Unlike some other studies (Mainardi, 1963a; Yanai & McClearn, 1972a, b) the results of the present investigation do not support the idea that female mice prefer the smells of male mice of other strains. However,

Table 14.3. *Strain preferences and sibling preferences for mice reared by various foster-parents*

Mice reared by	Strain preference (%)				Sibling preference (%)			
	C57		SEC		C57		SEC	
	Males	Females	Males	Females	Males	Females	Males	Females
Foster-parents of same strain	49.3 $N=10$ NS	47.5 $N=11$ NS	58.7 $N=11$ $P < 0.05$	62.6 $N=11$ $P < 0.01$	44.6 $N=10$ $P < 0.01$	57.0 $N=11$ $P < 0.01$	47.0 $N=11$ $P < 0.05$	49.2 $N=11$ NS
Foster-parents of other strain	49.2 $N=11$ NS	51.1 $N=11$ NS	57.3 $N=11$ $P < 0.01$	57.6 $N=11$ $P < 0.05$	53.0 $N=11$ $P < 0.05$	54.8 $N=11$ $P < 0.05$	53.6 $N=11$ $P < 0.05$	46.9 $N=12$ NS

Under 'Strain preferences', numbers significantly greater than 50 indicate preference for the same strain, while under 'Sibling preferences', numbers greater than 50 indicate a preference for siblings. Probability levels are for deviation from 50%. NS, not significant.

the outcome of these choice tests may be affected by several factors. Such factors could be (a) the conservatism of the test strain, (b) the individual variability in smell of the test strain which would affect the strain's diversity of early olfactory experience, and (c) the difference in smell between the stimulus strains used. If these factors are important, it would not be surprising that this type of experiment gives variable results. Differences in the testing methods used by different workers may also affect the outcome of such experiments, although where it has been examined there is a good correlation between the outcome of preference tests conducted using different methods (Yanai & McClearn, 1973; Huck & Banks, 1980*a, b*).

One interesting feature of the present results is that male mice showed significant preferences. Male C57 fostered on their own strain showed no significant strain preference while SEC males preferred their own strain. In-fostered males of both strains showed a significant preference for non-siblings. In-fostered males therefore showed a less conservative pattern of choice than did in-fostered females of their own strain. A similar suggestion has been made for Japanese Quail by Bateson (1980).

(2) *Effects of early experience*

The cross-fostering experiments were done to examine the role of early experience of parental strain on the subsequent olfactory preferences of the mice. In these experiments both in-fostered and cross-fostered mice were reared with siblings of their own strain.

Cross-fostering had no significant effect on females; none of the means differed significantly between in-fostered and cross-fostered females. This suggests that early experience of parental strain may be unimportant in determining olfactory preferences in females. Further experiments with individually cross-fostered females are needed to examine the role of early experience of littermates.

In males, cross-fostering did not affect strain preferences, although in both strains it caused a significant increase in preference for sisters; in-fostered males showed a significant preference for non-siblings whereas cross-fostered mates showed a significant preference for siblings. The effect on sibling preferences could be explained if the smells of parents were used when assessing the familiarity of a novel member of the same strain. The smell of a novel member of the same strain will be more familiar to that of in-foster-parents than to that of cross-foster-parents because the latter come from a different strain. In-fostered mice would therefore be more likely to judge a novel member of the same strain as slightly unfamiliar than would cross-fostered mice. However, if this suggestion is correct it is hard to see why strain preferences are unaffected since a novel member of the other strain should be more likely to be judged as slightly unfamiliar by a cross-fostered than by an in-fostered animal. It may be that littermates play a larger role than parents in the establishment of strain preferences, and further experiments with individually fostered males are needed.

It seems likely that the sibling recognition found in these experiments is based on early experience, as has been shown for Spiny Mice (Porter, Wyrick & Pankey, 1978) of other individuals. Sibling recognition by olfaction in inbred strains of mice has been demonstrated previously (Bowers & Alexander, 1967) but the mechanism by which inbred (and therefore presumably homozygous) mice of the same strain fed on the same diet can produce different smells is not understood. It may be that bacterial metabolism is involved (Gorman, Nedwell & Smith, 1974).

There are a number of reasons why inbred mice, notwithstanding their obvious advantages, may show rather different behaviour from wild mice. Inbreeding leads to random fixation of particular alleles in particular strains which may influence the smell of the strain, its pattern of choice of smells and the effects of early experience. Inbred strains may be poorly buffered againt the effect of the environment during development (Lerner, 1954), which may also affect the results of early experience. Data from wild House Mice would be very valuable in this context. Some work has been done with the related murid *Peromyscus* (Hill, 1974) and similar data from wild House Mice would be a useful complement to the results from inbred strains.

Summary

Early experience and sexual preferences in a number of rodent species are reviewed. First we examine works where early experience affects sexual preferences to the point, in some cases, of breaking the behavioural reproductive barriers between species. These effects in the case of altricial species were pursued through exposure to alternative stimuli to the parents. Precocial species were usually simply cross-fostered.

In the second part we review the effects of early experience on mating preferences in the House Mouse. The mouse as a possible model for these studies is extensively examined in terms of genetic differences and preferences for familiarity.

References

Alleva, E., D'Udine, B. & Oliverio, A. (1981). Effet d'une expérience olfactive précoce sur les préférences sexuelles de deux souches de souris consanguines. *Biology of Behaviour*, **6**, 73–8.

Anderson, P. K. (1964). Lethal alleles in *Mus musculus*: local distribution and evidence for isolation of deme. *Science*, **145**, 177–8.

Bateson, P. (1978). Sexual imprinting and optimal outbreeding. *Nature*, **273**, 659–60.

Bateson, P. (1979). How do sensitive periods arise and what are they for? *Animal Behaviour*, **27**, 470–86.

Bateson, P. (1980). Optimal outbreeding and the development of sexual preferences in Japanese Quail. *Zeitschrift für Tierpsychologie*, **53**, 231–44.

Beach, F. A. (1976). Sexual attractivity, proceptivity and receptivity in female mammals. *Hormones and Behaviour*, **7**, 105–38.

Beauchamp, G. K. & Hess, E. H. (1971). The effects of cross-species rearing on the social and sexual preferences of Guinea pigs. *Zeitschrift für Tierpsychologie*, **28**, 69–76.

Beauchamp, G. K. & Hess, E. H. (1973). Abnormal early rearing and sexual responsiveness in male Guinea pigs. *Journal of Comparative and Psychological Psychology*, **85**(2), 383–96.

Bowers, J. M. & Alexander, B. K. (1967). Mice: individual recognition by olfactory cues. *Science*, **158**, 1208–10.

Bronson, F. H. (1979). The reproductive ecology of the house mouse. *Quarterly Review of Biology*, **54**, 265–99.

Carter, C. S. (1972). Effects of olfactory experience on the behaviour of the Guinea pig (*Cavia porcellus*). *Animal Behaviour*, **20**, 54–60.

Crow, J. F. & Felstenstein, J. (1968). The effect of assortative mating on the genetic composition of a population. *Eugenetic Quarterly*, **15**, 85–97.

Crowcroft, P. & Rowe, P. F. (1963). Social organization and territorial behaviour in the wild house mouse (*Mus musculus* L.). *Proceedings of the Zoological Society of London*, **140**, 517–53.

Delong, K. T. (1967). Population ecology of feral house mouse. *Ecology*, **48**, 611–34.

Denenberg, V. H., Hudgens, G. A. & Zarrow, M. X. (1964). Mice reared with rats: modification of behavior by early experience with another species. *Science*. **143**, 380–1.

Doty, R. L. (1974). A cry for the liberation of the female rodent: courtship and copulation in *Rodentia*. *Psychological Bulletin*, **81**, 159–72.

D'Udine, B. & Partridge, L. (1981). Olfactory preferences of inbred mice (*Mus musculus*) for their own strain and for siblings: effects of strain, sex and cross-fostering. *Behaviour*, **78**, 314–24.

Gilder, P. M. & Slater, P. J. B. (1978). Interest of mice in conspecific male odours is influenced by degree of kinship. *Nature*, **274**, 364–5.

Godfrey, J. (1958). The origin of sexual isolation between bank voles. *Proceedings of the Royal Physiological Society of Edinburgh*, **27**, 47–55.

Gorman, M. L., Nedwell, D. B. & Smith, R. M. (1974). An analysis of the anal scent pockets of *Herpestes auropunctatus* (Carnivora: Viverridae). *Journal of Zoology*, *London*, **172**, 389–99.

Harper, L. V. (1970). Role of contact and sound in eliciting filial response and the development of social attachment in domestic Guinea pigs. *Journal of Comparative and Physiological Psychology*, **73**, 427–35.

Hayashi, S. & Kimura, T. (1978). Effects of exposure to males on sexual preference in female mice. *Animal Behaviour*, **26**, 290–5.

Hill, J. L. (1974). *Peromyscus*: effect of early pairing on reproduction. *Science*, **186**, 1042–4.

Huck, U. W. & Banks, E. M. (1980*a*). The effects of cross-fostering on the behaviour of two species of north american Lemmings, *Dicrostonyx groenlandicus* and *Lemmus trimucronatus*: I. Olfactory preferences. *Animal Behaviour*, **28**, 1046–52.

Huck, U. W. & Banks, E. M. (1980*b*). The effects of cross-fostering on the behaviour of two species of north american Lemmings, *Dicrostonyx groenlandicus* and *Lemmus trimucronatus*: II. Sexual behaviour. *Animal Behaviour*, **28**, 1053–62.

Kirchhof-Glazier, D. A. (1979). Absence of sexual imprinting in house mice cross-fostered to deermice. *Physiology and Behaviour*, **23**, 1073–80.

Kunkel, P. & Kunkel, I. (1964). Beiträge zur Ethologie des Hausmeerschweinschens (*Cavia apera* f. *porcellus*). *Zeitschrift für Tierpsychologie*, **21**, 602–41.

Lagerspetz, K. & Heino, T. (1970). Changes in social reactions resulting from early experience with another species. *Psychological Reports*, **27**, 255–62.

Lerner, I. M. (1954). *Genetic Homeostasis*. Oliver and Boyd: Edinburgh.

Lorenz, K. Z. (1937). The companion in the bird's world. *Auk*, **54**, 245–73.

McCarty, R. & Southwich, C. H. (1977). Cross-species fostering: effects on the olfactory preference of *Onychomys torridus* and *Peromyscus leucopus*. *Behavioural Biology*, **19**, 255–60.

McDonald, D. L. & Forslund, L. G. (1978). The development of social preferences in the voles *Microtus montanus* and *Microtus canicaudus*: effects of cross-fostering. *Behavioral Biology*, **22**, 457–508.

Mainardi, D. (1963a). Speziazioni nel topo: fattori etologici determinanti barriere riproduttive tra *Mus musculus domesticus* e *M. m. bactrianus*. *Istituto Lombardo (Rendiconti Scientifici)*, **B97**, 135–42.

Mainardi, D. (1963b). Eliminazione della barriera etologica all'isolamento riproduttivo tra *Mus musculus domesticus* e *M. m. bactrianus* mediante azione sull'apprendimento infantile. *Istituto Lombardo (Rendiconti Scientifici)*, **B97**, 291–9.

Mainardi, D. (1964). Relations between early experience and sexual preferences in female mice (a progress report). *Atti Associazione Genetica Italiana*, **9**, 141–5.

Mainardi, D., Marsan, M. & Pasquali, A. (1965a). Assenza di preferenze sessuali tra ceppi nel maschio di *Mus musculus domesticus*. *Instituto Lombardo (Rendiconti Scientifici)*, **B99**, 26–34.

Mainardi, D., Marsan, M. & Pasquali, A. (1965b). Causation of sexual preferences in the house mouse: the behavior of mice reared by parents whose odor was artificially altered. *Atti Società Italiana di Scienze Naturali Museo Civico Milano*, **104**, 325–38.

Murphy, M. R. (1980). Sexual preferences of male hamsters: importance of preweaning and adult experience, vaginal secretion, and olfactory or vomeronasal sensation. *Behavioral and Neural Biology*, **3**.

Oedberg, F. (1976). Failure to demonstrate imprinting on an artificial odour in two strains of mice. *Biology of Behaviour*, **1**, 309–27.

Porter, R. H., Deni, R. & Deane, H. M. (1977). Responses of *Acomys cahirinus* pups to chemical cues produced by a foster species. *Behavioral Biology*, **20**, 244–51.

Porter, R. H. & Etscorn, F. (1974). Olfactory imprinting resulting from brief exposure in *Acomys cahirinus*. *Nature*, **250**, 732–3.

Porter, R. H. & Etscorn, F. (1975). A primacy effect for olfactory imprinting in Spiny mouse. *Behavioral Biology*, **15**, 511–17.

Porter, R. H., Wyrick, M. & Pankey, J. (1978). Sibling recognition in spiny mice (*Acomys cahirinus*). *Behavioural Ecology and Sociobiology*, **3**, 61–8.

Quadagno, D. M. & Banks, E. M. (1970). The effect of reciprocal cross-fostering on the behaviour of two species of Rodents, *Mus musculus* and *Bayomys Taylori ater*. *Animal Behaviour*, **18**, 379–90.

Reimer, J. D. & Petras, M. L. (1967). Breeding structure of the house mouse, *Mus musculus*, in a population cage. *Journal of Mammalogy*, **45**, 88–9.

Rowe, F. P., Taylor, E. J. & Chudly, J. H. (1963). The number and movements of house mouse (*Mus musculus*) in the vicinity of four corn ricks. *Journal of Animal Ecology*, **32**, 87–97.

Smith, M. H. (1965). Behavioural discrimination shown by allopatric and sympatric males of *Peromyscus eremicus* and *Peromyscus californicus* between females of the same two species. *Evolution*, **19**, 430–5.

Yamazaki, K., Boyse, E. A., Miké, V., Thaler, H. T., Mathieson, B. J., Abbott, J., Boyse, J., Zayas, Z. A. & Thomas, L. (1976). Control of mating preferences in mice by genes in the major histocompatibility complex. *Journal of Experimental Medicine*, **144**, 1324–35.

Yamazaki, K., Yamaguchi, M., Andrews, P. W., Peake, B. & Boyse, E. A. (1978). Mating preferences of F2 segregants of crosses between MHC-congenic mouse strains. *Immunogenetics*, **6**, 253–9.

Yanai, J. & McClearn, G. E. (1972a). Assortative mating in mice: I. Female mating preference. *Behavior Genetics*, **2**, no. 2/3, 173–83.

Yanai, J. & McClearn, G. E. (1972b). Assortative mating in mice and the incest taboo. *Nature*, **238**, 281–2.

Yanai, J. & McClearn, G. E. (1973a). Assortative mating in mice: II. Strain differences in female mating preference, male preference, and the question of possible sexual selection. *Behavior Genetics*, **3**, no. 1, 65–74.

Yanai, J. & McClearn, G. E. (1973b). Assortative mating in mice: III. Genetic determination of female mating preference. *Behavior Genetics*, **3**, no. 1, 75–84.

V: COMPATIBILITY OF MATES

15

Re-mating in birds

IAN ROWLEY

The past fifty years have seen many intensive studies of birds that involved relatively short-lived, Northern Hemisphere species where the pair-bond was frequently and conspicuously renewed. Although many classics of ethology and population dynamics have come from such work, perhaps they have tended to over-emphasise the importance of courtship and to exaggerate the frequency with which new pairs are formed. In recent years several studies in other parts of the world have shown that many birds live for much longer than was previously suspected. Fogden (1972) found that many species in Sarawak had a minimum annual survival rate of around 86%; Snow & Lill (1974) showed similar figures for Trinidad, and Fry (1977) pointed out that Australian species tended to live far longer than their Northern Hemisphere counterparts. Rydzewski (1978) gathered together data from most parts of the world which confirmed that tropical and Southern Hemisphere birds are long-lived. It is, therefore, reasonable to assume that most birds that survive long enough to breed at all probably do so for more than one season. This means that a very large part of avian mate-choice is re-mating – mating for a second or subsequent reproductive effort.

This chapter reviews the value of re-mating with the same individual, the incidence of this in different monogamous species* and the associated problems – an important area which seems to have been neglected in favour of the more spectacular first pairings of strangers and virgins.

---

* Lack (1968) calculated that more than 92% of avian sub-families were monogamous. Since polygamy raises few problems in terms of re-mating that are not already shown by monogamous species and since polygamous mating systems have been comprehensively reviewed recently by Wittenberger (1979) they are not considered further here.

Terminology

I use the term mating as synonymous with copulation and pairing to cover the formation of a pair bond (*sensu* Hinde, 1964), usually a necessary precursor to mating except for promiscuous liaisons. So far as monogamous mate choice is concerned the major difference in mating systems is between those species that maintain *perennial* pair bonds and which consequently have no problem deciding with whom to mate each season, and those which have *seasonal* pair bonds that are formed at the start of each breeding season. Those individuals that form seasonal pair bonds and which survive to breed for a second time have two options for mate choice open to them – either they can re-mate with the same partner, which I call *re-uniting*, or they can choose a new mate and that I call *re-pairing*. In Table 15.6 I present such data on re-mating as I have been able to extract from the literature. In an attempt to standardise the data I consider only those pairs both members of which were individually identifiable. Between year one and year two a proportion of these pairs ceased to exist because one (or both) members died or otherwise disappeared; I follow Penney (1968) in calling this *splitting*. Re-pairing after loss of a partner is *mate-replacement* (see Fig. 15.1). Of those pairs, in which both members survive to year two, a proportion re-unite; those which do not are generally said to have *divorced*. The *divorce rate* is calculated as the % of pairs that survived to year two that did not re-unite; divorced individuals may either *re-sort* or remain solitary.

The advantages of re-uniting

Data are few and largely confined to sea birds but they do suggest that old-established pairs produce more young than new ones (Table 15.1). The advantages attributed to mating with the same partner as last time may be grouped under three headings: (1) physiological and behavioural characters associated with the age and experience of the partners; (2) established pairs achieving better breeding sites; and (3) the time saving involved in mating with a familiar partner.

Fig. 15.1. Terminology.

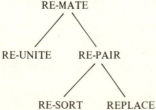

(*1*) *Advantages due to age or experience*

Most species suffer a heavy mortality of juveniles which leaves only individuals of higher quality to reach adulthood. Data are few but where they do exist they consistently show that older or more experienced adults produce more young (Table 15.2) until senescence intervenes. Most of the data come from colonial nesting sea birds and these have been recently reviewed by Ryder (1980); however there are sufficient examples from other species to support the generality of this concept and its importance (Perrins & Moss, 1974; Bryant, 1979; Rowley, 1981). Information about old age in animals is very scarce but does suggest that in long-lived species a reproductive decline (or even, cessation (Kummer, 1968)) may pre-date by several years the death of an individual.

A variety of factors lead to the choice of older or experienced partners as being more biologically efficient. Therefore re-uniting, which by definition *must* be mating with a non-novice, is favoured. These factors are:

(a) *Keeping company.* Many long-lived birds take one or two years to form their first pair bond (Penguins: Richdale, 1957: Albatrosses: Tickell, 1968: Swans: Minton, 1968) and during this time pairs do not lay eggs or even build a nest. Richdale (1951, p. 59) describes such penguins as 'keeping company'; during this time there is a considerable amount of swapping partners before a pair starts to breed. If a pair contemplating re-mating does not re-unite, then all this investment may be wasted if the 'new' pair has to start keeping company all over again.

Table 15.1. *A comparison of the productivity from old established and from newly formed pairs*

| | Fledglings per pair | | |
Bird	Established	New	% difference
Blue-faced Booby, *Sula dactylatra*[a]	0.74	0.48	43
Arctic Skua, *Stercorarius parasiticus*[b]	1.51	1.10	27
Kittiwake, *Rissa tridactyla*[c]	1.59	1.19	26
Red-billed Gull, *Larus novaehollandiae*[d]	0.92	0.81	12

[a] Kepler, 1969. [b] Wood, 1971. [c] Coulson, 1966. [d] Mills, 1973.

(b) *Egg size* increases with age in many species (Richdale, 1949; Mills, 1973) and although quality may vary with season as well as age (Schifferli, 1973) the size of the egg is generally assumed to reflect the reserves available for the embryo. Mills (1979) suggested that female Red-billed Gulls, *Larus novaehollandiae*, mated to older males produced larger eggs because such males were more assiduous in their courtship feeding of the female prior to egg laying, so that the age of both male and female partners may be significant.

(c) *Clutch size* has been shown to vary with age in several species of sea bird (Table 15.3) although many only lay one egg and so this factor is inoperative. Data on known-age passerines are few but show a similar trend (Bryant, 1979).

Table 15.2. *Number of fledglings raised per annum in relation to the experience of the female that reared them*

Bird	Experience of female	
	Novice	Experienced
Brown Pelican, *Pelecanus occidentalis*[a]	0.11	0.89
Gannet, *Sula bassana*[b]	0.52	0.82
Arctic Skua, *Stercorarius parasiticus*[c]	0.76	1.39
Kittiwake, *Rissa tridactyla*[d]	1.14	1.59
House Martin, *Delichon urbica*[e]	4.90	6.20
Splendid Wren, *Malurus splendens*[f]	1.62	3.41
Great Tit, *Parus major*[g]	0.94	1.45

[a] Blus & Keahey, 1978: table 1; [b] Nelson, 1966: table 15b; [c] Davis, 1976: table 1; [d] Coulson, 1966: table 6; [e] Bryant, 1979: table 2; [f] Rowley, 1981: table 14; [g] Perrins, 1979: table 25.

Table 15.3. *Influence of experience on clutch size*

Mean clutch size[a]	Breeding experience (years)		
	1	2–4	6–16
Kittiwake, *Rissa tridactyla*[b]	1.87	2.14	2.28
	(192)	(147)	(224)
Red-billed Gull,	1.64	1.92	1.96
Larus novaehollandiae[c]	(73)	(320)	(434)

[a] Sample size in parentheses. [b] Coulson, 1972: table 5; [c] Mills, 1973.

(d) *The laying date* tends to become earlier with increasing age or experience and particularly with the persistence of the pair bond. This is well shown for the gannet *Sula bassana* in Figure 15.2. If the pair bond is broken then laying reverts to a later date.

The importance of early laying varies with different species.

(i) For Arctic breeders the time when conditions are adequate for reproduction is brief and at a premium (Pitelka, Holmes & MacLean, 1974; Inglis, 1977).

(ii) For multi-brooded species an early start leaves time for later broods (Perrins, 1979).

(iii) In colonial nesters, early starters may achieve better sites and may be of better quality (Wooller & Coulson, 1977).

(iv) The penalty for late breeding is that only poor peripheral sites remain; birds in such sites sometimes suffer higher mortality presumably due to greater stress (Coulson, 1972).

(v) An increased risk of egg predation is incurred by late clutches which are out of phase with the colony as a whole (see review by Ryder, 1980).

Perrins (1970) drew attention to the importance of female nutrition prior to the formation of the eggs and it is probably the increased foraging efficiency of older females that enables them to lay down the necessary

Fig. 15.2. The relationship between age of female and the date upon which she lays, in the Gannet, *Sula bassana* (adapted from Fig. 52 in Nelson, 1978).

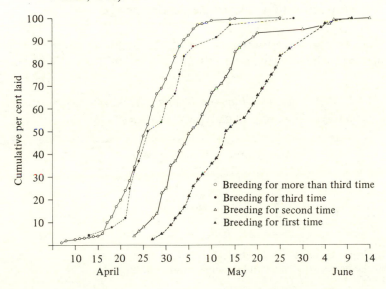

○ Breeding for more than third time
• Breeding for third time
△ Breeding for second time
▲ Breeding for first time

reserves sooner and start building their eggs earlier. That younger individuals are less-efficient foragers has been shown for several species (e.g. Orians, 1969; Recher & Recher, 1969; Dunn, 1972).

(e) *Hatching success* may vary with the age of the parents as is shown for the Yellow-eyed Penguin, *Megadyptes antipodes*, in Table 15.4. Two factors may influence this:

(i) Fertility of the male or female may increase either for physiological reasons or because of behavioural ineptitude at mating between novices.

(ii) Attentiveness during incubation may improve with time and experience. The Gannet provides a classic case and Nelson (1966) believes that some failures by young birds are due to their not manipulating the eggs correctly at the time of hatching. A Gannet egg is incubated between the webs of the feet and must be moved to the upper surface of the feet when pipping starts or else the chick is stood on and squashed. In Royal Penguins, *Eudyptes chrysolophus* it has been shown that older birds returning to breed are heavier due to greater reserves of subcutaneous fat. Without these reserves the males fail to defend their nest sites competently (Carrick & Ingham, 1970). It has been suggested (G. T. Smith, personal communication), that Royals without adequate reserves cannot delay their departure to sea after they have completed their incubation stint and that, unable to wait any longer for their relief to arrive (if it is late), they desert the egg.

(f) *Chick-raising* is yet another aspect of breeding that improves with age/experience. Ainley & Schlatter (1972) have shown that in the Adelie

Table 15.4. *Influence of age on hatching success of eggs in the Yellow-eyed Penguin*, Megadyptes antipodes

	Age of females (years)					
	2	3	4	5	6–13	14+
Number of eggs[a]	124	168	167	141	390	70
% hatching	32	77	87	91	92	77

(From Richdale, 1957: table 54.)

[a] Only eggs that were fully incubated are considered.

Penguin, *Pygoscelis adeliae*, the weight at fledging increased with the age of the parent as did the percentage of pairs that managed to rear two chicks (see Table 15.5).

(2) Quality of nest sites

In many species nest sites vary in quality and competition for good sites has long been recognised. With most sea birds, sites in the centre of the colony tend to be more productive; young birds pairing for the first time usually have to make do with peripheral sites but improve with time (Richdale, 1957; Coulson, 1972; Smith, 1974; Potts, Coulson & Deans, 1980).

Carrick (1972) with the Australian Black-backed Magpie, *Gymnorhina tibicen*, describes group formation and the progress, with time, up the ladder of territorial quality. I relate this in some detail since Carrick's paper is not readily available, nor known as widely as it deserves. Suitable magpie breeding habitat is scarce near Canberra and 19% of the population live in large non-breeding flocks. Four sorts of group are recognised; individuals first associate together as *open* groups in the non-breeding flock and progress through being *mobile* groups to *marginal* territories until they attain prime *permanent* territories when they become available. The productivity of these permanent territories far exceeds that of any other category – 0.56 fledglings per adult female compared to 0.09. Fig. 15.3 shows 38 permanent, seven marginal, four mobile and four open group territories. When the adult pair in permanent group four were killed on the road marginal group XLVI took over immediately. To test the quality of territories Carrick (1963) placed wooden trays on 10-ft poles in open group territories to provide the nest sites that were lacking; 25 groups failed

Table 15.5 *Influence of age on fledging success in the Adelie Penguin*, Pygoscelis adeliae

Age of parents (years)	Weight of fledgling (kg)	% of pairs with 2-chick broods
3	2.0	0
3	2.4	8
5	2.6	20
6–8	2.8	22

(From Ainley & Schlatter, 1972)

to respond but eight built nests, five laid eggs and two reared chicks. A full description of the formation and rise to breeding status of another group of magpies was given by Carrick (1970) and has been summarised by Rowley (1975, pp. 94–5).

Krebs (1971) showed with the Great Tit, *Parus major*, that there was

Fig. 15.3. Territories of Australian Magpies, *Gymnorhina tibicen*, in the breeding season of 1961. The four types of group were represented by 38 permanent (Arabic numerals), seven marginal (Roman numerals), four mobile (encircled) and four open (in parentheses) groups. Wooden trays on poles were presented to some open groups (see Carrick, 1963); five bred and two reared chicks with these 'improvements'. (Adapted from Fig. 3 of Carrick, 1972.)

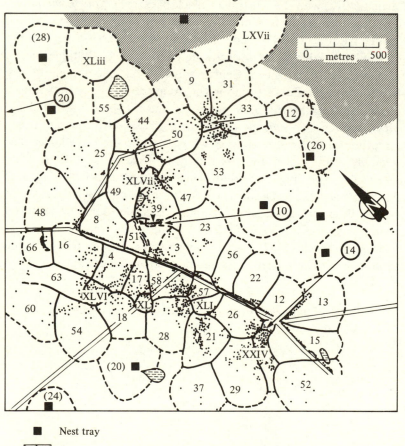

■ Nest tray

Trees

Non-breeder flock

Water

a reservoir of less-fortunate birds that rapidly took over the prime territories in Wytham Woods when he removed prime pairs.

Baeyens (1981) suggests that European magpies, *Pica pica*, have class I and class II territories and that young birds gain the latter as stepping stones to attaining vacant class I territories when they become available, sometimes breaking a pair bond to do so.

The warehouse Kittiwake, *Rissa tridactyla*, colony has been studied by Coulson and colleagues for more than 25 years and is discussed in detail in chapter 16. Sites in the centre of the colony are more productive and pairs there suffer fewer divorces than those on the edge. Edge males suffer a higher mortality rate (Coulson, 1972). Patterson (1965) and Hutson (1977) found similar peripheral effects with Black-headed Gulls, *Larus ridibundus*.

A study of Shags, *Phalacrocorax aristotelis*, on the Farne Islands has shown that nest-site quality and breeding experience were the two main factors affecting breeding success. Older birds returned to the colony earlier in the year, achieved better nest sites and raised more young. After the massive mortality in 1968 caused by the 'red-tide' (a toxic dinoflagellate bloom), the breeding performance of young Shags increased by 71% and that of older birds by 39%; both increases were attributed to changes in the quality of nest sites available to the survivors (Potts *et al.*, 1980).

(3) *Familiarity of partners*

In long-lived, experienced, birds, especially those with permanent pair bonds, courtship is brief and minimal, which is probably why copulation is so rarely observed in most of these species. The two partners already spend all day and every day together and side-by-side perform the variety of daily tasks – foraging, defending territory, preening or roosting – so that to a very large extent they are attuned to each other. Such birds certainly are not strangers needing elaborate courtship before the male can overcome his aggression towards an intruding female (*Corvus* spp.; Rowley, 1974).

Individuals that approach the breeding season already paired have a head start over birds that begin from scratch. This time saving may well result in the earlier egg laying of experienced birds and their consequent better breeding success (see above). Time may be crucial at high latitudes where climate severely limits the breeding season. Inglis (1977) describes Pink-footed Geese, *Anser brachyrhynchus*, arriving on their Icelandic breeding grounds not only already paired but with most copulation accomplished. He saw copulation once in 930 h over 46 days. Ryder (1967) describes a similar state of affairs for Ross' Goose, *Anser rossii*, on the Perry River.

Many seasonal breeders undergo a regression of the gonads and a massive post-nuptial moult after they have finished nesting. For spring breeders this process culminates in an autumnal recrudescence that may lead to heightened sexual activity depending on the species, the age of the individual and the nature of the season (Marshall & Coombs, 1957). In some cases autumnal nesting may take place but usually some factor (such as temperature or daylength) intervenes and breeding is delayed until spring. Most ornithologists make most of their observations during the breeding season and good field data on behaviour are rare outside this time. It does appear that many resident species may form pairs in the autumn (Coombs, 1960; Gorman, 1974), and that these persist through to the next breeding season. Data for migrants are fewer and confined largely to the waterfowl where ducks of the genus *Athya* pair routinely on the wintering grounds in southern North America (Weller, 1965).

Another value of familiarity between partners is stressed in yet another context, by Kunkel (1974) in his extensive review of mating systems found amongst tropical birds. Kunkel draws attention to the many tropical species that have very extended breeding seasons and points out that a member of such a species searching for a mate is faced with the problem of finding a conspecific at a compatible physiological state of readiness. Amongst other mechanisms to achieve successful mating amongst tropical birds Kunkel considers permanent pair bonds to be an efficient way of ensuring compatibility between partners, and considers this system to be common amongst many tropical families (Kunkel, 1974, Table 1).

Reasons for failure to re-unite

Despite the many advantages attributable to re-uniting with the same partner as last year, this course is not always practical or even possible. Whether or not a species usually re-mates depends largely on two factors – their longevity and their life style.

Longevity

Paramount amongst all the factors affecting mate choice for re-mating is the longevity of the species. Obviously the question of re-uniting old partners does not arise if one of them has died. Many of the small, much studied, passerines of the Northern Hemisphere suffer adult mortality rates around 50% per annum. Even where the annual adult survival is as high as 70% the probability that pairs will survive intact from one year to the next is only 0.49 (0.7 × 0.7). This means that any pair of a seasonally-bonded species with less than 70% survival is faced with odds that are worse than even that a partner will have failed to survive. It is reasonable to assume that selection would not favour mate fidelity in species exhibiting high adult mortality for despite the benefits accruing to re-uniting the cost of waiting for the non-return of a dead mate could well mean that opportunities for re-pairing are forgone when prospective new mates are lost after being rebuffed. If one sex outnumbers the other, as frequently happens, the more numerous sex cannot afford to pass up the opportunity to re-pair for too long or else there may be no available candidates left.

At the other extreme those species with long life spans and many years of reproductive activity stand to gain most from pairs remaining together and perfecting their reproductive technique.

Life styles

Although the life style of a species may vary between populations and between cohorts of different ages, within any one population a particular life style is characteristic and influences the pattern of mate choice. This, together with longevity, largely decides the frequency of re-uniting that takes place.

If the movements associated with juvenile dispersal and immature flocks are disregarded, different species of bird may be categorised as living in one (or more) of three basic life-styles: they may be *residents*, spending all their adult life in one locality; they may be *migratory* in the strict sense defined by Lack (1954) to involve regular movement twice a year between two restricted geographical areas, a breeding and a wintering one; or they may be *nomadic* wandering far and wide in response to unpredictable climatic, cyclic, or seasonal conditions. Despite these fundamental differences all birds lay eggs that require incubation in a stationary nest. Even migrants and nomads must, therefore, cease travelling for long enough to hatch eggs and to raise young to a stage where they can accompany their parents or take care of themselves.

As with many attempts at classification these three life styles are not clear-cut entities but tend to merge one into the other and to vary widely in detail.

Table 15.6 presents data gleaned from the literature grouped according to lifestyle. Only species where more than ten pairs of individually identifiable birds have been studied are included. From one year to the next a proportion of these birds disappear and are never seen again; this loss

Table 15.6. *The persistence of pair-bonds in birds*

Species	Number of breeding pairs		In year two		divorced (%)	References
	In year one	Split[a] (%)	both alive	re-united		
Residents						
(i) Mute Swan, *Cygnus olor*	535	27	389	292	5	Minton, 1968
Lesser Sheathbill, *Chionis minor*	45	27	33	33	0	Burger, 1980
Greater Kestrel, *Falco rupicoloides*	37	24	28	26	7	Kemp, in litt.
Australian Raven, *Corvus coronoides*	221	27	161	161	0	Rowley, 1973
(ii) Superb Wren, *Malurus cyaneus*	27	78	6	6	0	Rowley, 1965
Splendid Wren, *Malurus splendens*	52	52	25	25	0	Rowley, 1981
(iii) Galah, *Cacatua roseicapilla*	177	47	92	85	8	Rowley, unpublished
Major Mitchell's Cockatoo, *C. leadbeateri*	45	11	40	40	0	Rowley, unpublished
Feral Pigeon, *Columba livea*	7	29	5	5	0	Murton, Thearle & Coombs, 1974
(iv) Song-thrush, *Turdus philomelos*	11	100	0	0	0	Davies & Snow, 1965
Blackbird, *Turdus merula*	50	64	18	16	11	Snow, 1958
Robin, *Erithacus rubecula*	24	79	7	6	14	Lack, 1940
(v) Natal Robin, *Cossypha natalensis*	19	32	13	9	31	Farkas, 1969
Flightless Cormorant, *Nannopterum harrisi*	—	(13)	151	18	88	Harris, 1979
Skylark, *Alauda arvensis*	—	—	36	17	53	Delius, 1965
Marsh Tit, *Parus palustris*	16	69	5	4	20	Southern & Morley, 1950
Great Tit, { UK	329	66	109	77	29	Harvey, Greenwood & Perrins, 1979; Kluijver, 1951
Parus major { Holland	—	(> 50)	71	55	23	

Migrants

Species						Reference
Shelduck, *Tadorna tadorna*	—	—	112	83	27	Patterson (in litt).
Stilt Sandpiper, *Micropalama himantopus*	25	56	11	11	0	Jehl, 1973
Dunlin, *Calidris alpina*	—	(27)	43	31	28	Soikkeli, 1967
Western Sandpiper, *Calidris mauri*	—	(50)	13	8	38	Holmes, 1971
Swift, *Apus apus*	41	34	27	27	0	Weitnauer, 1947
Welcome Swallow, *Hirundo neoxena*	25	48	13	12	8	Park, 1981
House Martin, *Delichon urbica*	127	83	21	0	100	Bryant, 1979, and in litt.
Song-sparrow, *Melospiza melodia*	200	85	30	8	73	Nice, 1937
Field sparrow, *Spizella pusilla*	25	92	2	1	50	Best, 1977
Prairie Warbler, *Dendroica discolor*	154	92	13	6	54	Nolan, 1978
House Wren, *Troglodytes aedon*	215	88	26	11	58	Kendeigh, 1941

Nomads

Species						Reference
Adelie Penguin, *Pygoscelis adeliae*	277	40	165	138	16	Penney, 1968
Adelie Penguin, *Pygoscelis adeliae*	193	60	77	24	44	Le Resche & Sladen, 1970
22 pairs did not breed leaving: 55						
Rock-hopper Penguin, *Eudyptes chrysocome*	25	44	14	13	7	Warham, 1963
Yellow-eyed Penguin, *Megadyptes antipodes*	737	27	539	442	18	Richdale, 1957
Little Penguin, *Eudyptula minor*	158	12	139	115	17	Reilly & Cullen, 1981, and in litt.
Wandering Albatross, *Diomedea exultans*	64	17	53	53	0	Tickell, 1968
Waved Albatross, *D. irrorata*	310	(5)	—	272	—	Harris, 1973
Laysan Albatross, *D. immutabilis*	341	3	330	323	2	Rice & Kenyon, 1962
Buller's Mollymawk, *D. bulleri*	—	—	400	400	0	Richdale & Warham, 1973

343

Table 15.6—*continued*

Species	Number of breeding pairs					References
	In year one	Split[a] (%)	In year two		Divorced (%)	
			both alive	re-united		
Northern Fulmar, *Fulmarus glacialis*	—	—	443	422	5	Ollason & Dunnet, 1978
Northern Fulmar, *Fulmarus glacialis*	54	2	53	51	4	Macdonald, 1977
Fairy Prion, *Pachystila turtur*	223	56	98	96	1	Richdale, 1965
Sooty Shearwater, *Puffinus griseus*	83	77	32	19	41	Richdale, 1963
Manx Shearwater, *P. puffinus*	—	—	175	158	10	Brooke, 1978
Northern Gannet, *Sula bassana*	149	23	126	96	15	Nelson, 1978
Masked Booby, *S. dactylatra*	56	25	42	23	45	Kepler, 1969
Great Skua, *Stercorarius skua*	294	9	267	263	1	Wood, 1971
Glaucous-winged Gull, *Larus glaucescens*	13	23	10	7	30	Vermeer, 1963
Silver Gull, *L. novaehollandiae* (N.Z.)	153	10	138	125	9	Mills, 1973
Silver Gull, *L. novaehollandiae* (W. Australia)	50	18	41	40	2	Nicholls, 1974 and personal communication
Common Kittiwake, *Rissa tridactyla*	458	11	408	295	38	Coulson, 1966
Oystercatcher, *Haematopus ostralegus*	83	20	66	58	12	Harris, 1967
White-tailed Black Cockatoo, *Calyptorhynchus funereus*	126	41	74	73	1	Saunders, 1982
Corella, *Cacatua tenuirostris*	16	12	14	13	7	Smith, personal communication
Little Raven, *Corvus mellori*	107	31	74	68	8	Rowley, 1973
Australian Shelduck, *Tadorna tadornoides*	—	—	63	42	33	Riggert, 1977

[a] Figure in parentheses indicates % mortality in species where data for 'splitting' were not available.

is generally accepted as being synonymous with death, but we do know that in a few cases some individuals survived outside the study area, unrecognised. I have used the term 'split' to indicate pairs that have been broken through this non-reappearance of one (or both) parties (after Penney, 1968). The percentage of pairs splitting is shown in Table 15.6; it is higher than the mortality figure. Column 3 of Table 15.6 shows the number of pairs both members of which survived from year one to year two; a long-lived pair contributes for each year that the two birds survive. Those pairs which do not re-unite although their partner is alive are said to have divorced (by general usage); where two pairs swap partners this counts as two divorces.

(a) *Residents* live in five ways and species are grouped accordingly in Table 15.6.

(i) Some species live in all-purpose territories (= exclusive areas) that provide all the requirements of the pair throughout the year, and of their family until the young disperse. Such species have the least problem in maintaining their pair bonds since male and female are always together. Divorce is rare and perennial monogamy is the commonest mating system, pairs enduring so long as both partners survive.

Many long-lived species take several years to reach sexual maturity and immatures with unpaired adults tend to live in relatively footloose flocks that serve as reservoirs from which casualties in the breeding population can be replaced. Such mate replacement may pose special problems and the field of candidates for mate choice may be far smaller than is generally realised. In the case of *Corvus coronoides* loss of a female from an established pair may be made good within hours at the height of the breeding season (Territory 1–4, Fig. 15.4): certainly in time for the new

Fig. 15.4. Constancy of pair bonds in the Australian Raven, *Corvus coronoides* (part of Fig. 4 of Rowley, 1973).

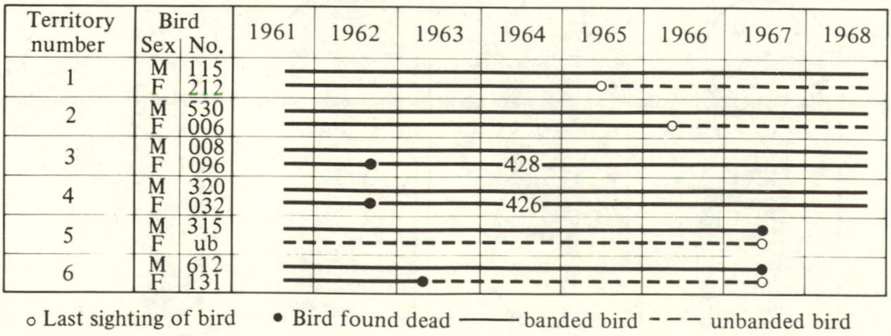

Territory number	Bird Sex	No.	1961	1962	1963	1964	1965	1966	1967	1968
1	M	115								
	F	212								
2	M	530								
	F	006								
3	M	008								
	F	096			428					
4	M	320								
	F	032			426					
5	M	315								
	F	ub								
6	M	612								
	F	131								

o Last sighting of bird   • Bird found dead ——— banded bird − − − unbanded bird female sometimes to help raise her predecessor's nestlings. The male appears to have no difficulty in defending his territory and attracting a new mate at the same time. However if the male dies (Territory 5 & 6, Figs. 15.4), breaking the pair bond, the surviving female, although rapidly supplied with suitors, appears unable to re-mate and to defend territory; her new consort, of course, has no idea of the territory boundaries and the conflict between courting the 'widow' and learning the bounds of the real estate, appears to be too much. Widowed female *C. coronoides*, therefore, withdraw to the flock of unmated birds where they forge a new pair bond, and at a later season may achieve territorial status again (Rowley, 1973).

(ii) In the tropics and southern temperate regions several resident territorial species tend to live in groups containing more than two adults (*Turdoides* spp.: Zahavi 1974; Gaston, 1977, 1978; *Corcorax melano-rhamphus*: Rowley, 1978; *Malurus* spp.: Rowley, 1965, 1981; *Corvinella corvina*: Grimes, 1980). Divorce is unknown in such groups; not only do pair bonds survive well, but replacement of casualties is usually from

Fig. 15.5. Re-uniting (dark shading) and replacement by inheritance (medium) or succession (light), in the Splendid Wren, *Malurus splendens*. Cross-hatched areas were unoccupied for a season following a major calamity such as a fire. (Data from Rowley 1981, updated.)

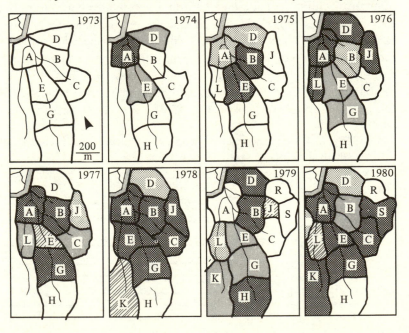

within the group and therefore immediate and requiring minimal introduction by way of courtship. Where such a replacement by *inheritance* is
not available within a group, replacement by a neighbouring supernumerary
may take place quickly as is shown in Fig 15.5 (= '*succession*').

(iii) Some resident species have a permanent nest-site territory to which
they return daily (usually to roost) although they spend most of their time
foraging in a locally nomadic flock. Such species maintain long-lasting
monogamous pair bonds and divorce is rare. Replacement of casualties
is generally rapid and from within the local flock (Fig. 15.6), so that the
range of candidates for mate choice is restricted. Galahs, *Cacatua
roseicapilla*, replaced during a breeding-season do not breed that year.
Major Mitchell's Cockatoo, *C. leadbeateri*, may even spend their first
season together 'keeping company' without laying eggs (Rowley, unpublished data).

(iv) In a few species of residents the pairs break up after the young are
reared and males and females maintain separate territories throughout the

Fig. 15.6. Local foraging movements made by breeding Galahs,
Cacatua roseicapilla, showing restricted range of candidates for mate
replacement.

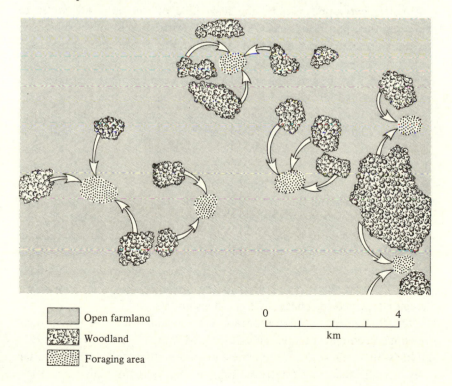

☐ Open farmland

▨ Woodland

▦ Foraging area

0   4

km

non-breeding season (e.g. Robins, *Erithacus rubecula*: Lack, 1939; Blackbirds, *Turdus merula*: Snow, 1958). Whether due to high mortality, to females moving further than males (even migrating in the case of the robin), or to the difficulties of transforming an enemy who has been occupying the next-door territory into a mate when it comes time to breed, pair bonds in Robins and Blackbirds are surprisingly transitory.

(v) Some resident species cease to defend a particular area (= territory) after the young are fledged and may spend the non-breeding season foraging over a home range shared with several other pairs (Great Tit, *Parus major*: Hinde, 1952; Chaffinch, *Fringella coelebs*: Marler, 1956; Steller's Jay, *Cyanoccita stelleri*: Brown, 1963; Skylark, *Alauda arvensis*: Delius, 1965; Bicoloured Antbird, *Gymnopithys bicolor*: Willis, 1967; Natal Robin, *Cossypha natalensis*: Farkas, 1968). The extent to which the pair bond is maintained in these local flocks appears to vary widely and probably influences the divorce rate. Some of these species (Willis, 1967) form pairs in the flock and then take up territory together whilst in the others the males take up territories and attract mates to them (Delius, 1965).

(b) *Migrants* appear to be the least able of the three life styles to maintain their pair bonds (see Table 15.6), partly because of the increased mortality due to the hazards of long distance travel and partly to a tendency for each sex to travel each way in separate waves, with males arriving back at the breeding site a week or more before the females. An extreme case is that of the Pochard, *Anas ferina*, and the Tufted Duck, *A. fuligula*, where the two sexes occupy separate winter quarters after migrating (Salmonsen, 1968). Nisbet & Medway (1972) found that male and female Eastern Great Reed Warblers, *Acrocephalus orientalis*, occupied different habitats in winter. Price (1981) found that individual Greenish Warblers, *Phylloscopus trochipodes*, of each sex maintained their own territories throughout the winter and that they returned to the same winter territories the next year. White Wagtails, *Motacilla alba*, have been studied as individually colour-banded migrants on their winter quarters in Israel and Zahavi (1971) found that if food was provided pairs established and defended territories. Zahavi considered that these pair-bonds were unlikely to be the same ones as operated at the breeding sites since males and females departed in separate waves, days apart.

Not all migrants travel in separate waves; some waders arrive on their breeding grounds together (Huxley & Montague, 1926; Lind, 1961; Holmes, 1966) but since most partners migrate south at different times after they have finished breeding, it is unlikely that breeding pairs spend the winter together. Recently data on the site fidelity of migrant waders in their winter quarters have been presented (papers in Pitelka, 1979) but I have been unable to locate any evidence of mate fidelity there.

Most ducks are short-lived, breed when one year old, and do not maintain permanent pair bonds. However, the shelduck tribe do form long-lasting bonds and in some species these survive the spectacular moult migrations that occur immediately after breeding is completed although the sexes appear to travel both ways, separately and without their families (*Tadorna tadorna*: Patterson, Young & Tompa, 1974; Patterson, *in litt.*). Migratory swans and geese both tend to travel with their progeny of the last nesting and to maintain long-lasting pair bonds throughout the winter (Raveling, 1969; Cook, 1976; Evans, 1979; Scott, 1980) and presumably these pairs re-mate. Some geese that nest in the Arctic arrive back at their breeding grounds already paired (Ryder, 1967; Kistchinski, 1971; Inglis, 1977).

The few data for the migatory passerines that I have been able to unearth emphasise that more than 80% of pairs are split from one season to the next and that divorce takes place amongst the survivors in more than 50% of cases from the four North American species studied. It appears that males show great site fidelity but that the females are much more variable in this regard, so that the chances of a male re-uniting are very small.

Contrary to the American experience the only true migrant to have been studied in Australia, the Welcome Swallow, *Hirundo neoxena*, appears to suffer less splitting and to maintain its pair bonds surprisingly well (Park, 1981). We do not know, yet, where these birds winter, but this evidence suggests that their journey is not very arduous or dangerous.

(c) *Nomads* are the wanderers: birds that, once breeding is completed, may travel thousands of kilometres to find the right conditions for feeding or until the urge to breed arises again. Nomads may be divided into (i) the true *opportunists* that will respond to optimal conditions of food and climate and settle to breed wherever these occur (Ibis: Carrick, 1962; Woodswallows: Immelmann, 1962; Ducks: Frith, 1962), or (ii) those that show *site fidelity* such as sea birds that return to traditional breeding sites which may be either colonial (Gulls) or territorial (Oystercatchers).

(i) So far as the maintenance of pair bonds is concerned no good data exist for the opportunistic species since no-one has invested the time and effort necessary to colour band individuals in situations where they are never likely to be encountered again. Most probably mortality is high and the lifespan relatively short so that few pair bonds will survive from one breeding to the next.

(ii) With species that return to traditional sites (philopatry) good data are available particularly in the case of the Yellow-eyed Penguin studied by Richdale from 1936 to 1948, the Black-legged Kittiwake studied by Coulson since 1954 (and continuing), the study of the Adelie Penguin at Cape Crozier (1962–1972) and of the Little Penguin, *Eudyptula minor*, that has been running since 1968 (Reilly & Cullen, 1981). Other, less long-term studies are included in Table 15.6 which shows that both mortality and divorce tend to be higher amongst nomads than residents.

In many of the coastal and inland philopatric nomads the pairs return to their breeding site together at the start of a new season and show a high incidence of re-uniting (Herring Gulls, *Larus argentatus*: Tinbergen, 1956; Oystercatcher, *Haematopus ostralegus*: Harris, 1967; Little Raven, *Corvus mellori*: Rowley, 1973; White-tailed Black Cockatoos, *Calyptorhynchus funereus*: Saunders, 1979). Unfortunately little is known about the relationship between individuals away from the breeding area except that Tinbergen (1956) said that gulls formed pairs in 'clubs' before moving to the breeding area. In the White-tailed Black Cockatoo, Saunders found that the young of the previous year stayed with its parents right through the winter, and I am sure this accounts for the low divorce rate in that species. The Silver Gull is of particular interest because it illustrates the variability that may occur within a species. The Western Australian population may breed two or three times in the year (Nicholls, 1974; Wooller & Dunlop, 1979), whilst the New Zealand race breeds only once a year (Mills, 1973). Only one pair of 41 that survived for a year divorced in Western Australia ($= 2\%$) compared with a 9% divorce rate in New Zealand. This probably reflects a greater tendency for the former to remain together throughout the year. A tantalising snippet from south-eastern Australia (Carrick, 1972) describes a pair, the female of which was resident whilst the male travelled some 500 km to his winter quarters, which further illustrates the variability that can occur within a population.

The nomadic, seasonally breeding, pelagic seabirds provide some fascinating contrasts and comparisons. Because they travel a long way to feed, incubation and foraging stints tend to be prolonged and so the pair lacks the repeated co-operative exchanges of other species and the consequent reinforcement of the pair bond. Albatrosses show a remarkably low divorce rate (0–2%) especially when it is considered that many can raise young only every other year (see Table 15.6). This constancy of pair bond appears to be the consequence of a very long time spent keeping company before the pair begins serious nesting and egg production. One can only assume that companions are changed quite frequently during this time and that compatible partners emerge and only then begin to nest. With

Yellow-eyed Penguins, Adelie Penguins and Kittiwakes overall divorce rates are much higher (16–28%) than in Albatrosses. Le Resche & Sladen (1970) showed that young Adelies split and divorced much more frequently than older birds (see Table 15.7). Functionally, therefore, these first breeding attempts may be regarded as an extension of the 'keeping company' period.

Pelagic penguins demonstrate the problems of nomads trying to maintain pair bonds. Fig. 15.7 shows the pattern of parental behaviour in the Adelie Penguin and emphasises the little time that the pair spends together during the year: there is nowhere near so great an opportunity for pair-bond reinforcement as occurs with most passerines. In most of the pelagic nomads the males tend to return to the nest site first and to show mate fidelity only secondarily. The strength of this fidelity was beautifully demonstrated by Penney (1962) with the Adelie Penguin; he and his assistants could pick up incubating penguins and swap birds that were near neighbours, each settling contentedly on the egg it found at the new site. When the female returned from sea to take her turn at incubating she went straight to her correct site (but wrong mate) and was soundly pecked; she then moved to her correct mate, changed over and proceeded to rear the 'wrong' egg!

Discussion

This review shows that provided both partners survive, their reproductive success is likely to be greatest if they re-mate with the bird they bred with last season, but that not all species manage to find last year's

Table 15.7. *Comparison of splitting and mate fidelity between young and old Adelie Penguins*, Pygoscelis adeliae

	Pairs year one	Split		Pairs year two				
				Both alive	Re-united	Divorced		
		N	%			N	%	
Old pairs	277	112	40	165	138	27	16	Penney, 1968
Young pairs	193	166	60	77 (but 22 did not breed)				
				55	34	24	44	Le Resche & Sladen, 1970[a]

[a] Table V1 of this paper presents an incorrect arrangement of the figures: the divorce rate could have been 56% but the point to be made is the same.

partner with equal ease. Residents that maintain some form of territory all the year round as a pair have least problem (Raven, Galah, Major Mitchell, Mute Swan, Feral Pigeon and Sparrow) – their mate is present all day, every day. Species that abandon their breeding territory once the young are fledged face greater difficulties if the pair bond is to persist – they must show fidelity either to mate alone (Great Tit, Oystercatcher, Little Raven) or to their family (Bewick's Swan, Pink-footed, Canada, and Snow Geese and Black Cockatoos).

The greatest difficulty occurs in those species that only pair for the breeding season. It appears that male and female separate after breeding and enter a post-nuptial moult with regression of the gonads that very probably leads to a virtually asexual existence until the next breeding

Fig. 15.7. Average schedule of presence and absence in the colony for breeding males and females of the Adelie Penguin, *Pygoscelis adeliae.* (A) over 1959–1960 season, (B) nesting routine showing the small amount of overlap between parents. (Adapted from Penney, 1968.)

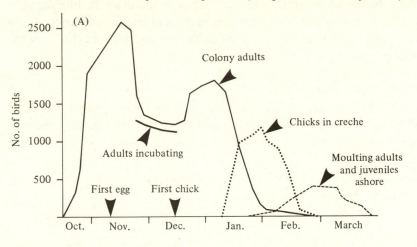

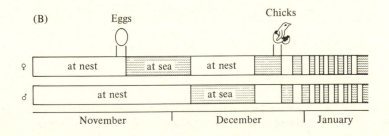

season comes round. Relationships between such individuals in the non-breeding season may vary from outright territorial aggression, as between individual Robins and Blackbirds (irrespective of sex), through various flock dominance hierarchies, to the state described by Zahavi (1971) with pairs forming on the non-breeding grounds presumably because two birds could defend a limited food source better than one.

The urge to breed reawakens in such seasonal breeders at different times in different species but whenever it occurs those cases where the pair bond has been broken are faced with the same problem namely 'has the mate of last year survived?' This is the point where mortality as a species-specific characteristic becomes extremely important. Natural selection for mate fidelity does not seem to have occurred in those species that suffer high mortality. Instead selection in such birds appears to have been towards site fidelity, particularly in the male, and whether or not a pair re-unites depends on the female returning to the nest site that she used the previous year and to a lesser extent on *when* she returns.

With longer-lived species the picture is different. It is harder to find any pattern and there does not appear to be any one explanation for the wide variation in divorce rates found in species with apparently similar ecology. Coulson (1966) and others, have suggested that swapping partners could be a response to poor success in breeding the previous year; data are adequate for thorough analysis in only a very few species (Table 15.8). In the Kittiwake and Manx Shearwater such divorce is particularly evident

Table 15.8. *Comparison of the divorce rates following reproductive success or failure*

	Rate of divorce following previous years' breeding	
	Success	Failure
Little Penguin, *Eudyptula minor*[a]	15% (84)	20% (55)
Manx Shearwater, *Puffinus puffinus*[b]	5% (138)	27% (37)
Flightless Cormorant, *Nannopterum harrisi*[c]	89% (36)	91% (46)
Kittiwake, *Rissa tridactyla*[d]	17% (281)	52% (44)

[a] Reilly & Cullen, 1981; [b] Brooke, 1978; [c] Harris, 1979; [d] Coulson, 1966.

amongst failed breeders but figures from the Little Penguin suggest that differences are not significant in that species. Nesting failure, particularly at the egg stage, means that the seasonal pair bond is broken earlier and has less opportunity for reinforcement through the joint raising of a family. The non-bonded period is correspondingly lengthened and I suggest it is this, rather than a specific assessment of breeding capacity, that achieves a re-sorting of partners. I have included the anomalous Flightless Cormorant, *Nannopterum harrisi*, in Table 15.8 for its apparent reversal of the trend; this is due to the male partner of successful pairs taking his fledglings to sea to teach them how to forage, whilst the females frequently re-mate and may breed several times in a year (Harris, 1979).

The period of keeping company and a certain amount of mate re-sorting is an important aspect of mate choice. Biologists should beware the stud-breeders' simple outlook – that male plus female equals offspring. Aviculturalists have long been alert to the importance of compatibility in birds and of the need to provide captive birds with a choice of partners to achieve successful breeding. There is no reason to suppose that wild birds are any less choosey, and what we label 'divorce' is, in reality, mate choice being exercised by individuals attempting to re-mate.

I would like to suggest that for long-lived birds the major part of the addition to the population in any one year may come from a relatively few, very successful, pairs. And that those pairs reach this pinnacle of success over a period of years during which they may (1) re-sort partners until compatibility is attained, (2) improve their breeding performance by experience, and (3) enhance their breeding opportunities by achieving better nest sites. Within any one species the relative importance of these three factors will vary.

Summary

Many species of tropical and southern temperate birds are longlived and therefore re-mating is an important aspect of their mate choice. To re-unite with the mate of a previous season has many advantages but the ease with which such individuals find each other varies according to life style and longevity. Residents that maintain pair bonds all the year round have few problems in this regard. Migrants that sever their seasonal pair bonds after breeding may travel long distances separately and tend to have been selected for philopatry rather than mate fidelity. A review of those studies that present data from individually marked birds over several seasons is presented.

Many people helped in the preparation of this chapter by discussion, by suggesting titles that I had overlooked, and by supplying data in a form suitable for my review: I thank them for their patience and apologise for not listing them all by name. I hope that those authors whose work I have overlooked will appreciate the size of the literature search involved and that they and those who consider I have misconstrued their data will take the trouble to write and inform me. The figures were prepared by C. P. S. de Rebeira of the Division of Wildlife Research, CSIRO.

References

Ainley, D. G. & Schlatter, R. P. (1972). Chick-raising ability in Adelie Penguins. *Auk*, **89**, 559–66.

Baeyens, G. (1981). Functional aspects of serial monogamy: the magpie pair-bond in relation to its territorial system. *Ardea*, **69**, 145–66.

Best, L. B. (1977). Territory quality and mating success in the Field Sparrow (*Spizella pusilla*). *Condor*, **70**, 192–204.

Blus, L. J. & Keehey, J. A. (1978). Variation in reproductivity with age in the Brown Pelican. *Auk*, **95**, 128–34.

Brooke, M. de L. (1978). Some factors affecting the laying date, incubation and breeding success of the Manx Shearwater, *Puffinus puffinus*. *Journal of Animal Ecology*, **47**, 477–95.

Brown, J. L. (1963). Aggressiveness, dominance and social organisation in the Steller Jay. *Condor*, **65**, 460–84.

Bryant, D. M. (1979). Reproductive costs in the House Martin (*Delichon urbica*). *Journal of Animal Ecology*, **48**, 655–75.

Burger, A. E. (1980). An analysis of the displays of Lesser Sheathbills *Chionis minor*. *Zeitschrift für Tierpsychologie*, **52**, 381–96.

Carrick, R. (1962). Breeding, movements, and conservation of Ibises (Threskiornithidae) in Australia. *CSIRO Wildlife Research* **7**, 71–88.

Carrick, R. (1963). Ecological significance of territory in the Australian Magpie *Gymnorhina tibicen*. In *Proceedings of the XIIIth International Ornithological Congress*, vol. **2**, ed. C. G. Sibley, pp. 740–53. A.O.U.: Louisiana.

Carrick, R. (1970). Follow the band. *Australian Bird Bander*, **8**, 62–3.

Carrick, R. (1972). Population ecology of the Australian Black-backed Magpie, Royal Penguin, and Silver Gull. In 'Population Ecology of Migratory Birds: a Symposium', *United States Department of the Interior, Wildlife Research Report* **2**, 41–89.

Carrick, R. & Ingham, S. E. (1970). Ecology and population dynamics of antarctic sea birds. In *Antarctic Ecology*, vol. **1**, ed. M. W. Holdgate, pp. 505–25. Academic Press: New York.

Cooke, F. G. (1976). Sections on reproduction of the Snow Goose/Blue Goose, *Anser coerulescens*, in *Handbook of North American Birds*, vol. **2**, ed. R. S. Palmer, pp. 143–8. Yale University Press: New Haven.

Coombs, C. J. F. (1960). Observations on the Rook *Corvus frugilegus* in southwest Cornwall. *Ibis*, **102**, 394–419.

Coulson, J. C. (1966). The influence of the pair-bond and age on the breeding biology of the Kittiwake Gull *Rissa tridactyla*. *Journal of Animal Ecology*, **35**, 269–79.

Coulson, J. C. (1972). The significance of the pair-bond in the Kittiwake. In *Proceedings of the XVth International Ornithological Congress*, ed. K. H. Voous, pp. 424–33. Brill: Leiden.

Davies, P. W. & Snow, D. W. (1965). Territory and food in the Song Thrush. *British Birds*, **58**, 161–75.

Davis, J. W. F. (1976). Breeding success and experience in the Arctic Skua *Stercorarius parasiticus* (L). *Journal of Animal Ecology*, **45**, 531–5.

Delius, J. D. (1965). A population study of Skylarks, *Alauda arvensis. Ibis*, **107**, 466–92.

Dunn, E. K. (1972). Effect of age on the fishing ability of Sandwich Terns, *Sterna sandvicensis. Ibis*, **114**, 360–6.

Evans, M. E. (1979). Aspects of the life cycle of the Bewick's Swan, based on recognition of individuals at a wintering site. *Bird Study*, **26**, 149–52.

Farkas, T. (1969). Notes on the biology and ethology of the Natal Robin *Cossypha natalensis. Ibis*, **111**, 281–92.

Fogden, M. P. L. (1972). The seasonality and population dynamics of equatorial forest birds in Sarawak. *Ibis*, **114**, 307–43.

Frith, H. J. (1962). Movements of the Grey Teal, *Anas gibberifrons* Müller (Anatidae). *CSIRO Wildlife Research*, **7**, 50–70.

Fry, C. H. (1977). The evolutionary significance of co-operative breeding in birds. In *Evolutionary Ecology*, ed. B. Stonehouse & C. Perrins, pp. 127–35. Macmillan: London.

Gaston, A. J. (1977). Social behaviour within groups of Jungle Babblers *Turdoides striatus. Animal Behaviour*, **25**, 828–48.

Gaston, A. J. (1978). Ecology of the Common Babbler *Turdoides caudatus. Ibis*, **120**, 415–32.

Gorman, M. L. (1974). The endocrine basis of pair-formation behaviour in the male Eider *Somateria mollissima. Ibis*, **116**, 451–65.

Grimes, L. G. (1980). Observations of group behaviour and breeding biology of the Yellow-billed Shrike (*Corvinella corvina*). *Ibis*, **122**, 166–92.

Harris, M. P. (1967). The biology of Oystercatchers, *Haematopus ostralegus* on Skokholm Island, South Wales. *Ibis*, **109**, 180–93.

Harris, M. P. (1973). The biology of the Waved Albatross (*Diomedea irrorata*) of Hood Island, Galapagos. *Ibis*, **115**, 483–510.

Harris, M. P. (1979). Population dynamics of the Flightless Cormorant *Nannopterum harrisi. Ibis*, **121**, 135–46.

Harvey, P. H., Greenwood, P. J. & Perrins, C. M. (1979). Breeding area fidelity of Great Tits (*Parus major*). *Journal of Animal Ecology*, **48**, 305–13.

Hinde, R. A. (1952). The behaviour of the Great Tit (*Parus major*) and some related species. *Behaviour*, Suppl. II, 1–201.

Hinde, R. A. (1964). Section on pair formation. In *A New Dictionary of Birds*, ed. A. Landsborough Thomson, pp. 581–2. Nelson: London.

Holmes, R. T. (1966). Breeding ecology and annual cycle adaptations of the Red-backed Sandpiper (*Calidris alpina*) in northern Alaska. *Condor*, **68**, 3–46.

Holmes, R. T. (1971). Density, habitat, and the mating system of the Western Sandpiper (*Calidris mauri*). *Oecologia (Berlin)*, **7**, 191–208.

Hutson, G. D. (1977). Agonistic display and spacing in the Black-headed Gull, *Larus ridibundus. Animal Behaviour*, **25**, 765–73.

Huxley, J. S. & Montague, F. A. (1926). Studies on the courtship and sexual life of birds. The Black-tailed Godwit, *Limosa limosa* (L). *Ibis 12th series*, **2**, 1–25.

Immelmann, K. (1963). Drought adaptations in Australian desert birds. *Proceedings of the XIIIth International Ornithological Congress*, vol. **2**, ed. C. G. Sibley, pp. 649–57. A.O.U.; Louisiana.

Inglis, I. R. (1977). The breeding behaviour of the Pink-footed Goose; behavioural correlates of nesting success. *Animal Behaviour*, **25**, 747–64.

Jehl, J. R. (1973). Breeding biology and systematic relationships of the Stilt Sandpiper. *Wilson Bulletin*, **85**, 115–47.

Kendeigh, S. C. (1941). Territorial and mating behaviour of the House Wren. *Illinois Biological Monographs*, **18**(3), 1–120.

Kepler, C. B. (1969). The breeding biology of the Blue-faced Booby, *Sula dactylatra personata*, on Green Island, Kure. *Publications of Nuttall Ornithological Club*, **8**, 1–97.

Kistchinski, A. A. (1971). Biological notes on the Emperor Goose in northwest Siberia. *Wildfowl*, **22**, 29–34.

Kluijver, H. N. (1951). The population ecology of the Great Tit, *Parus m. major*. *Ardea*, **39**, 1–135.

Krebs, J. R. (1971). Territory and breeding density in the Great Tit, *Parus major* L. *Ecology*, **52**, 2–22.

Kummer, H. (1968). *Social Organisation of Hamadryas Baboons, a Field Study*. Karger: Basel.

Kunkel, P. (1974). Mating systems of tropical birds: the effects of weakness or absence of external reproduction-timing factors, with special reference to prolonged pair bonds. *Zeitschrift für Tierpsychologie*, **34**, 265–307.

Lack, D. (1939). The behaviour of the Robin. *Proceedings of the Zoological Society of London A*, **109**, 169–200.

Lack, D. (1940). The behaviour of the Robin: population changes over four years. *Ibis*, (14), **4**, 299–324.

Lack, D. (1954). *The Natural Regulation of Animal Numbers*. Oxford University Press: Oxford.

Lack, D. (1968). *Ecological Adaptations for Breeding in Birds*. Methuen: London.

Le Resche, R. E. & Sladen, W. J. L. (1970). Establishment of pair and breeding-site bonds by young known-age Adelie Penguins (*Pygoscelis adeliae*). *Animal Behaviour*, **18**, 517–26.

Lind, H. (1961). Studies on the behaviour of the Black-tailed Godwit (*Limosa limosa* (L)). Munksgaard: Copenhagen.

Macdonald, M. A. (1977). Adult mortality and fidelity to mate and nest-site in a group of marked Fulmars. *Bird Study*, **24**, 165–8.

Marler, P. (1956). Behaviour of the Chaffinch *Fringella coelebs*. *Behaviour*, Supplement, **5**, 1–184.

Marshall, A. J. & Coombs, C. J. F. (1957). The interaction of environmental, internal and behavioural factors in the rook (*Corvus f. frugilegus* Linnaeus). *Proceedings of the Zoological Society, London*, **128**, 545–89.

Mills, J. A. (1973). The influence of age and pair-bond on the breeding biology of the Red-billed Gull *Larus novaehollandiae scopulinus*. *Journal of Animal Ecology*, **42**, 147–62.

Mills, J. A. (1979). Factors affecting the egg size of Red-billed Gulls *Larus novaehollandiae scopulinus*. *Ibis*, **121**, 53–67.

Minton, C. D. T. (1968). Pairing and breeding of Mute Swans. *Wildfowl*, **19**, 41–60.

Murton, R. K., Thearle, R. J. P. & Coombs, C. F. B. (1974). Ecological studies of the Feral Pigeon *Columba livia* var. III Reproduction and plumage polymorphism. *Journal of Applied Ecology*, **11**, 841–54.

Nelson, J. B. (1966). The breeding biology of the Gannet *Sula bassana* on the Bass Rock, Scotland. *Ibis*, **108**, 584–626.

Nelson, J. B. (1978). *The Sulidae Gannets and Boobies*. Oxford University Press: Oxford.

Nice, M. M. (1937). Studies in the life-history of the Song Sparrow 1. A population study of the Song Sparrow. *Transactions of the Linnean Society, New York*, **4**, 1–247.

Nicholls, C. A. (1974). Double brooding in a Western Australian population of the Silver Gull, *Larus novaehollandiae* Stephens. *Australian Journal of Zoology*, **22**, 63–70.

Nisbet, I. C. T. & Lord Medway (1972). Dispersion, population ecology and migration of Eastern Great Reed Warblers *Acrocephalus orientalis* wintering in Malaysia. *Ibis*, **114**, 451–94.

Nolan, V. (1978). The ecology and behaviour of the Prairie Warbler *Dendroica discolor.* *American Ornithological Union Monographs,* **26,** 1–595.

Ollason, J. C. & Dunnet, G. M. (1978). Age, experience and other factors affecting the breeding success of the Fulmar, *Fulmarus glacialis* in Orkney. *Journal of Animal Ecology,* **47,** 961–76.

Orians, G. H. (1969). Age and hunting success in the Brown Pelican (*Pelecanus occidentalis*). *Animal Behaviour,* **17,** 316–19.

Palmer, R. S. (1975). *Handbook of North American Birds,* vol. 3. Yale University Press: New Haven.

Park, P. (1981). A colour-banding study of Welcome Swallows breeding in southern Tasmania. *Corella,* **5,** 37–41.

Patterson, I. J. (1965). Timing and spacing of broods in the Black-headed Gull *Larus ridibundus. Ibis,* **107,** 433–59.

Patterson, I. J., Young, C. M. & Tompa, F. S. (1974). The Shelduck population of the Ythan estuary, Aberdeenshire. *Wildfowl,* **25,** 16–28.

Penney, R. L. (1962). Voices of the Adelie. *Natural History,* **71,** 16–25.

Penney, R. L. (1968). Territorial and social behaviour in the Adelie Penguin. *Antarctic Bird Studies,* **12,** 83–131.

Perrins, C. M. (1970). The timing of birds' breeding seasons. *Ibis,* **112,** 212–55.

Perrins, C. M. (1979). *British Tits.* Collins: London.

Perrins, C. M. & Moss, D. (1974). Survival of young Great Tits in relation to age of female parent. *Ibis,* **116,** 220–4.

Pitelka, F. A. (1979). Shorebirds in marine environments. *Studies in Avian Biology,* **2,** 1–261.

Pitelka, F. A., Holmes, R. T. & Maclean, S. F. (1974). Ecology and evolution of social organization in arctic sandpipers. *American Zoologist,* **14,** 185–204.

Potts, G. R., Coulson, J. C. & Deans, I. R. (1980). Population dynamics and breeding success of the Shag, *Phalacrocorax aristotelis,* on the Farne Islands, Northumberland. *Journal of Animal Ecology,* **49,** 465–84.

Price, T. (1981). The ecology of the Greenish Warbler, *Phylloscopus trochiloides* in its winter quarters. *Ibis,* **123,** 131–44.

Raveling, D. G. (1969). Social classes of Canada Geese in winter. *Journal of Wildlife Management,* **33,** 304–18.

Recher, H. F. & Recher, J. A. (1969). Comparative foraging efficiency of adult and immature Little Blue Herons (*Florida caerulea*). *Animal Behaviour,* **17,** 320–2.

Reilly, P. N. & Cullen, J. M. (1981). The Little Penguin *Eudyptula minor* in Victoria. II: Breeding. *Emu,* **81,** 1–19.

Rice, D. W. & Kenyon, K. W. (1962). Breeding cycles and behaviour of Laysan and Black-footed Albatrosses. *Auk,* **79,** 517–67.

Richdale, L. E. (1949). The effect of age on laying dates, size of eggs and size of clutch in the Yellow-eyed Penguin. *Wilson Bulletin.* **61,** 91–8.

Richdale, L. E. (1951). *Sexual Behaviour in Penguins.* University of Kansas: Lawrence.

Richdale, L. E. (1957). *A Population Study of Penguins.* Oxford University Press: Oxford.

Richdale, L. E. (1963). Biology of the Sooty Shearwater, *Puffinus griseus. Proceedings of the Zoological Society of London,* **141,** 1–117.

Richdale, L. E. (1965). Breeding behaviour of the Narrow-billed Prion and the Broad-billed Prion on Whero Island, New Zealand. *Transactions of the Zoological Society of London,* **27,** 87–155.

Richdale, L. E. & Warham, J. (1973). Survival, pair-bond retention and nest-site tenacity in Buller's Mollymawk. *Ibis,* **115,** 257–63.

Riggert, T. (1977). The biology of the Mountain Duck on Rottnest Island, Western Australia. *Wildlife Monograph,* **52,** 1–67.

Rowley, I. (1965). The life-history of the Superb Blue Wren, *Malurus cyaneus. Emu*, **64**, 251–97.

Rowley, I. (1970). The genus *Corvus* (Aves: Corvidae) in Australia. *CSIRO Wildlife Research*, **15**, 27–71.

Rowley, I. (1973). The comparative ecology of Australian corvids II. Social organisation and behaviour. *CSIRO Wildlife Research*, **18**, 25–65.

Rowley, I. (1974). Display situations in two Australian ravens. *Emu*, **74**, 47–52.

Rowley, I. (1975). *Bird Life*. Collins: Sydney.

Rowley, I. (1978). Communal activities among White-winged Choughs *Corcorax melanorhamphus. Ibis*, **120**, 178–97.

Rowley, I. (1981). The communal way of life in the Splendid Wren *Malurus splendens. Zeitschrift für Tierpsychologie*, **55**, 228–67.

Ryder, J. P. (1967). The breeding biology of Ross' Goose in the Perry River region, Northwest Territories. *Canadian Wildlife Service Report*, No. 3. 56 pp.

Ryder, J. P. (1980). The influence of age on the breeding biology of colonial nesting seabirds. In *Behaviour of Marine Animals: Current Perspectives in Research*, vol. **4**, ed. J. Burger, B. L. Olla & H. E. Winn, pp. 153–68. Plenum Press: New York.

Rydzewski, W. (1978). The longevity of ringed birds. *The Ring*, **8**, 218–62.

Salmonsen, F. (1968). The moult migration. *Wildfowl*, **19**, 5–24.

Saunders, D. A. (1982). Breeding biology of the Short-billed form of the White-tailed Black Cockatoo *Calyptorhynchus funereus. Ibis*, **124**, 422–55.

Saunders, D. A. (1979). *The Biology of the Short-Billed Form of the White-Tailed Black Cockatoo*, Calyptorhynchus funereus latirostris Carnaby. *Unpublished Ph.D. thesis, University of Western Australia*.

Schifferli, L. (1973). The effect of egg weight on the subsequent growth of nestling Great Tits *Parus major. Ibis*, **115**, 549–58.

Scott, D. K. (1980). Functional aspects of the pair-bond in winter in Bewick's Swans (*Cygnus columbianus bewickii*). *Behavioral Ecology and Sociobiology*, **7**, 323–7.

Smith, G. T. (1974). An analysis of the function of some displays of the Royal Penguin. *Emu*, **74**, 27–34.

Snow, D. W. (1958). *A Study of Blackbirds*. Allen and Unwin: London.

Snow, D. W. & Lill, A. (1974). Longevity records for some neotropical land birds. *Condor*, **76**, 262–7.

Soikkeli, M. (1967). Breeding cycle and population dynamics in the Dunlin (*Calidris alpina*). *Annales Zoologici Fennici*, **4**, 158–98.

Southern, H. N. & Morley, A. (1950). Marsh Tit territories over six years. *British Birds*, **43**, 33–47.

Tickell, W. L. N. (1968). The biology of the Great Albatrosses, *Diomedea exulans* and *Diomedea epomorphora. Antarctic Bird Studies*, **12**, 191–212.

Tinbergen, N. (1956). On the functions of territory in gulls. *Ibis*, **98**, 401–11.

Vermeer, K. (1963). The breeding ecology of the Glaucous-winged Gull (*Larus glaucescens*) on Mandarte Island, British Columbia. *Occasional Papers of the British Columbia Provincial Museum*, **13**. 104 pp.

Warham, J. (1963). The Rockhopper Penguin *Eudyptes chrysocome* at Macquarie Island. *Auk*, **80**, 229–56.

Weller, M. W. (1965). Chronology of pair formation in some nearctic *Aythya* (Anatidae). *Auk*, **82**, 227–35.

Weitnauer, E. (1947). Am Neste des Mauerseglers, *Apus apus apus* (L). *Ornithologische Beobachter*, **44**, 133–82.

Willis, E. O. (1967). The behaviour of Bicolored Antbirds. *University of California Publications in Zoology*, **79**, 1–132.

Wittenberger, J. F. (1979). The evolution of mating systems in birds and mammals. In

Social Behaviour and Communication, vol. **3** of *Handbook of Behavioural Neurobiology*, ed. P. Marler & J. G. Vandenbergh, pp. 271–349. Plenum Press: New York.

Wood, R. C. (1971). Population dynamics of breeding South Polar Skuas of unknown age. *Auk*, **88**, 805–14.

Wooller, R. D. & Coulson, J. C. (1977). Factors affecting the age of first breeding of the Kittiwake, *Rissa tridactyla. Ibis*, **119**, 339–49.

Wooller, R. D. & Dunlop, J. N. (1979). Multiple laying by the Silver Gull, *Larus novaehollandiae* Stephens, on Carnac Island, Western Australia. *Australian Wildlife Research*, **6**, 325–35.

Zahavi, A. (1971). The social behaviour of the White Wagtail *Motacilla alba alba* wintering in Israel. *Ibis*, **113**, 203–11.

Zahavi, A. (1974). Communal nesting by the Arabian Babbler. *Ibis*, **116**, 84–7.

16

Mate choice in the Kittiwake Gull

J. C. COULSON AND C. S. THOMAS

Introduction

The Kittiwake Gull, *Rissa tridactyla*, is typical of sea birds in that it has a high survival rate and is long lived. At sexual maturity, Kittiwakes have an expectation of breeding for over six years (Coulson & White, 1959) and it is therefore likely that both members of the breeding pair will survive from one breeding season to the next. In some Kittiwake colonies, the adult birds leave immediately breeding is finished and the last young are fledged (Belopol'skii, 1961; Salomonsen & Gitz-Johansen, 1950) but in those at the southern end of the species range, some of the breeding birds may remain in the colony for some weeks or even months after the last young have fledged. Whilst in these southern colonies, there is some changing of mate after the young fledge, these changes appear to be temporary and do not necessarily correspond to the pairs formed in the next breeding season. Obviously there is no prospect of this behaviour occurring in northern colonies. Since there is no evidence that members of a pair remain together during the winter months, when the species is oceanic, mate choice may be assumed to take place at the start of each breeding season when the colony is re-occupied. This can be either the re-forming of pairs from previous years or the formation of new pairs.

It might be expected that a bird returning to the colony in the spring would have a large number of individuals of the opposite sex from which to choose a mate. From our data on a colony of colour-ringed individuals we have shown that the choice is much more limited, mainly because both time and space introduce considerable constraints on the number of possible mates which are available to birds occupying a particular nest site.

In the sections which follow, we pay particular attention to the factors that influence mate choice in the Kittiwake.

361

Study area and methods

Most of this investigation has been made on a colony of about 100 breeding pairs which nest on the window ledges of a warehouse at North Shields, England (Coulson, 1966, 1968; Coulson & Wooller, 1976). Since 1954, every breeding bird in the colony, as well as many potential recruits have been marked with a unique combination of coloured leg-bands. In this situation, unmarked birds are recruits or potential recruits. Each year, the basic breeding biology of each pair is recorded: time of return, identity of mate, site occupied, time of egg laying, clutch size and breeding success. Accordingly we have built up a considerable series of information concerning individual birds.

Once a Kittiwake has nested, it rarely, if ever, changes its colony, the

Fig. 16.1. The mean date of return to the colony of female Kittiwakes in relation to their breeding experience (age). On average, birds breeding for the first time are the last to arrive at the colony. The vertical lines indicate the 95% confidence intervals.

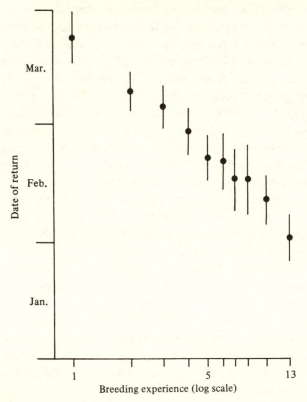

only exception being where considerable disturbance results in the colony as a whole moving to a new site. In an extensive search for breeding birds which had changed their colony, Coulson & Wooller (1976) found that 23% of non-breeders marked in the study colony had moved elsewhere whilst not a single breeding bird nested away from the place in which it had first bred. The faithfulness to the colony has enabled us to determine the survival rates of male and female Kittiwakes (sexed from their body measurements, behaviour or the sex of their mates) from the rate of disappearance of marked breeding birds (Coulson & Wooller, 1976).

Mate choice

It is convenient to consider mate choice in two sections; choice of mates by first breeders and that of birds which have bred previously and therefore have the possibility of retaining their mate from the previous year.

First mate choice

Kittiwakes which are about to breed for the first time are characterised by appearing in the colony later than the established breeding birds (Fig. 16.1). In our study colony, many breeding birds returned between January and February whilst those prospecting do not appear until March, April or even later (Coulson, 1959). Some birds visit a series of colonies before choosing the one in which they intend breeding and often prospecting takes place in the summer before first breeding. The late arrival of young birds results in a tendency for these individuals to mate with others of a similar age or breeding experience (Table 16.1). The exception to this rule lies in the small number of old birds (usually females) which take young partners (see p. 372).

In a stable Kittiwake colony, some 17% of breeding birds are nesting

Table 16.1. *The influence of date of arrival at the breeding colony of male and female Kittiwakes about to breed for the first time upon the percentage which obtain another first breeder as a mate*

Date of return of prospector	Prospecting males		Prospecting females	
	%	No.	%	No.
January–February	29.4	17	50.0	8
February–March	40.7	59	52.5	40
April–May	55.9	43	80.0	35

for the first time and most of the mate choice amongst these individuals takes place after the older birds have already obtained mates. The usual pattern of mate choice is that the male obtains a nest site and then attracts a female to the ledge. Nest sites in the centre of the colony (see Coulson, 1968, 1971) are more attractive to both males and females. A male on the edge of the colony may wait several weeks to obtain a mate whilst one at a physically similar site in the centre obtains a mate within days. The social context of the site plays an important part in the ease with which the male obtains a mate, and there is severe competition amongst males for the central sites. Males which nest in the centre of the colony are both longer lived and reproductively more successful in each year than those which nest on the edge (Table 16.2).

First breeders move from colony to colony when prospecting and since they form the largest age group, first-breeding males have a large number of females from which to attract and choose a mate; a number and choice which is never achieved again during the life span of the bird.

Subsequent mate choice

After the first breeding season, an appreciable proportion of the birds re-mate with the same partner although about 44% take a new mate. Two major causes of mate change have been identified – the partner from the previous breeding season has died during the intervening time or the pair have undergone 'divorce' (that is, both members of the previous pair survive and return to the colony but take new partners). In a small number of cases, the female misses a breeding season, often after the first breeding attempt (Wooller & Coulson, 1977).

Table 16.2. *The breeding performance and survival rates of male Kittiwakes nesting in the centre and on the edge of the breeding colony*

	Central nesters	Edge nesters	Difference (%)	Significance of difference
Clutch size	2.21	2.08	6.3	$\chi^2_2 = 18.3$, $P < 0.001$
Chicks hatched/year	1.64	1.49	10.1	$\chi^2_3 = 10.0$, $P < 0.05$
Chicks fledged/year	1.43	1.31	9.2	$\chi^2_3 = 6.4$, n.s.
Sample size	570	412		
Annual survival rate	0.838*	0.792*	4.6	$t = 2.14$, $P < 0.05$
Sample size	707	614		

* From Coulson & Wooller (1976).
n.s., not significant.

Death of mate

The data on survival rates have been taken mainly from Coulson & Wooller (1976). The survival rate (the proportion of birds which survive from one breeding season to the next) of adult Kittiwakes decreases as the ages of the birds increase (Fig. 16.2). Consequently, a higher proportion of older birds lose their mates between one breeding season and the next. In recent years, the mortality rate of birds in this colony has increased and hence this factor has become more important. Most of the mortality takes place during the winter months when the birds are away from the colony and when, presumably, the pair bonds do not exist. The mortality rate is higher in the male Kittiwake than the female and hence more females with previous breeding experience are searching for mates than experienced males.

Divorce

The rate of divorce is highest amongst young breeding birds and decreases markedly amongst older individuals (Fig. 16.3).

The main cause of the break-up of the pair bond changes from divorce amongst younger birds to mortality of the mate in older individuals (Fig. 16.4).

Fig. 16.2. The annual survival rates of female Kittiwakes in relation to their age. The standard error is indicated by the vertical lines. (From Coulson & Thomas, 1980.)

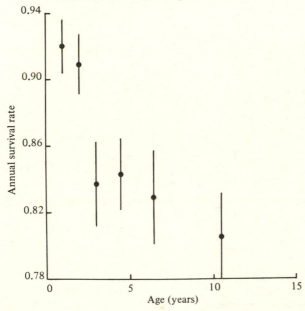

Persistence of the pair bond

The duration of the pair bond of birds forming pairs before 1969 is shown in Fig. 16.5. Essentially the duration of the pair bond corresponds to that expected from a constant annual rate of changing mate but there are more pairs which remain together for more than 11 years than would be expected from this simple model. A more detailed analysis of the proportion of pairs which divorce, in relation to age and pair status (Table 16.3) shows that the divorce rate decreases with both age and previous pair status. This suggests that a prior association between two birds enhances the probability that those individuals will remain together in the future and this effect is clearly demonstrated in Table 16.4 where divorce rate is shown in relation to the past duration of the pair bond for four age categories.

Fig. 16.3. The divorce rate of female Kittiwakes in relation to their age. Note the progressive decrease in divorce rate with increasing breeding experience (age). (From Coulson & Thomas, 1980.)

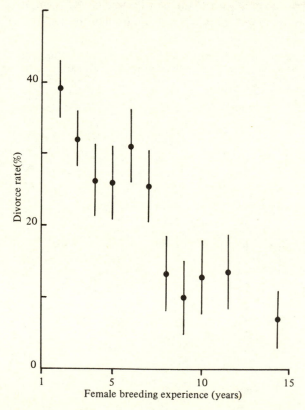

The effect of mate retention

The retention of the same mate from one breeding season to the next results in a 7% increase in clutch size, and a 12% increase in the number of chicks fledged per pair (based on 1206 pair-years). Clearly there is an advantage in retaining the same mate, particularly one with whom a bird has bred successfully. Divorce is correlated with the failure of a pair to rear young in a breeding season (Table 16.5; see also Coulson, 1966, 1972) and it would appear an appropriate strategy for unsuccessful pairs to change partners as this may increase the probability of their being successful in the future. Much of the failure in breeding amongst Kittiwakes appears to be associated with the level of compatibility of the members of the pair during the incubation period (Coulson, 1972). Individual pairs develop their own rhythm of sharing incubation, using one, two, three or

Fig. 16.4. The cause of mate change amongst female Kittiwakes in relation to their age. (From Coulson & Thomas, 1980.)

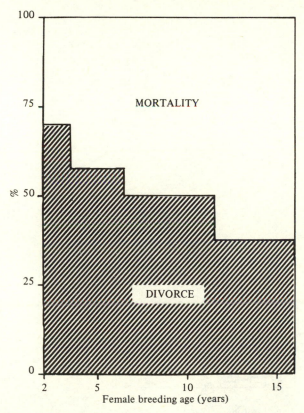

Table 16.3. *The relationship between age, pair status and the probability of divorce*

Pair first formed	Female breeding age now (years)						
	1	2	3	4 and 5	6 and 7	8 to 11	12 to 18
This year	0.39	0.41	0.43	0.30	0.32	0.27	0.25
One or more years ago	—	0.23	0.21	0.28	0.14	0.09	0.00
Sample sizes							
This year	152	70	47	67	48	37	12
One or more years ago	0	52	52	109	71	100	33

Derived from Coulson & Thomas (1980).

Fig. 16.5. The duration of the pair bond (in years) in Kittiwake pairs formed before 1969. The results are expressed as a percentage of the total number of pairs considered. Note the decay curve suggesting that about half of the pair bonds break up each year. (From Coulson & Thomas, 1980.)

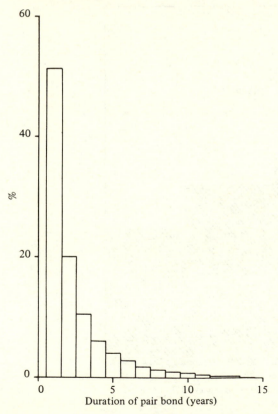

four shifts per day. Unlike many other birds, failure to hatch the eggs is more important than chick mortality as a cause of breeding failure in the Kittiwake (Coulson & White, 1958; Cullen, 1957; Maunder & Threlfall, 1972; Swartz, 1966).

Although the correlation between failed breeding and subsequent mate change clearly exists, many failed breeders have been found to retain their mates in the next breeding season and there are a number of instances of successful breeding being followed by divorce. We do not envisage divorce as a deliberate decision on the part of the failed breeders but that it stems from failed breeders leaving the colony earlier (often before some young

Table 16.4. *The influence of the prior association between the two members of the pair upon the probability of divorce*

No. of years pair together	Female breeding age now (years)			
	1	2–3	4–7	8–19
1	0.39	0.42	0.31	0.27
2–3	—	0.22	0.30	0.12
4–7	—	—	0.12	0.04
8–19	—	—	—	0.00
Sample size				
1	152	117	115	49
2–3	—	104	111	63
4–7	—	—	69	49
8–19	—	—	—	21

Table 16.5. *The probability of a pair undergoing divorce before next year in relation to female breeding age and breeding success this year*

No. of chicks fledged this year	Female breeding age this year (years)			
	1	2–3	4–7	8–19
(a) None	0.49	0.34	0.29	0.11
(b) At least one	0.36	0.29	0.25	0.11
Difference (a)–(b)	0.13	0.05	0.04	0.00
Sample sizes				
(a) None	35	32	34	27
(b) At least one	114	185	248	144

have fledged) and returning at a less-consistent time in the following spring (Table 16.6). This results in a much increased likelihood that one of the pair will obtain a new mate before its partner from the previous year returns, the earlier-returning bird behaving in much the same way as a bird whose mate has died.

Mate choice by previous breeders

The difference in the date of return to the colony of newly-forming breeding pairs is, on average 17 days, suggesting that this is approximately the amount of time taken for mate selection and pair formation to occur. The strong correlation between date of return to the colony and age, reported in Fig. 16.1, suggested that on average, birds arrive back at the colony approximately 10 days earlier in each successive year of their lives. These two factors will contribute to the tendency for birds to mate with a partner of a similar breeding age and also restrict the amount of time and the number of females which are available in the colony for a male arriving back at a particular time.

Kittiwakes exhibit a strong attachment to the nest site from the previous year (Coulson & Thomas, 1980). This effect is dominated by the male so that when divorce occurs, it is usual for the female to move to a new site. Only in cases where the male has died does the female more frequently retain the previous nest site (Fig. 16.6).

It is revealing to examine the distance moved by females which change their nest site (and their mate). Potentially, one might have expected the birds to redistribute throughout the colony, particularly one the size of that in which the study was made. However, this is not so and most of the females take a new mate within a few metres of their original site. This is easily measured in the uniformly placed windows of the study colony.

Table 16.6. *The time of return of members of a pair in the following breeding season in relation to whether they re-pair or form a new partnership*

	Difference in date of return (days)	% within 4 days	Sample size
Same pair	12.6	39	493
Divorce			
Last year's pair	23.9	17	119
This year's pair	16.8	31	119

On average, females which change mate and nesting site move only 1.5 windows horizontally and 0.7 windows vertically. For most nest sites in the colony, there are between nine and 14 males within this area and the female, on average, finds her mate amongst this small number. However, since about 56% of males retain their mate from the previous breeding season, it may be assumed that the number of males requiring a new partner in this area is between four and eight. Since males usually retain their previous nest site, it is evident that females requiring a new mate are considered by and attracted to a small number of males close to their previous nesting site and that they are, for one reason or another, unavailable to males elsewhere. In practice, the selection of mates by males seeking new partners is even further restricted temporally. Table 16.7 shows the numbers of females which are available to take a new mate in relation to the date of return of the birds to the colony (divided into 20-day periods). A similar pattern can be found amongst the males. On average, the two birds forming a new pair arrive back at the colony within 17 days of each other. When the male arrives, many of the females, which may be potential mates because of their physical proximity in the colony, have either returned already and taken new mates or are not due to return for some days. Only 22% of the females in the colony arrive back in each of the periods of the first 20 days in January and March. This suggests that most males which have previously bred choose their new mate from only two or three females (22% of a maximum of 12).

Fig. 16.6. The proportions of male and female Kittiwakes changing nest site in successive years according to whether they retain the same mate, divorce or their mate of the previous year had died. (From Coulson & Thomas, 1980.)

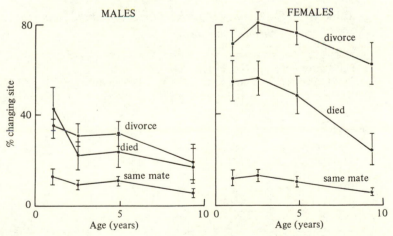

Throughout life, the mortality rate of male Kittiwakes is higher than that of females (Coulson & Wooller, 1976) and this results in an appreciably higher proportion of old females (which have bred for more than nine years) in the population. These birds do not follow the pattern of young and mid-aged Kittiwakes pairing with a mate of the same or similar age (Fig. 16.7), simply because of the shortage of such aged males. Typically, these females do not take a slightly younger male as a partner but normally choose a bird about to breed for the first time. The dominant role in nest site selection is reversed and this change in behaviour appears to stem from the extreme reluctance of the old females to move nest site, in contrast to the behaviour of young females (Fig. 16.6). Thus it appears that the 'matriarchal dominance' of these old females leads to a situation in which the only potential mates are young males who have not attained a nest site. This effect is also assisted by the old females often remaining unpaired for several weeks after their return, again indicating the difficulty which these individuals experience in attracting, or being attracted to, an older male.

Conclusions

In studies on the significance of the pair bond in the Kittiwake, it has been shown that retention of the same mate in subsequent years is associated with higher breeding success and production of young. It would appear that there is a selective advantage in retaining the same mate. However, if this is so, the reason why some birds change their mate requires examination. Whilst the death of their previous partner forces some birds to take a new mate, others change mate although their previous partner

Table 16.7. *The number of females first seen in the colony in each 20-day period through the spring*

Days after 31st December	No. of females first seen	Percentage
1–20	217	22
21–40	173	18
41–60	156	16
61–80	210	22
81–100	134	14
101–120	59	6
121–140	23	2
Total	972	

is still alive and in the colony. This change is associated with failure to breed successfully in the previous breeding season and seems to operate through the two birds arriving back at the colony at markedly different times. Previously successful pairs tend to return at more similar dates than members of unsuccessful pairs. Essentially the divorce system appears to result from one of the partners returning earlier than the other and responding in the same manner as a bird whose mate has died, that is, waiting a short time and then seeking a new mate.

Choice of colony, nest site and mate all appear to be leisurely processes in birds which have never bred and since these tend to take place in the summer when the established breeders have already built nests, and are often incubating eggs or even feeding young. Inexperienced birds are more likely to pair up together. In older birds this tendency persists due both to the retention of previous mates and to a marked age effect influencing the date of return to the colony. The main exception to this pattern occurs in old females where there are virtually no males of a similar age and this,

Fig. 16.7. The age of the members of each pair in each year of the study. The diagonal lines enclose the birds of the same age (breeding experience). (From Coulson & Thomas, 1980.)

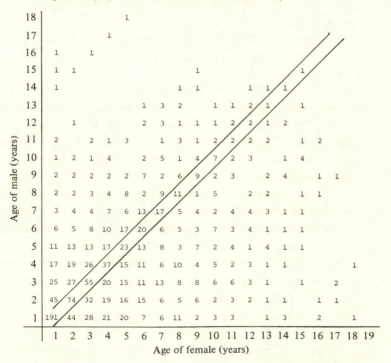

compounded with a much greater tendency for these females to retain their nesting site, results in their taking young, inexperienced males as their partners.

Whilst there appears to be much scope for genuine choice of a mate in birds about to breed for the first time, this is much reduced in experienced breeders since a male takes a new mate from the females which had nested in very close proximity to it in the previous year. Since an appreciable proportion of the neighbours retain the same mate, and the time of return is spread over several weeks or even months, the number of females available to an individual male requiring a new mate is small, perhaps only two or three birds, and clearly there is only little scope for choice. Nevertheless, females taking new mates in central sites in the colony breed more successfully than similar individuals near the periphery of the colony. This difference could arise through a form of social stimulation which affects central birds to a greater extent. Alternatively, it could result in individuals of better quality being recruited to the centre of the colony from the non-breeding population. This difference persists because the new mates do not move appreciable distances within the colony and very rarely from the centre to the periphery of the colony.

Summary

1 Mate choice is markedly different in young Kittiwake Gulls about to breed for the first time and in older ones which have bred previously.

2 Young birds about to breed for the first time often visit several colonies and since they form the largest age class, there is a large choice of mate for both sexes. These first-breeding birds usually pair up together, mainly as a result of their late arrival in the colony, by which time many of the experienced breeders have already established pair bonds.

3 In Kittiwakes with previous breeding experience, many pairs are re-established from the previous year. In others, mate change occurs due either to the death of the previous partner or to divorce (where the previous mate is still alive and in the colony). The mortality rate of both sexes increases with age whereas divorce rate decreases with age and the number of years in which the pair has existed. A few pairs persist for more than 12 breeding seasons.

4 Increased breeding success occurs in birds which retain their mate from the previous year. Divorce is correlated with failure to breed successfully in the previous year and this appears to stem from

an element of incompatibility in some pairs, particularly during incubation.

5 In experienced breeders, mate choice is reduced by: (i) some birds re-forming the same pair as in previous years: (ii) the females finding a new mate close to their previous nest-site; and (iii) the considerable variation in time of return and mate selection by birds of different age groups. As a result of these restrictions, an experienced breeding male may have a choice of only two or three females from which to find a new mate.

6 Despite this limited choice by established breeding birds, those nesting centrally in the colony breed more successfully than comparable birds nesting near the periphery. This could result from a form of social stimulation or, alternatively, from a marked selection of fit and less-fit individuals at the time of first breeding, which apparently stems from competition in nest-site selection and mate choice by the male.

We wish to acknowledge the assistance given by Smith's Dock Co. Ltd and, more recently, Mr J. Pepper of Jim Marine Ltd, for access to the colony of Kittiwakes nesting on the warehouse at North Shields. We are also grateful to G. Brazendale, Dr A. Hodges, Dr R. Wooller and J. Chardine for their assistance and records on the Kittiwakes nesting on this building.

References

Belopol'skii, L. O. (1961). *Ecology of Sea Colony Birds of the Barents Sea.* Israel Program for Scientific Translation: Jerusalem.

Coulson, J. C. (1959). The plumage and leg colour of the Kittiwake and comments on the non-breeding population. *British Birds,* **52,** 189–96.

Coulson, J. C. (1966). The influence of the pair-bond and age on the breeding biology of the Kittiwake Gull *Rissa tridactyla. Journal of Animal Ecology.* **35,** 269–79.

Coulson, J. C. (1968). Differences in the quality of birds nesting in the centre and on the edges of a colony. *Nature,* **217,** 478–9.

Coulson, J. C. (1971). Competition for breeding sites causing segregation and reduced young production in colonial animals. *Proceedings of the Advanced Study Institute on Dynamics in Populations* (Osterbeek, 1971), pp. 257–68.

Coulson, J. C. (1972). The significance of the pair-bond in the Kittiwake. *Proceedings of the XVth International Ornithological Congress,* pp. 424–33. Brill: Leiden.

Coulson, J. C. & Thomas, C. S. (1980). A study of the factors influencing the duration of the pair-bond in the Kittiwake Gull, *Rissa tridactyla. Proceedings of the XVIIth International Ornithological Congress,* pp. 822–33. Berlin.

Coulson, J. C. & White, E. (1958). Observations on the breeding of the Kittiwake. *Bird Study,* **5,** 74–83.

Coulson, J. C. & White, E. (1959). The post-fledging mortality of the Kittiwake. *Bird Study,* **6,** 97–102.

Coulson, J. C. & Wooller, R. D. (1976). Differential survival rates among breeding Kittiwake Gulls *Rissa tridactyla* (L.). *Journal of Animal Ecology,* **45,** 205–13.

Cullen, E. (1957). Adaptations in the Kittiwake to cliff-nesting. *Ibis*, **99**, 275–302.
Maunder, J. E. & Threlfall, W. (1972). The breeding biology of the Black-legged Kittiwake in Newfoundland. *Auk*, **89**, 789–816.
Salomonsen, F. & Gitz-Johansen, A. (1950). *The Birds of Greenland*. Munksgaard: Copenhagen.
Swartz, L. G. (1966). Seacliff birds of Cape Thompson. In *Environment of Cape Thompson Region, Alaska*, ed. N. J. Wilimovsky & J. N. Wolfe, pp. 611–78. U.S. Atomic Energy Commission: Oak Ridge, Tennessee.
Wooller, R. D. & Coulson, J. C. (1977). Factors affecting the age of first breeding of the Kittiwake *Rissa tridactyla*. *Ibis*, **119**, 339–49.

17

Mate choice in humans as an interpersonal process

STEVE DUCK AND DOROTHY MIELL

A paper with this title may well provoke the reader to ask: 'Well what else could human mate choice be, if not an interpersonal process?'. Nevertheless much work on human mate choice can be accused of treating it as an *event* rather than a *process* – as a moment of decision based on some centrally important cue, rather than an extended negotiation during which one or both persons persuade the other and communicate strategically in ways guided by a desire to establish the full and complex working relationships that marriage embodies. Accordingly the present chapter will work towards a 'process view' by way of the earlier existing research.

Several early lines of social psychological enquiry stress the overriding and long-lasting effects of features of persons that are not interpersonally negotiated or interpersonally evolved. Such studies have concerned the influence of an individual's relatively static characteristic such as personality or physical attractiveness. Some other views have been based on the Freudian suggestion that individuals may seek as marital partners those other persons who resemble their opposite-sex parents: that is to say, a man will seek as a wife someone who resembles his mother in physical appearance and a woman will seek as a husband someone who resembles her father (see Murstein, 1971, for a discussion). Other variations on a similar theme suggest that individuals carry around in their minds some impression of their own attractiveness to other people and they simply seek as mates someone who falls within the range of their own level of attractiveness (Berscheid & Walster, 1974). There are several versions of this particular view: one suggests that individuals will therefore seek other individuals whose physical attractiveness level is about the same as their own (Murstein, 1977): another view suggests that an individual's self-esteem will be the guiding influence in selection of mates such that a male with high self-esteem and self-confidence will choose more attractive female mates than would a male with low self-esteem (Stroebe, 1977). In this instance, then, the relevant features of the male are *esteem* rather than physical attractiveness but the tendency is still to regard physical attractiveness in the female as the deciding feature and, hence, some pre-existing property of persons as the major causal force in human mate choice.

Research based on many of the foregoing ideas has been carried out in a variety of ways. Again emphasising that we are dealing at this point with a literature which concerns itself with an *individual's* properties – and the static properties of an individual at that – we shall now go on to sketch out briefly some of the main types of research which have been done from this particular starting point. We shall be selective of the research here and we are not intending to give a representative review so much as an indication of the flavour and style of some of the work which has been done. Readers will judge from the way in which we have led up to this point that we regard this kind of research as essentially outmoded and relatively useless in the search for a better understanding of how mate choice proceeds. However, such work was the basis of early investigations of human mate choice and as such it deserves to be considered in a way which leads us to a better understanding of how and why present day research evolved.

An important early distinction which must be made is between those studies which concern themselves with dating choice or choice of partners at the early stages of courtship and those studies which concern the properties of individuals who have already entered marriage. As may be perhaps expected, many of the studies of dating choice are more concerned with physical characteristics of the relevant individuals whereas studies of established marital partners are, on the whole, more concerned with aspects of personality (Murstein, 1976). In both styles of research, however, the emphasis falls upon those characteristics which each individual brings to the relationship and there is very little discussion of how the influence of these factors is negotiated, any more than there is discussion of how other interpersonal influences may come to exert directional force upon the relationship.

Taking first some studies of dating choice, which may be presumed to constitute the early stages of courtship and, hence, have some bearing on the ultimate choice of marital partner, we shall concentrate on the work which deals with the so-called 'matching hypothesis'. This hypothesis (briefly stated) suggests that the male partner will be influenced by his level of self-esteem in his choice of female dating partner (Stroebe, 1977). Males with high self-esteem (whatever their own physical attractiveness) will tend to seek out females of high physical attractiveness, whereas males of low self-esteem (whatever their own physical attractiveness) will tend to be satisfied with partners of lower physical attractiveness levels.

The classic way of studying such a hypothesis is to invite a male subject to take part in an experiment and by various manipulations of test scores to induce this individual to believe that he has performed exceptionally well or else exceptionally badly on some test which measures personal capacities. Thus, for example, in a study by Walster, Aronson, Abrahams & Rottman (1966) subjects were invited to take part in an intelligence test and were subsequently given false feedback which indicated that they had scored well above or well below the average for a student population on the test. Such false feedback is intended to create in the subjects a temporary state of raised or lowered self-esteem and constitutes the independent variable in the study. The subject is then taken for a cup of coffee by the experimenter who by 'coincidence' happens to meet a female friend. This female friend is, in fact, a confederate of the experimenter and has been dressed and made up in a way which makes her look physically attractive on the one hand or physically unattractive on the other hand! Here, therefore, we meet the other variable in the study and it can be readily perceived that the purpose of the study is to see whether the male makes more or fewer attempts to invite the confederate for a date as a result of the level of self-esteem temporarily induced by the earlier part of the experiment. The general finding of this study was that individuals who have had their self-esteem temporarily raised were more plucky in their relationships with the confederate who was made up to look attractive. However, several subsequent studies have cast doubt upon this particular interpretation and the most important variable in these circumstances is now thought to be fear of rejection on the male's part rather than attractiveness on the female's part (Stroebe, 1977).

However difficult it may be to interpret these studies, it is particularly obvious that they are not throwing a great deal of light on the ultimate process of courtship and its eventual outcome. Other researchers have, therefore, taken a different style of approach to the problems of initiation of courtship and have concerned themselves with the physical appearance of the partners alone. Murstein (1971, 1977) has developed a theory which places a greater emphasis on the developmental processes of courtship and places only its first emphasis on physical-stimulus properties of the individuals concerned. In this theory, known as Stimulus-Value-Role theory, Murstein suggests that individuals first try to match up their physical appearance one with the other and to choose partners whose physical appearance is comparable in attractiveness. Subsequent parts of the theory concern the developments which take place once this matching of physical appearance has taken place satisfactorily. Murstein (1976, 1977) has presented data to support the early stages of his theory by means of independent ratings of the photographs of married and courting couples. From such evidence, it seems to be the case that married and courting couples are indeed more similar to one another in attractiveness level than would be predicted by chance alone. The other parts of the theory are less well substantiated but begin to make us think of the possibility that other processes can take over – once the business of sorting on the basis of physical attractiveness has been completed. Murstein (1977) argues that the values of the two partners will become important after this first sorting has taken place and partners will then begin to establish for themselves whether they share a similar value system. Murstein's theory thus provides a link between the static approach of those who investigate physical attractiveness and a more continuous process of courtship which is hinted at by other workers.

The main emphasis which is found in work on married couples who have *completed* courtship is based on similarity or complementarity of personality. In the first case, workers have sought to establish whether marital partners have greater similarity of personality characteristics, somehow measured, than other people do. The evidence on this hypothesis is equivocal and there is no satisfactory resolution of the conflicts. There are, however, several important points to bear in mind: first, the influence of the stage at which courtship or marriage is assessed (see Duck, 1977, chapter 6, for a discussion). We should not naively assume that the same aspects of personality, the same relationship between two personalities, and the same relationship between different aspects of the two personalities hold across all recorded time in a given relationship. On the contrary, some courtship partners pay little attention to one another's personality in early stages, and some forms of interrelationship between personalities have to be negotiated in complex ways over an extended period (for instance, in adopting the behavioural roles of husband and wife, or in adjusting to the new roles of parenthood).

The second point relates to this first one above. Personality can be measured in various ways simultaneously: for instance, someone can be an extrovert, Capricornian, with a high need for Achievement, with low intra-punitiveness and be kind to animals but strict with his children. Accordingly one should not be amazed (though many researchers have been) when workers using different measures of personality record different results. It is a simple fact that some personality dimensions are more appropriate for use with newly acquainted couples (for instance, those assessing general sociability, like Extroversion–Introversion). Others are better suited for the context of long-term relationships (for instance, personality needs in the context of marriage). Thus the choosing of one's personality measures is not a merely capricious methodological business but something with strong *theoretical* reverberations (Duck, 1977).

When these two points (stage of relationship; type of personality measure) are taken together it is clear that many combinations of inappropriate measures and stages of relationship could be created to confuse the picture of personality's influence on human mate choice. Small wonder, then, that results have been equivocal and conflicting. It appears to be the case that marriage partners are very similar on certain values and certain particulars of personality characteristics but other investigators have demonstrated quite conclusively that this is not a general characteristic of all marital relationships. Marriage partners differ from one another on almost as many values and personality characteristics as they share similarity as indicated by a variety of investigators (e.g. Day, 1961; Levinger, Senn & Jorgensen, 1970).

Taking a different line, Winch (1958) argued that many married couples manifested complementarity of personality characteristics. In brief, the best example of this is a case where one partner is dominant and the other is submissive. In this two partners are complementary because one of them is high on one need (dominance) whilst the other is high on another (submissiveness). Other instances of complementarity can be found where one individual is high on a given need and the other person is low (for example where one person is highly dominating and the other person is low in dominance). This proposal has some intuitive plausibility in view of the fact that complementarity on certain needs will make a marriage easier to conduct. Clearly individuals who are equally dominant will spend a good deal of their married life arguing about who should control things, whereas individuals who are complementary on dominance needs will find that their relationship works that much more easily.

This analysis can be seen to provide clues as to why complementarity should be important: it is because it makes the negotiation of the relationship that much more easy to carry out. Therefore this work (extremely briefly reviewed as it has been) would seem to indicate that the value and importance of personality characteristics in mate choice lie in the negotiation of roles *for the conduct of the relationship*. The importance of personality characteristics, therefore, comes not from their bare significance to the individual, nor from the dry relationship which they have to the other partner's personality characteristics, but from the implications which they have for the conduct and negotiation of the relationship by the two partners involved. Once this basic point is accepted in outline, it now becomes more feasible to explore mate choice and the courtship process as interpersonal activities which have to be negotiated over a period of time and then carried into effect by the two partners concerned.

In work with a similar background of ideas, Huston and colleagues (1981) have carried out studies of the ways in which partners describe their courtship experiences. Huston, Surra, Fitzgerald & Cate (1981) carried out retrospective interviews with individuals who are married, and recorded the influence of key events on the progress of courtship and the partners' confidence that the eventual outcome of the relationship would be marriage. By interviewing both partners and by assessing the importance of particular key events, Huston and his colleagues have been able to discover four different styles of process by which mate choice is naturally effected by humans. The research thus takes the emphasis away from models based on the compatibility of personal characteristics of the partners. It moves towards the description of mate choice as an interpersonal process which is based on idealisation (that is, the tendency to view the course of the relationship in simple terms, to represent its trajectory as a smooth one, and to describe its path as a steady incline towards deep intimacy). When one keeps contemporary records of relationship growth, however, (as Duck & Miell, 1981, have done) then it becomes clear that things are not so simple. In day-to-day records people identify the ups and downs of relational life that we all experience, but in looking back on the relationship's progress these vicissitudes are given no representation at all. Subjects' graphs are simple curves, without detail. The accounts given by the subjects in Huston et al. (1981) showed a similar tendency to idealisation, although Huston did not have the data to do more than speculate that this was occurring. He did, however, note the significance placed by his subjects on particular interpersonal events and episodes. Many of these appear likely to be more influenced by the partners' immediate needs and desires rather than by some pre-existing individual values or traits. For example, some couples create commitment to each other by means of deeply personal interaction extended over a long period of time whereas for other individuals it may result from a series of misunderstandings. It could even be evolved through the influence of quarrels and conflict – and the resolution of these threatening states of affairs (Braiker & Kelley, 1979). Many subjects in a series of experiments have reported that the resolution of conflict is a major propulsive force in the evolution of their courtship.

The interpersonal process of conflict negotiation and resolution is, evidently, of fundamental significance to the development of courtship along satisfactory lines and is completely independent of the pre-existing personal characteristics that the partners bring to the relationship.

By graphing the development of different courtships, and proposing a neat four-category classification system, Huston and co-workers (1981) are able to demonstrate that the processes which accompany the development of relationships towards marriage are not uniform for all couples. Some courtships are short and move rapidly towards marriage. Such courtships are characterised by low levels of love and maintenance behaviours at early stages of the relationship followed by rapid increases in love and commitment. Other couples who are involved in long protracted courtship report high levels of love and maintenance activities early in their relationship but also high levels of conflict. Partners in prolonged relationships report considerable amounts of love for their partners before certainty of marriage is reached, even though these partners did not perform activities together as extensively as did partners in accelerated courtships. This suggests that prolonged relationships require extensive maintenance to sustain the feelings of love and that partners may find it necessary to focus on the emotional aspects of the relationship by resolving problems or by self-disclosing about their feelings.

However one interprets these findings it is clear that the Huston studies emphasise the need for researchers to look for differences in the paths which lead couples towards marriage and to seek out the meaning of courtship and marriage for the partners involved. It is certainly clear from the studies which Huston has carried out that the negotiation of courtship and the interpersonal processes which affect the evolution of the relationship are far more significant than those static personal pre-existing characteristics which individuals bring to a potential relationship.

Huston's approach and the general flavour of an interpersonal research style in the development of courtship is certainly a much more profitable line of enquiry for workers seeking to understand human mate choice as it occurs in real time, and such notions accord with our own work on friendship choice. Briefly stated, our own work indicates that people reach established deep friendships through a series of negotiated manoeuvres whose purpose is to establish the amount of personality similarity that exists between them at deep levels. According to our own work on the development of friendship (Duck, 1973, 1977; Miell, Duck & La Gaipa, 1979; Duck & Miell, 1981; and in press), acquainting individuals use processes of inference and guesswork to assess the nature and topography of their partner's personality, filtering out at any stage those persons who do not measure up. Thus, for instance, individuals attend to one another's physical appearance at an early stage, not merely for its own intrinsic interest or value, but also because of the clues that it gives about the person lying beneath it. Persons' physical styles partly and imperfectly indicate their natures as people and, if a style is all you can see of the persons when you first meet them, it makes sense for you to use it as the basis for personality inferences from which you can form a temporary judgement about your likely compatibility. One would expect people to replace such temporary assumptions by the somewhat safer judgements that can be based on growing knowledge of attitudes and beliefs as the relationship proceeds to increase the partners' knowledge of one another. Some of our other work suggests that this does indeed occur as predicted, although it leads to relationship difficulties where one's original judgements are subsequently shown to have been wrong (Duck & Craig, 1978).

By attending to a sequence of differently-based information about a partner the person is able to 'filter out' at the various stages those persons who would be unsuitable intimates (Duck, 1977). Conversely, individuals satisfying the filtering criteria adequately and successfully will be permitted to enter into the fuller negotiation of a satisfactory working relationship that is the ultimate end point of acquaintance between people who provide each other with satisfactory amounts of personality support.

In a series of studies of the growth of relationships we first showed that personality factors took on different weights at different stages in the relationship, as predicted by the above model, and we subsequently concerned ourselves with the daily activities that allowed these personality factors to exert their influences. Thus Duck & Craig (1978) measured the personalities of acquaintances by three different means and then followed the friendships through for an eight-month period. We were able to show that very general measures of personality predicted the friendship choices made at early points of measurement (one month) but that by eight months such predictions could not be made on that basis. Only very detailed and specific personality measures were good predictors at that stage.

In a more recent study, Duck & Miell (1981; and in press) kept daily records of the social activities of acquaintances and friends with the hope of detecting changes in the patterns of behaviour used to indicate growing intimacy. We found some strange caution in the process of acquaintance. For instance, friends tended to meet in public places for a greater proportion of the time up until about six weeks of acquaintance, when they began to meet much more often in private. Also, friends took a considerable time to reach a stage where their main interpersonal activity was the sharing of a significant number of secrets and private pieces of knowledge. It surprised us that the time to reach such a stage was so extended, but it probably underlines the significance and difficulty of the processes of social negotiation that are involved in establishing a working relationship. Being supportive of a partner's personality is not enough: in the real world of people rather than of personality profiles, relationships have to be constructed and made to work. That is not simply a business of selecting promising material (although that is important): it is a matter of negotiating and creating a workable piece of social machinery.

In the context of both friendship choice and mate choice, such suggestions have a much more satisfactory 'feel' to them than the primitive ideas of early work which proposed a super-regnant influence of a particular personal feature of acquainting individuals. Friendship choice and mate choice are formed and channelled by the way in which partners communicate to each other the extent of overlap between their personalities. They are, therefore, very much processes of gradual disclosure and social negotiation. It is entirely apt, therefore, to describe human mate choice as an interpersonal process.

Summary

The present chapter argues that human mate choice is a process of interpersonal negotiation performed by the two partners involved. Such a view is supported by a review of representative early research which assumed that mate choice resulted simply from the apposition of two suitable personalities. In taking a contrary position we present evidence that the construction of a relationship is an interpersonal process involving communication, discussion, and creative evolution of a working social unit. We argue that human mate choice is just such an interpersonal process.

We are grateful to Robert A. Hinde for his thought-provoking discussion of the paper.

References

Berscheid, E. & Walster, E. H. (1974). A little bit about love. In *Foundations of Interpersonal Attraction*, ed. T. L. Huston, pp. 355–81. Academic Press: New York.

Braiker, H. B. & Kelley, H. H. (1979). Conflict in the development of close relationships. In *Social Exchange in Developing Relationships*, ed. R. L. Burgess & T. L. Huston, pp. 135–68. Academic Press: New York.

Day, B. R. (1961). A comparison of personality needs of courtship couples and same-sex friendships. *Sociology and Social Research*, **45**, 435–40.

Duck, S. W. (1973). *Personal Relationships and Personal Constructs: A Study of Friendship Formation.* John Wiley & Sons: London.

Duck, S. W. (1977). *The Study of Acquaintance.* Teakfields (Saxon House): Farnborough.

Duck, S. W. & Craig, G. (1978). Personality similarity and the development of friendship: A longitudinal study. *British Journal of Social and Clinical Psychology,* **17**, 237–42.

Duck, S. W. & Miell, D. E. (1981). Charting the development of relationships. Paper presented at *One day Conference on Long Term Relationships,* Oxford, November 1981.

Duck, S. W. & Miell, D. E. (in press). Towards a comprehension of friendship development and breakdown. In *The Social Dimension: European Perspectives on Social Psychology,* ed. H. Tajfel. Cambridge University Press: Cambridge.

Huston, T. L., Surra, C. A., Fitzgerald, N. M. & Cate, R. M. (1981). From courtship to marriage: mate selection as an interpersonal process. In *Personal Relationships 2: Developing Personal Relationships,* ed. S. W. Duck & R. Gilmour, pp. 53–88. Academic Press: London.

Levinger, G., Senn, D. J. & Jorgensen, B. W. (1970). Progress toward permanence in courtship: a test of the Kerckhoff-Davis hypothesis. *Sociometry,* **33**, 427–33.

Miell, D. E., Duck, S. W. & La Gaipa, J. J. (1979). Interactive effects of sex and timing of self-disclosure. *British Journal of Social and Clinical Psychology,* **18**, 355–62.

Murstein, B. I. (1971). A theory of marital choice and its applicability to marriage adjustment. In *Theories of Attraction and Love,* ed. B. I. Murstein, pp. 100–51. Springer: New York.

Murstein, B. I. (1976). *Whom Will Marry Whom? Theories and Research in Marital Choice.* Springer: New York.

Murstein, B. I. (1977). The Stimulus-Value-Role (SVR) Theory of dyadic relationships. In *Theory and Practice in Interpersonal Attraction,* ed. S. W. Duck, pp. 105–27. Academic Press: London.

Stroebe, W. (1977). Self-esteem and interpersonal attraction. In *Theory and Practice in Interpersonal Attraction,* ed. S. W. Duck, pp. 79–104. Academic Press: London.

Walster, E. H., Aronson, K., Abrahams, D. & Rottman, L. (1966). Importance of physical attractiveness in dating behaviour. *Journal of Personality and Social Psychology,* **4**, 508–16.

Winch, R. F. (1958). *Mate-Selection: a Study of Complementary Needs.* Harper and Row: New York.

VI:HORMONAL MECHANISMS

18

Hormonal mechanisms of mate choice in birds

J. B. HUTCHISON AND R. E. HUTCHISON

Introduction

Hormones are well known to be closely related to sexual behaviour. But whether sex hormones have any specific role in the establishment and expression of mating preferences, which can be distinguished from their more general actions on reproductive behaviour, does not appear to be known. The few studies addressed to these problems have been concerned with preferences in the female. In a number of mammalian species, oestrous females show a preference for intact as opposed to castrated males in choice tests (reviewed by Johnston, 1979). Anoestrous females show no such preference. While this experimental approach indicates perception on the part of the female of male characteristics, which evidently depend on testicular hormones, it does not answer the more complex question of whether there are subtle individual differences in preferences for potential mates in sexually active animals. These might depend both on the effect of hormones on learning the characteristics of conspecifics and family members in early development, and subsequently recognising features in adulthood which are themselves hormone-dependent secondary sexual characteristics. The studies of Beach on socio-sexual relationships in dogs (Beach, 1970; Beach & LeBoeuf, 1967) are unique in tackling this question directly. Choice tests showed that oestrous Beagle bitches consistently preferred to mate with some apparently normal sexually active dogs, but not with others. Beach (1969, p. 989) drew the important conclusion that 'although ovarian hormones are *necessary* for the bitch's engagement in coital relations, the mere presence of these hormones is not always *sufficient* to guarantee the behavioral result. Superimposed upon the background of physiological oestrus is a system of preference that leads a female to accept some males and at least partially reject others'. Interestingly, Beach found that the bitches showed different preferences in a social context when they were anoestrus, suggesting that oestrus does impose a completely different set of conditions for behavioural interactions.

The evolutionary perspective provided by sociobiology has stimulated new interest in the processes underlying mate choice. Several characteristics that are potentially important in determining choice of mate have been identified (see Halliday, this volume). Some of these, including identification of species and sex, fertility, genetic type and parental quality are closely integrated into the reproductive cycle. If these characteristics are to influence choice of mate, they must be assessable by the chooser (Searcy, 1982). Secondary sexual characters such as plumage patterning, olfactory signals or morphological structures which could have signal value in the choice of a mate are likely to be influenced by hormones. For example, in *Xenopus laevis*, the South African Clawed Toad, androgen induces development of black, rough nuptial pads, enlarged brachial musculature and vocalisations (Hutchison, 1964; Kelley & Pfaff, 1976) which could serve in mate assessment. Although it is difficult to measure the degree to which any of these secondary sexual structures is involved in choice of mate, an even more challenging problem is to identify hormone-dependent behaviour patterns which have specific functions in assessment of qualities in potential mates. In the context of the reproductive cycle, there could be a sequence of choices each requiring different mechanisms. For example, the initial choice might be of species and sex. Once this has been established, reproductive condition might be an important character in assessing the potential fertility of a mate. Each choice is likely to be separated in time and involve different criteria.

The aims of this paper are to consider whether hormones influence behaviour associated with choosing a conspecific mate in appropriate reproductive condition to ensure efficient reproduction and viable offspring. Since we shall also discuss possible modes of action of hormones on mechanisms of mate choice, our material is restricted to behavioural systems that are likely to be influenced by hormones. This paper will, therefore, be concerned with mate choice in male birds, because there is evidence that courtship displays are used in assessment of sex and species of a potential mate (Davies, 1970). There is also no doubt that patterns of male courtship behaviour in birds are extremely sensitive to steroidal sex hormones (reviewed by Hutchison, 1976a). Finally, some indication is emerging of the mode of action of androgen on the avian brain.

Mechanisms of hormone action

In theory, hormones could affect choice of mate in at least three ways. First, hormones could influence mechanisms involved in the learning of conspecific characteristics which are later used in identifying a potential mate. Sexual imprinting, which has been extensively studied in birds (reviewed by Immelmann, 1975; Bateson, 1978a), appears to be a special process in early development which may be affected by foetal or post-hatching hormones. Second, hormones could influence adult behaviour involved in making the choice by direct action on the mechanisms acquired in early development. Third, hormones could result in changes in behavioural interactions with a potential mate which, at critical periods in the reproductive cycle, allow assessment of mate characteristics indicating reproductive condition. In the examples to be discussed below, the first two processes would permit identification of species and sex, the second would allow recognition of reproductive condition in the potential mate to avoid delay in the reproductive cycle and inadequate preparation for rearing the young.

Hormones for mate choice

Which hormones are likely to be involved in choice of mate by the male, and how are they controlled? This question has to be considered carefully, because it could refer to hormonal effects within the female which influence signals to which the male responds, or to hormonal effects within the male. Only the latter problem will be addressed here. In the case of androgens, the question is further complicated, because the primary androgen in most vertebrates, testosterone, is a precursor or 'pre-hormone' for a variety of androgenic metabolites which may themselves be biologically active and influence behaviour (Zigmond, 1975). The most conspicuous of these steroids, 5α-dihydrotestosterone (Fig. 18.1) is involved mainly in the development of secondary sexual characters such as the cock's comb, but can have significant behavioural effects. Testosterone and one of its androgenic metabolites, androstenedione, are substrates for the formation of oestrogen by the aromatase enzyme in the target tissues on which these androgens act (Naftolin *et al.*, 1975). Therefore, as will be made clear later, it can be extremely important to identify whether a particular hormonal effect on behaviour is oestrogen- or androgen-dependent. Androgens are secreted not only by the interstitial cells of the testes, but also by the adrenal cortex. This is a by-product of glucocorticoid synthesis which can in theory have behavioural consequences, but in practice there is no indication that in male birds adrenal androgens have any physiological role in the control of behaviour. A further complication in understanding the role of avian androgens is that appreciable concentrations of the metabolite of testosterone, 5α-dihydrotestosterone, are found in the blood plasma of many species. This metabolite is potentially important in view of its androgenic potency. But whether it has behavioural actions is still a matter of controversy (Hutchison, 1978; Adkins-Regan, 1981). Finally, not many studies using radio-immunoassay methods for measuring hormone concentrations in avian blood plasma have completely separated testosterone from 5α-dihydrotestosterone. The inclusive term 'androgen' will be used here to indicate total testosterone and androgenic metabolites in the blood.

There is now considerable evidence that concentration of androgen in avian blood plasma is influenced by environmental factors such as light and food resources (Wingfield, 1980; Farner & Wingfield, 1980) or social stimuli (Feder, Stoney, Goodwin & Reboulleau, 1977). These factors act on the neuroendocrine system in the hypothalamus to stimulate release of neurohormones and ultimately gonadotrophins which regulate interstitial cell production of androgen in the testes (Davies & Follett, 1975). In view of the action of environment on the neuroendocrine system, testicular output of androgens is likely to differ between males with different

Fig. 18.1. Principal pathways of androgen metabolism in the brain that are relevant to hormone-dependent behaviour associated with mate choice.

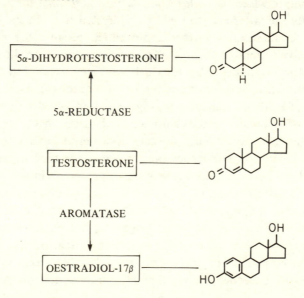

individual histories. However, there is no evidence that rapid elevation in peripheral androgen, such as results from sexual interaction causes changes in male behaviour though it could be essential for the production and transport of viable spermatozoa in the reproductive tracts (Lincoln, 1974).

Mode of hormone action

Before considering whether androgens influence mate choice directly, it is useful to review briefly what is known of the physiological effects of these hormones on behaviour. Androgens influence hypothalamic areas of the brain involved in the control of reproductive behaviour in birds (reviewed by Hutchison, 1978). This is probably the most important route of action on male behaviour. For example, crystalline implants of androgen are effective in restoring courtship behaviour in castrated male doves (*Streptopelia risoria*) when placed in the preoptic-anterior hypothalamic area of the brain, but not in adjacent brain areas (Hutchison, 1967). In addition, studies of the fate of isotopically labelled testosterone indicate that the hormone is concentrated mainly in this brain area. So the current view is that the brain contains target cells for androgen which are closely associated with sexual behaviour. There is also a good deal known about the action of androgen at the cellular level. The general model proposes the following sequence of events: (a) the androgen being lipid-soluble passes through the cell membrane; (b) it binds to cytoplasmic receptor proteins specific for the particular steroid; and (c) the bound complex is translocated to the cell nucleus and ultimately initiates protein synthesis and this somehow triggers the target cell into specified function (McEwen, Krey & Luine, 1978). The fact that androgens are extensively metabolised by enzymes in the target cells in the brain adds an additional difficulty in attempting to understand the action of these hormones on behaviour.

Direct effects of androgen on mate choice

Is there any evidence that androgens have any direct effect on the acquisition or learning of characters that are later identified during choice of mate? Specific social experience is required for sexual imprinting during sensitive periods in early development (Immelmann, 1972; Bateson, 1978a). Elevations in plasma androgen may be correlated with these sensitive periods. But this is not necessarily evidence for a causal effect of androgen on sexual imprinting.

Laboratory studies indicate that choice of mate by adult male Japanese Quail is determined both by early experience of siblings (Bateson, 1978b,

1980) and by association with certain colour morphs (Gallagher, 1976). The period when sexual imprinting occurs in Japanese Quail appears to extend from days 6 to 20 after hatching (Gallagher, 1977). At this stage the adult-type plumage is developing (Bateson, 1979). Although the stability of the mating preference depends on the age of exposure and conditions of rearing (Gallagher, 1978; Gallagher & Ash, 1978; Bateson, 1980) male Japanese Quail tend to show a consistent preference for the brown colour morph. The initial question to be considered is whether hormones have any direct effect on behaviour associated with the expression of a mating preference irrespective of any possible action in early development.

Androgen in the expression of mate choice

Whether androgens are associated directly with choice of mate in the male adult can be tested experimentally in an apparatus which allows the male to indicate his preference for brown or white females, but prevents him from mating with the object of his choice (apparatus described by Bateson, 1980). In other words, the act of choosing a mate is divorced from the performance of copulatory behaviour. The positive correlation between preference for brown females (Fig. 18.2) and plasma concentration of androgens indicates that the hormones may influence preference for a mate

Fig. 18.2. Relationship between plasma level of androgen (combined testosterone and 5α-dihydrotestosterone) and preference for a brown or white female shown during a choice test by intact sexually active males reared with brown females. The preference is shown as the difference between the periods of time spent near the brown female (D_b) and the white female (D_w). $rs = 0.69$; $P < 0.01$.

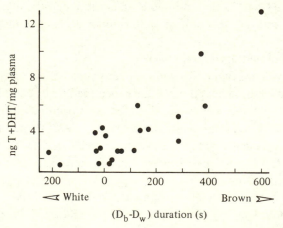

$(D_b\text{-}D_w)$ duration (s)

directly. Males in which gonadal hormones have been eliminated by castration immediately after hatching spend the same amount of time near the stimulus females as intact males. However, they show no consistent preference for either colour morph (Fig. 18.3). Males castrated on the day of hatching consistently prefer the brown morph when treated systemically with testosterone as adults (Hutchison & Bateson, in prep.). Testosterone is required, therefore, for the expression of the colour preference in adulthood.

Although the choice is made independently of the performance of copulatory behaviour in the test apparatus, an important question is how mechanisms underlying choice of mate by the male relate to other aspects of sexual behaviour. Presumably, choice of mate normally precedes copulatory behaviour and is, therefore, separated in time from hormone-dependent processes underlying copulation. But is the the choice of mate related closely to other elements of sexual behaviour which precede copulation such as courtship? In Japanese Quail, the amount of 'strutting', which is presumed to be a courtship pattern and is known to be hormone-dependent, is positively correlated with the strength of the preference for the brown morph. Does androgen influence mate choice as an indirect consequence of its action on strutting, or does the hormone act directly on mate choice mechanisms? Strutting in the testing apparatus

Fig. 18.3. Choice between brown and white females shown by brown males reared with brown females. The preference ratio consists of the duration near the brown female (D_b) as a ratio of the total time near brown and white females ($D_b + D_w$). The chance level is 0.5. Each individual's score was compared with chance level (*$P < 0.05$, **$P < 0.01$).

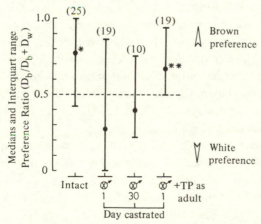

usually occurs after the choice has been made. This suggests that androgen could influence recognition processes underlying choice of mate directly. To speculate further along these lines without more data is obviously dangerous, but strutting could be an indication to the female or other males that a positive choice has been made by the male. These experiments do not show that a *learned* preference is involved, and this aspect is discussed in more detail below.

Androgen in the acquisition of preference

Are androgens implicated in the early learning of characteristics which are used later when a choice of mate is made? In Japanese Quail, androgen levels are elevated before hatching on the eighth and fifteenth days of incubation. But the concentrations of plasma androgen are very low (1.0–1.25 ng/ml plasma) relative to the adult (10–15 ng/ml plasma) (Ottinger & Brinkley, 1979; Ottinger & Bakst, 1981). Androgen levels rise initially during the post-hatching period on day 18 (Ottinger & Bakst, 1981) which is roughly coincident with the period when sexual imprinting occurs in Japanese Quail. Presumptive interstitial cells do appear in the testes during early embryonic development. But steroidogenic activity occurs only two to three weeks after hatching at a period which corresponds to the pre-adult surge in testosterone (Haffen, Scheib, Guichard & Cedard, 1975; Ottinger & Bakst, 1981). The origin of the androgen measured during the early post-hatching period is still unknown, but it is likely to be testicular. Levels of androgen measured in the adrenals of chick embryos have been shown to be higher than in the testes (Tanabe, Nakamura, Fujioka & Doi, 1979). But after hatching, these concentrations are lower than in the testes. Therefore, the adrenals are unlikely to contribute testosterone when sexual imprinting is thought to occur in Japanese Quail; though an equivalent study has not been carried out in this species.

Testicular androgen present during the early post-hatching period does not affect the mating preference for the brown morph, because males castrated immediately after hatching show preferences similar to those of intact males, providing that androgen therapy is given in adulthood. Further experiments (Hutchison & Bateson, 1982) have provided evidence that the expression of an *acquired* preference for a novel white colour morph is influenced by androgen. These experiments are based on the finding that intact, sexually active brown males reared singly with the white colour morph show a preference for this morph in adulthood (Gallagher, 1976; Hutchison & Bateson, 1982). These males had evidently learnt the characteristics of the white morph during development.

Males castrated at hatching and treated with testosterone as adults also showed this preference, whereas untreated castrated males did not (Hutchison & Bateson, 1982). Testicular hormones do not appear, therefore, to be involved in the acquisition of a preference for the white morph during early development. However, testosterone is required for the male to express a preference in adulthood.

At present, it is difficult to speculate on the way in which androgen acts to influence this mating preference. A direct action of testosterone on the brain is likely, but this is impossible to verify unless the steroid is applied directly to the brain. Whether testosterone itself or a metabolite formed elsewhere act on brain mechanisms associated with the preference, and how this can be distinguished from the action of hormones on hypothalamic mechanisms of mating behaviour has still to be determined. Since retrieval of learned information in chicks is influenced by testosterone (Andrew, 1980), androgen may link characteristics learned during development with mechanisms required for the expression of the preference in adult Quail.

Indirect effects of androgen on mate choice

Androgens could play a part in choosing a mate in the appropriate reproductive condition for efficient breeding. Ensuring that a potential mate is in the correct stage of reproductive development is especially important in birds where the reproductive cycles of the male and female have to be synchronised very closely. This is necessary to ensure that fertilisation occurs in correct relation to the development of the hard-shelled egg which has to be fertilised before the shell is laid down (Hinde, 1965, 1970; Hutchison, 1977). The building of a nest and incubation also have to be in synchrony with egg-laying. Lehrman (1965) showed clearly that there is a reciprocal relationship between the male and female dove. The behaviour of the male influences the endocrine system of the mate, which in turn influences its behaviour and finally the endocrine system and behaviour of the original bird. Reproductive development in the male during the cycle depends, therefore, on a sequence of transitions in behaviour which is related to endocrine factors and the behaviour of the female.

Mate choice in the dove

The initial courtship behaviour of the male dove consists of a rapid alternation between two types of behaviour which result in different female responses (Hutchison, 1970). First, aggressive courtship patterns either drive the female away if she is sexually inactive or induce her to retreat if she is sexually active. If she is sexually active then male nest soliciting behaviour attracts the female to a presumptive nest site where she also shows nest soliciting. Male courtship observed in a laboratory situation consists, therefore, of an expression of two motivational systems: aggressive and nest-oriented behaviour (Hutchison, 1970). Over time, there is a transition in behaviour. With continual interaction, the male's behaviour changes quite rapidly so that he begins to show more nest soliciting. Within a matter of a day, the male's behaviour consists almost exclusively of this pattern (Lovari & Hutchison, 1975). The transition to nest soliciting is much slower if the male shows a preponderance of aggressive courtship. If the males are chosen for aggressiveness in courtship (Hutchison & Lovari, 1976), the whole reproductive cycle is delayed and nest building is rudimentary. Ovulation and egg laying occur after a significantly longer period than normal, indicating that ovarian development is either delayed or reversed (Fig. 18.4). This is an extreme example

Fig. 18.4. (a) Differences in latency to egg-laying (*$P < 0.05$), and therefore in length of reproductive cycle between males which showed aggressive courtship without the nest-oriented component (P) and a group which displayed full aggressive and nest-oriented courtship (PS). (b) Androgen levels differed between P and PS groups – individual testosterone levels are shown. (Data derived from Hutchison & Katongole, 1975.)

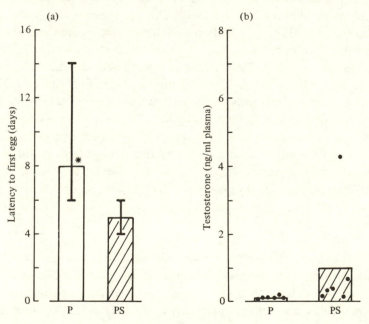

of asynchrony imposed by the experimental conditions. Aggressive court-ship probably has the function of both identifying the sex of a potential mate and driving off females that are either not reproductively active, or are not in the correct endocrine condition essential in this species for rapid and efficient completion of the reproductive cycle.

Do courtship patterns have any other function in choice of mate? In a species such as the Barbary Dove, where the male contributes to the parental care of the young, it is crucial that the eggs are fertilised by his own sperm if his time and energy spent in parental care are not to be wasted (Trivers, 1972). Following this hypothesis, it is also essential that the male dove eliminates the effects of cuckoldry by driving off any females inseminated by another male (Erickson & Zenone, 1976, 1978), or delays the female reproductive development until sperm from previous insemina-tions is no longer viable (Zenone, Sims & Erickson, 1979). Female displays of nest soliciting, which result in increased aggressive courtship in the male (Erickson & Zenone, 1976), may provide an indication to the male of whether she has been inseminated previously by another male. The nest-soliciting behaviour of the female is known to be enhanced by male courtship (Cheng, 1973) and could signal advanced ovarian development. However, the female shows little nest soliciting in the presence of highly aggressive males and this is known to delay female reproductive develop-ment (Hutchison & Lovari, 1976). Therefore, for the signal to be effective the male must display some nest soliciting to allow the female in turn to display nest soliciting. Then the male can assess whether the female is in the appropriate physiological condition for successful reproduction.

In summary, if we follow the functional arguments put forward so far, the transition from aggressive to nest-oriented courtship is important in the initial choice of mate by the male. Aggressiveness must be sustained for long enough to identify species and sex of a potential mate, and whether she is sexually active. Yet the transition in his behaviour to nest soliciting must occur soon enough to allow the female to signal her reproductive condition.

Hormonal factors

Courtship displays in the male dove depend upon testicular androgen acting directly on the preoptic–anterior hypothalamic area of the brain (Hutchison, 1967). Does the transition between aggressive and nest-oriented courtship also depend on the action of sex hormones in the brain? It can be suggested that the transition requires a 'switch' from one hormone-sensitive control system to another. Studies with injected and intracerebrally implanted steroids have provided evidence for this hypothesis (Hutchison, 1976*b*). Castrated males implanted with testosterone show both aggressive and nest-oriented courtship – behaviour which resembles that of an intact male undergoing initial courtship. Oestrogens, usually regarded as female hormones, have very specific effects in the castrated male dove which replicate the post-transition phase when nest soliciting is displayed in the absence of aggressive courtship. This effect is striking and can be obtained with the naturally occurring oestrogen, oestradiol-17β (Hutchison, 1970), or the synthetic oestrogen, diethyl-stilboestrol (Hutchison, Steimer & Duncan, 1981) which is highly specific in its binding to oestrogen receptors in target brain cells (Chamness, King & Sheridan, 1979). There is good evidence, therefore, that oestrogen may be very important in determining when and to what degree the male shows nest soliciting. The transition itself could depend on increasing oestrogen during courtship interactions with the female. A problem with this hypothesis, however, is that the male's blood plasma contains no oestradiol (Koronbrot, Shomberg & Erickson, 1974).

Where does the oestrogen come from? One possibility is that oestradiol is formed in the target area in the brain where testosterone is effective for courtship – the preoptic and anterior hypothalamic regions. An aromatase

Fig. 18.5(a). Localisation of aromatase activity in the male dove brain. Areas 1 (area basalis) and 3 (anterior hypothalamus) are immediately rostral and caudal to 2 (preoptic area). Testosterone is converted to oestradiol-17β in the preoptic area. Conversion is minimal in adjacent areas. (Data from Steimer & Hutchison, 1980.)

Fig. 18.5(b). Preoptic aromatase activity is markedly increased by intramuscular injections of testosterone propionate (black bars) in castrated doves compared with saline-treated controls. The inductive effect of androgen is specific to the preoptic area (POA) and does not occur in the area basalis (AB). (Data derived from Steimer & Hutchison, 1981.)

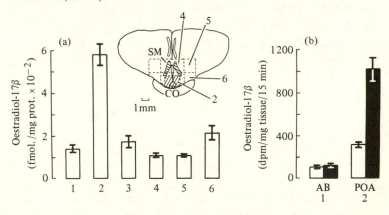

system has been found which is highly active in converting testosterone to oestradiol (Fig. 18.5(a)); it is precisely localised in the preoptic area (Steimer & Hutchison, 1980), and is likely to occur in the target cells which take up testosterone. Since injected androgen increases preoptic aromatase activity markedly (Fig. 18.5(b), Steimer & Hutchison, 1981a), the enzyme itself appears to be influenced by hormonal condition. This would in turn regulate the availability of oestradiol in target areas associated with nest soliciting. The preoptic aromatase system could function as a 'regulator' of the timing of the transition, the setting of which would depend on hypothalamic androgen level. Recently, it has been shown that plasma testosterone levels rise soon after the initial courtship interactions (O'Connell, Reboulleau, Feder & Silver, 1981). The surge in testosterone could set in motion a cascade of events which increases the availability of behaviourally effective oestradiol in the brain and ultimately the transition towards increased nest-oriented behaviour. Therefore increase in one hormone could, according to the model proposed in Fig. 18.6, set in motion the enzymatic changes involved in converting one hormone to another. Each hormone would be associated directly with a particular complex of behaviour patterns in the male.

The tight organisation of behavioural and hormonal events in the male dove, and the synchronisation of male and female cycles pose unique problems in neuroendocrine control. However, the preoptic aromatase system could have the necessary responsiveness to hormonal and environmental conditions to modulate the action of androgen in a changing behavioural situation. Perhaps the aromatase system and other enzymes

Fig. 18.6. Hypothetical series of events underlying transitions in male behaviour. A hormone (H_1) is required in the regulation of male behavioural interactions of type A with the female. Increase in H_1 changes brain enzyme activity (E_1) specific for the metabolism of the hormone and results in formation of a second hormone (H_2) required for a different (type B) male interaction with the female. A series of hormonal and enzymatic changes could underlie further transitions in male behaviour.

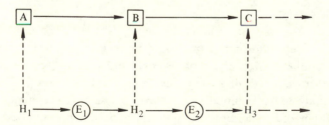

in the dove brain which metabolise androgens, such as the 5β-reductase system (Hutchison & Steimer, 1981; Steimer & Hutchison, 1981*b*), are designed to provide a degree of plasticity in hormone regulation within target areas of the brain associated with behaviour. Reproductive synchrony and the consequent behavioural mechanisms required for choice of mate may be factors which have shaped these androgen metabolising enzymes in the dove brain during evolution.

Conclusions

In the context of the reproductive cycle, mate choice is likely to consist of a sequence of choices over time which involve different hormonal mechanisms. Initial choice could be for species, sex and individual type. Subsequent choices for reproductive condition would be important in assessing potential fertility of a mate. Androgen in the adult male can be shown experimentally to be directly involved in the expression of a learned preference for a particular type of female. Testicular hormones do not influence acquisition of the preference during early development under conditions in which mate choice has been studied so far. It would appear, therefore, that learning of the features on which the sexual preference later depends is not affected by sex hormones. But adult levels of these hormones may influence the 'retrieval' of learned features required for the choice. Androgens also have an indirect action on the choice of mate by the male at later stages in the reproductive cycle. This indirect effect results in transitions in male behaviour which in turn induce changes in behaviour of the female allowing male assessment of fertility, reproductive condition and the possibility of previous insemination. Under these conditions where a complex series of interactions is required for the male to make a choice, androgen may be converted in the brain to other hormones, such as oestrogens, which influence transitions in male behaviour. The brain enzymes responsible for the conversions appear to have the necessary plasticity in responsiveness to hormonal and environmental conditions to modulate the action of androgen during the cycle.

Summary

Two examples are discussed which illustrate possible differences in the influence of hormones on mate choice in male birds. The first example identifies a direct action of androgen in Japanese Quail on mating preferences acquired during early development. Testosterone is shown experimentally to be required for the expression of a preference for a particular type of female. But testicular hormones are not involved in the acquisition of this preference during development. The second example illustrates an indirect action of androgen in the male Barbary Dove resulting in changes in behavioural interaction with a potential mate which, at particular stages in the reproductive cycle, allow assessment of fertility. A physiological model is proposed which attributes the behavioural transitions during the reproductive cycle to changes in androgen metabolism within the brain.

We thank Frank Beach for providing us with unpublished information. We are also grateful to Peter Marler, Carl Erickson and the Editor of this volume for their comments on the manuscript.

References

Andrew, R. J. (1980). The functional organization of phases of memory consolidation. In *Advances in the Study of Behavior*, 2nd edn, pp. 337–67. Academic Press: New York.

Adkins-Regan, E. (1981). Effect of sex steroids on the reproductive behavior of castrated male ring doves (*Streptopelia* sp.). *Physiology & Behavior*, **26**, 561–5.

Bateson, P. P. G. (1978a). Early experience and sexual preferences. In *Biological Determinants of Sexual Behaviour*, ed. J. B. Hutchison, pp. 29–53. John Wiley: Chichester.

Bateson, P. (1978b). Sexual imprinting and optimal outbreeding. *Nature*, **273**, 659–60.

Bateson, P. (1979). How do sensitive periods arise and what are they for? *Animal Behaviour*, **27**, 470–86.

Bateson, P. (1980). Optimal outbreeding and the development of sexual preferences in Japanese Quail. *Zeitschrift für Tierpsychologie*, **53**, 231–44.

Beach, F. A. (1969). Locks and Beagles. *American Psychologist*, **24**, 971–89.

Beach, F. A. (1970). Coital behaviour in dogs. VIII. Social affinity, dominance and sexual preference in the bitch. *Behaviour*, **36**, 131–48.

Beach, F. A. & LeBoeuf, B. J. (1967). Coital behaviour in dogs. I. Preferential mating in the bitch. *Animal Behaviour*, **15**, 546–58.

Chamness, G. C., King, T. W. & Sheridan, P. J. (1979). Androgen receptor in the rat brain – assays and properties. *Brain Research*, **161**, 267–76.

Cheng, M.-F. (1973). Effect of estrogen on behavior of ovariectomised ring doves (*Streptopelia risoria*). *Journal of Comparative Physiology and Psychology*, **83**, 234–9.

Davies, D. T. & Follett, B. K. (1975). The neuroendocrine control of gonadotropin release in the Japanese quail. II. The role of the anterior hypothalamus. *Proceedings of the Royal Society of London*, Series B, **191**, 303–15.

Davies, S. J. J. F. (1970). Patterns of inheritance in the bowing display and associated behaviour of some hybrid *Streptopelia* doves. *Behaviour*, **36**, 187–214.

Erickson, C. J. & Zenone, P. G. (1976). Courtship differences in male ring doves: avoidance of cuckoldry? *Science*, **192**, 1353–4.

Erickson, C. J. & Zenone, P. G. (1978). Aggressive courtship as a means of avoiding cuckoldry. *Animal Behaviour*, **26**, 307.

Farner, D. S. & Wingfield, J. C. (1980). Reproductive endocrinology of birds. *Annual Review of Physiology*, **42**, 457–72.

Feder, H. H., Storey, A., Goodwin, D. & Reboulleau, C. (1977). Testosterone and "5α-dihydrotestosterone" levels in peripheral plasma of male and female ring doves (*Streptopelia risoria*) during the reproductive cycle. *Biology of Reproduction*, **16**, 666–77.

Gallagher, J. E. (1976). Sexual imprinting: effects of various regimens of social experience on mate preference in Japanese quail, *Coturnix coturnix japonica*. *Behaviour*, **57**, 91–114.

Gallagher, J. E. (1977). Sexual imprinting: a sensitive period in Japanese quail (*Coturnix coturnix japonica*). *Journal of Comparative and Physiological Psychology*, **91**, 72–8.

Gallagher, J. E. (1978). Sexual imprinting: variables influencing the development of mate preference in *Coturnix coturnix japonica*. *Behavioral Biology*, **24**, 481–91.

Gallagher, J. E. & Ash, M. (1978). Sexual imprinting: the stability of mate preference in Japanese quail (*Coturnix coturnix japonica*). *Animal Learning and Behavior*, **6**, 363–5.

Haffen, K., Scheib, D., Guichard, A. & Cedard, L. (1975). Prolonged sexual bipotentiality of the embryonic quail testis and relation to sex steroid biosynthesis. *General and Comparative Endocrinology*, **26**, 70–8.

Hinde, R. A. (1965). Interaction of internal and external factors in integration of canary reproduction. In *Sex and Behavior*, ed. F. A. Beach, pp. 381–415. J. Wiley: New York.

Hinde, R. A. (1970). *Animal Behaviour: a synthesis of Ethology and Comparative Psychology* (2nd edn). McGraw-Hill: New York.

Hutchison, J. B. (1964). Investigations on the neural control of clasping and feeding in *Xenopus laevis* (Daudin). *Behaviour*, **24**, 47–65.

Hutchison, J. B. (1967). Initiation of courtship by hypothalamic implants of testosterone propionate in castrated doves (*Streptopelia risoria*). *Nature*, **216**, 591–2.

Hutchison, J. B. (1970). Differential effects of testosterone and oestradiol on male courtship in Barbary doves (*Streptopelia risoria*). *Animal Behaviour*, **18**, 41–52.

Hutchison, J. B. (1976a). Hypothalamic mechanisms of sexual behaviour, with special reference to birds. In *Advances in the Study of Behaviour*, vol. **6**, eds. J. S. Rosenblatt, R. A. Hinde, E. Shaw & C. Beer, pp. 159–318. Academic Press: New York.

Hutchison, J. B. (1976b). Hormones and brain mechanisms of sexual behaviour: a possible relationship between cellular and behavioural events in doves. In *Perspectives in Experimental Biology*, vol. **1**, *Zoology*, ed. P. Spencer Davies, pp. 417–36. Pergamon Press: Oxford and New York.

Hutchison, J. B. (1978). Hypothalamic regulation of male sexual responsiveness to androgen. In *Biological Determinants of Sexual Behaviour*, ed. J. B. Hutchison, pp. 277–319. John Wiley: Chichester.

Hutchison, J. B. & Katongole, C. B. (1975). Plasma testosterone in courting and incubating male Barbary doves (*Streptopelia risoria*). *Journal of Endocrinology*, **65**, 275–6.

Hutchison, J. B. & Lovari, S. (1976). Effects of male aggressiveness on behavioural transitions in the reproductive cycle of the Barbary dove. *Behaviour*, **59**, 296–318.

Hutchison, J. B. & Steimer, Th. (1981). Brain 5β-reductase: a correlate of behavioral sensitivity to androgen. *Science*, **213**, 244–6.

Hutchison, J. B., Steimer, Th. & Duncan, R. (1981). Behavioural action of androgen in the dove: effects of long-term castration on response specificity and brain aromatization. *Journal of Endocrinology*, **90**, 167–78.

Hutchison, R. E. (1977). Temporal relationships between nesting behaviour, ovary and oviduct development during the reproductive cycle of female budgerigars. *Behaviour*, **60**, 278–303.

Hutchison, R. E. (1978). Hormonal differentiation of sexual behavior in Japanese quail. *Hormones and Behavior*, **11**, 363–87.

Hutchison, R. E. & Bateson, P. (1982). Sexual imprinting in male Japanese quail. The effects of castration at hatching. *Developmental Psychobiology*, **15**, 471–7.

Immelmann, K. (1972). Sexual and other long-term aspects of imprinting in birds and other species. In *Advances in the Study of Behavior*, vol. **4**, ed. D. S. Lehrman, R. A. Hinde & E. Shaw, pp. 147–74. Academic Press: New York.

Immelmann, K. (1975). Ecological significance of imprinting and early learning. *Annual Review of Ecology and Systematics*, **6**, 15–37.

Johnston, R. E. (1979). Olfactory preferences, scent marking and "proceptivity" in female hamsters. *Hormones and Behavior*, **13**, 21–39.

Kelley, D. B. & Pfaff, D. W. (1976). Hormone effects on male sex behavior in adult South African clawed frogs, *Xenopus laevis*. *Hormones and Behavior*, **7**, 159–82.

Korenbrot, C. C., Shomberg, D. W. & Erickson, C. J. (1974). Radioimmunoassay of plasma estradiol during the breeding cycle of ring doves (*Streptopelia risoria*). *Endocrinology*, **94**, 1126–32.

Lehrman, D. S. (1965). Interaction between internal and external environments in the regulation of the reproductive cycle of the ring dove. In *Sex and Behavior*, ed. F. A. Beach, pp. 355–80. J. Wiley: New York.

Lincoln, G. A. (1974). Luteinising hormone and testosterone in man. *Nature*, **252**, 232–3.

Lovari, S. & Hutchison, J. B. (1975). Behavioural transitions in the reproductive cycle of Barbary doves (*Streptopelia risoria* L.). *Behaviour*, **53**, 126–50.

McEwen, B. S., Krey, L. C. & Luine, V. N. (1978). Steroid hormone action in the neuroendocrine system: when is the genome involved? *The Hypothalamus*, ed. S. Reichlin, R. J. Baldessarini & J. B. Martin, pp. 255–68. Raven Press: New York.

Naftolin, F., Ryan, K. J., Davies, I. J., Reddy, V. V., Flores, F., Petro, D., Kuhn, M., White, R. J., Takoaka, Y. & Wolin, L. (1975). The formation of estrogens by central neuroendocrine tissue. *Recent Progress in Hormone Research*, **31**, 295–316.

O'Connell, M. E., Reboulleau, C., Feder, H. H. & Silver, R. (1981). Social interactions and androgen levels in birds. 1. Female characteristics associated with increased plasma androgen levels in the male ring dove (*Streptopelia risoria*). *General and Comparative Endocrinology*, **44**, 454–64.

Ottinger, M. A. & Bakst, M. R. (1981). Peripheral androgen concentrations and testicular morphology in embryonic and young male Japanese quail. *General and Comparative Endocrinology*, **43**, 170–7.

Ottinger, M. A. & Brinkley, H. J. (1979). Testosterone and sex related physical characteristics during the maturation of the male Japanese quail (*Coturnix coturnix japonica*). *Biology of Reproduction*, **20**, 905–9.

Searcy, W. A. (1982). The evolutionary effects of mate selection. *Annual Review of Ecology and Systematics*, **13**, in press.

Steimer, Th. & Hutchison, J. B. (1980). Aromatization of testosterone within a discrete hypothalamic area associated with the behavioral action of androgen in the male dove. *Brain Research*, **192**, 586–91.

Steimer, Th. & Hutchison, J. B. (1981*a*). Androgen increases formation of behaviourally effective oestrogen in dove brain. *Nature*, **292**, 345–7.

Steimer, Th. & Hutchison, J. B. (1981*b*). Metabolic control of the behavioural action of androgens in the dove brain: testosterone inactivation by 5β-reduction. *Brain Research*, **209**, 189–204.

Tanabe, Y., Nakamura, T., Fujioka, K. & Doi, O. (1979). Production and secretion of sex steroid hormones by the testes, the ovary, and the adrenal glands in embryonic and young chickens (*Gallus domesticus*). *General and Comparative Endocrinology*, **39**, 26–33.

Trivers, R. L. (1972). Parental investment and sexual selection. In *Sexual Selection and the Descent of man, 1871–1971*, ed. B. Campbell, pp. 136–79. Aldine: Chicago.

Wingfield, J. C. (1980). Fine temporal adjustment of reproductive functions. In *Avian Endocrinology*, ed. A. Epple & M. Stetson, pp. 367–89. Academic Press: New York.

Zenone, P. G., Sims, M. E. & Erickson, C. J. (1979). Male ring dove behavior and the defence of genetic paternity. *American Naturalist*, **114**, 615–26.

Zigmond, R. E. (1975). Binding metabolism and action of steroid hormones in the central nervous system. In *Handbook of Psychopharmacology*, ed. L. L. Iversen, S. D. Iversen & S. H. Snyder, vol. **5**, pp. 239–328. Plenum Press: New York.

19

Endocrine determinants and constraints on sexual behaviour in monkeys

ERIC B. KEVERNE

Sexual behaviour in social groups of monkeys is rarely equitably distributed. Male dominance is frequently reported to have a marked influence on which males display sexual behaviour (Carpenter, 1942; Hall, 1967; Struhsaker, 1967; Bernstein, 1976) and although dominance hierarchies in females are less readily determined from overt aggressive encounters, there are nevertheless reports which suggest that females of high social rank have priority over access to males (Drickamer, 1974; Sade *et al.*, 1977; Dunbar, 1980), and reproduce more often (Dunbar & Dunbar, 1977; Abbott & Hearn, 1978). The purpose of this paper is to consider the extent to which the secretions of the endocrine system play a part in this unequal distribution of sexual behaviour in social groups of monkeys. Studies of hormones and behaviour have inevitably relied heavily on laboratory primates and it is unfortunate that few species have received investigation in depth. Hence, this paper concerns itself mainly with two species of Old World Monkey, the Rhesus and Talapoin Monkey, both of which live in social groups composed of large numbers of both adult males and females. These two species provide good examples of the way in which mating is related to an individual's status in the social hierarchy.

Gonadal hormones and the sexual behaviour of male monkeys in the social group

It is quite clear that the structure and composition of monkey groups has marked effects on both gonadal and adrenocortical hormones. A number of studies have shown that the levels of sexual and aggressive behaviour in high-ranking males correlate with high levels of testosterone (Bernstein, Rose & Gordon, 1977; Rose, Holaday & Bernstein, 1971; Keverne, Meller & Martinez-Arias, 1978). In addition, members of

407

differing primate species show adrenocortical responses to social manipula-tions (Leshner & Candland, 1972; Mendoza, Coe, Lowe & Levine, 1979) and to the receipt of aggression (Chamove & Bowman, 1978; Sassenrath, 1970; Scallet, Suomie & Bowman, 1981).

In sexual behaviour, studies have inevitably focused on the significance of gonadal hormones and it was found that testosterone levels increased in adult males that became sexually active when introduced to attractive females (Rose, Gordon & Bernstein, 1972; Eberhart, Keverne & Meller, 1980). In contrast, when males were introduced singly into well-established social groups whose members attacked and defeated them, their testosterone levels fell dramatically (Rose, Bernstein & Gordon, 1975). It is therefore important to establish whether the primate groups' organisation and an individual monkey's role in it modify behaviour in any way by an action on steroid hormones. Thus, the question arises as to whether males of high social rank inhibit the sexual behaviour of subordinates by suppressing their testosterone secretion? In order to answer this question it is necessary to understand exactly what, if any, the effects of testosterone are on the sexual behaviour of male monkeys, and this is best assessed away from the social influences of the group, in heterosexual pair tests. In pair tests of monkeys, testosterone alone does not appear to determine whether or not a male is sexually active. Male Rhesus Monkeys may continue to show sexual interest and mate with females years after they have been castrated (Resko & Phoenix, 1972; Wilson, Plant & Michael, 1972; Phoenix, Slob & Goy, 1973). However, there is a general decline in the frequency of intromission and ejaculations, and these are restored by the administration of testosterone. Testosterone in the Rhesus Monkey appears therefore to influence the sexual performance of the male, rather than his sexual interest in the female. Thus, while increased levels of testosterone in high-ranking males may enhance their sexual performance, it seems unlikely that suppressed levels of testosterone in subordinate males can account for their sexual inactivity. In fact, the sexual inactivity of low-ranking males is itself incomplete, for although mating is restricted, subordinates continue to display interest in the females as judged from the inspections they make of the females' perineal region. Moreover, the administration of testosterone to subordinate male Talapoin Monkeys in the social group fails to stimulate their sexual activity (Dixson & Herbert, 1977). This is not because low-ranking males are without the opportunity to mate females, since female sexual solicitations increase toward low-ranking males when they receive testosterone. While the treatment of low-ranking males with testosterone does not stimulate their mating, it does increase the aggression they receive from other males.

Thus aggressive behaviour, the direction of which defines the dominance hierarchy, may be a factor inhibiting the sexual activity of subordinates. If this were indeed the case, then one might predict that removal of higher-ranking males would enable the subordinates to mate with impunity. This approach has been tested in a number of social groups of Talapoin Monkeys containing four adult males and four or five adult females. The results were somewhat surprising, for in the absence of dominant males, subordinates seldom mated with females and when they did so, not only was their performance low, but their sexual behaviour was entirely initiated by the females. One of the consequences of social subordination in male Talapoin Monkeys is the elevation of the stress hormones cortisol and prolactin (Keverne, 1979; Eberhart & Keverne, 1979). Compared with males living in social isolation, both cortisol and prolactin levels increased dramatically when subordinate males were with the female group (Keverne, Eberhart & Meller, 1982). This occurred even though aggressive behaviour was significantly reduced because dominant males were absent. In contrast to this, dominant males, when moved back into the social group of females in the absence of other males, experienced a decrease in prolactin while cortisol remained low.

Hence, although we see no significant difference between the levels of stress hormones cortisol and prolactin in 'dominant' and 'subordinate' males in isolation, moving into the social group produces markedly different hormonal profiles in these animals. Whereas the stress hormones decrease in the dominant male, they increase significantly in the subordinate, an increase which cannot be explained solely on the basis of aggression received. However, while aggressive behaviour *per se* may not be inhibiting the sexual behaviour of subordinates, their inability to cope with sexual opportunities may well be related to their past experiences of defeat and the potential for this to be reinforced at any time.

The social hierarchy therefore provides some indication as to the behavioural propensities of an individual, the expression of which may be related to that individual's coping ability reflected in the increased secretion of cortisol and prolactin. In dominant males with marked increases in plasma testosterone we observe high levels of sexual perform-ance, and in the social group when all the males are present, dominant males receive the highest levels of sexual invitations from the females. It is possible that the high testosterone of dominant males may enhance their arousal and perception of females, as well as their attractiveness to females (Keverne, 1979), while subordinates would remain unattractive, and so reduce the aggression they might otherwise provoke from the dominant males. In reproductive terms, high levels of testosterone are known to be important in initiating and maintaining spermatogenesis (Steinberger, 1971). Hence, the behavioural and endocrine strategies of subordinate males might be viewed as part of their adaptation to minimise the cost of staying in a social group, while maintaining the potential for reproduction should the opportunity arise. However, when the opportunity does arise, by removal of dominant males, we see that the subordinate fails in the short term to cope adequately with these opportunities. His behaviour is that of an anxious male with low sexual performance and high levels of stress hormones. Clearly then, this male, possibly because of his past experience of chronic subordination, experiences great problems in coping with mate choice, even when dominant males are temporarily absent. With this in mind, a different perspective falls on the functional significance of the females' sexual skin swelling. As well as falling into the category of a non-behavioural cue enhancing the females' attractiveness, it may well provide a handicap to the males' performance, particularly that of anxious males. Males that cannot readily sustain a potent erection would be more likely to experience intromission difficulties, and a high mount-to-ejaculation ratio would result, as is the case with subordinate males. Hence, the females' sexual skin swelling, in addition to attracting males, may serve to select between high- and low-ranking males on the basis of their performance.

Female hormones and the behaviour of heterosexual pairs of monkeys

Although the behaviour of male monkeys may continue long after castration, the same is not true for female monkeys. Removal of the females' ovaries results in a rapid (approximately two weeks) decline in sexual interactions. Moreover, when heterosexual pairs of Rhesus Monkeys are allowed to interact in a laboratory situation, a striking feature of their sexual interaction is the cyclicity in male sexual behaviour with respect to the ovarian secretory activity in the female (Michael & Herbert, 1963; Czaja & Bielert, 1975). During the folicular phase of the menstrual cycle, when oestrogen secretion predominates, sexual interactions gradually increase, reaching a peak just prior to ovulation (Michael, Herbert & Welegalla, 1967). In the luteal phase of the cycle, when progesterone predominates, sexual interactions decline as the female becomes progressively less attractive (Michael, Saayman & Zumpe, 1968).

It would appear, therefore, that sexual interactions in the female primate are more strongly under the influence of ovarian hormones. In order to evaluate what part these hormones play in determining both the females' motivation to mate, and which females are mated with, it is necessary to investigate their sites of action. The usual approach to understanding the effects of a given hormone is to remove its secreting gland and then replace the hormone. This kind of approach owes a lot to traditions developed in physiological psychology and is best carried out by routinely pairing animals together away from the complexities of the social group.

Removal of the ovaries, and hence oestrogen and progesterone, makes the female Rhesus Monkey less attractive, which in the laboratory may be characterised by a complete sexual disinterest in the female by males (Michael & Welegalla, 1968). Oestrogen replacement, but not progesterone, restores female attractiveness while progesterone given to oestrogen-treated females antagonises this effect (Michael, Saayman & Zumpe, 1967). The problem arises, however, when one tries to dissect out which components of female attractiveness are primarily being influenced, and when this invariably turns out to be more than one, then the question arises as to which is more important. Thus oestrogen may enhance non-behavioural aspects of female attractiveness (sexual skin colour or swelling, and vaginal secretions and pheromones) and may also increase sexual motivation which can be measured from changes in soliciting, a behaviour which may itself enhance the females' attractiveness. However, many females do not show obvious increases in sexual invitations around their ovulatory period when male sexual behaviour is highest (Michael & Welegalla, 1968). In fact, paradoxically, they often show decreases. Such is the interest of the male at this time that females have little opportunity to make sexual invitations, and the initiative is firmly with their male partner. It would appear, therefore, that oestrogen is primarily influencing non-behavioural aspects of female attractiveness. If, however, the female is given some degree of independence from the dominating influence of the male, and control over the interaction is in her hands, then we see that oestrogen also influences her motivational behaviour. This point is illustrated when a female monkey is given a lever to press which controls access to a partitioned male. Oestrogen given to ovariectomised females increases their rate of pressing for access to the males (Keverne, 1976). Therefore oestrogen also increases the females' sexual motivation, and although this has little opportunity for expression within the constraints of pair testing, one can envisage that such a behavioural back-up could become important for arousing sexually sluggish males.

Of course, it could be argued that this lever-pressing behaviour is not related to increased sexual motivation resulting from an action of oestrogen on the brain, but reflects a stronger social inclination of the female, or even an improved motor performance. However, since oestrogen is without significant effect on female lever pressing for other females, or for food reward, this seems an unlikely explanation. Of course, the ultimate proof could be provided by implanting minute amounts of oestrogen into discrete regions of the brain. If this were carried out on ovariectomised unattractive females, then one might predict that oestrogen implanted directly into those regions of the brain concerned with sexual motivation (anterior hypothalamus and medial preoptic region) would increase female sexual invitations without enhancing the non-behavioural aspects of female attractiveness normally produced by the somatic action of oestrogen. Unfortunately, although this approach has been attempted, the results proved singularly unsuccessful because of failure to hit the appropriate neural site, and because the implants themselves were sufficiently large to raise peripheral oestrogen concentrations (Michael, 1971).

The importance of behavioural cues to compensate for loss of non-behavioural aspects of attractiveness is further illustrated when female monkeys are treated with progesterone. Administration of progesterone to ovariectomised oestrogen-treated females results in a loss of male sexual interest (mounting attempts and ejaculations) while female sexual invitations increase (Baum, Everitt, Herbert & Keverne, 1976). However, this increase in female sexual invitations is not due to a behavioural action of this hormone on the brain, since giving low doses of progesterone directly into the vagina produces exactly the same behavioural effect without reaching detectable levels in the plasma, and hence the brain (Baum et al., 1977). Here, then, we not only have an example of how a hormone can produce a behavioural change which is secondary to changes in non-behavioural aspects of attractiveness, but we can see how the female's attempts to sustain male interest by increasing her solicitations fail with the decline in non-behavioural aspects of her attractiveness.

If one has to decide therefore, which is more important in determining the males' sexual behaviour, observations such as these lead to the inevitable conclusion that it is the non-behavioural aspects of the females' attractiveness emanating from the vagina, at least within the confines of the laboratory cage. This ineffectiveness of sexual solicitations in the absence of non-behavioural aspects of attractiveness is further illustrated when ovariectomised females are given testosterone. Such treatment of the female Rhesus Monkey markedly increases sexual solicitations, but in the absence of female oestrogens, such invitations go unheeded by the male, and result in little or no sexual interaction (Trimble & Herbert, 1968).

So far, I have considered the actions of the ovarian hormones, oestrogen and progesterone, and have shown that they influence female attractiveness and soliciting behaviour. No mention has been made of the female's receptive behaviour, mainly because the female monkey is prepared to receive the male throughout her menstrual cycle (Michael & Zumpe, 1970; Keverne, 1976). However, removal of the main source of female androgens, the adrenals, does affect the receptive behaviour of Rhesus Monkeys (Everitt, Herbert & Hamer, 1972), but in Stumptail Macaques even this procedure is without effect on female sexual receptiveness (Baum, Slob, de Jong & Westbroek, 1978). In ovariectomised female Rhesus Monkeys given oestradiol, removal of the adrenal androgens markedly decreases the number of invitations these females make to males, and significantly increases the number of refusals they make of male advances. These unreceptive aspects of sexual behaviour are reversed by low doses of testosterone replacement given either by injection or by direct implantation into the anterior hypothalamus (Everitt & Herbert, 1975). Since adrenal androgens are more or less constantly secreted throughout the menstrual cycle, the female monkey becomes permanently receptive (but variably attractive). This large degree of emancipation of the female's brain from the influence of ovarian hormones on sexual behaviour may be viewed as an evolutionary development of some significance. We no longer have a brain which is governed by the cyclic control of oestrus, but one which appears to be permanently receptive. It is this relegation of the gonadal hormones to a permissive role and ascension of social organisation to a determining role in sexual behaviour that I wish to consider next.

Female hormones and behaviour in the social group

In captive groups of Talapoin Monkeys, ovariectomising the females eliminates sexual interactions, just as it does in Rhesus Monkeys when they are brought together as heterosexual pairs, even though female solicitations persist. Oestrogen replacement to all the females restores the sexual skin-swelling and vaginal secretions, and sexual behaviour is reinstated. However, such sexual behaviour is not distributed equally among the group, even though these non-behavioural aspects of attractiveness appear to be similar among all females. The higher-ranking females receive most sexual attention while lower-ranking females receive little, and in some groups may even be totally excluded (Bowman, Dilley & Keverne, 1978). Why then are sexual interactions not evenly distributed; is it because high-ranking females are aggressively inhibiting the behaviour of those of lower rank? This appears not to be the case, since overt aggression is extremely low among these females (one attack per week). Low-ranking females do not, however, have the same opportunities; their use of the cage space is restricted and they make considerably fewer sexual solicitations than high-ranking females. Thus, one major difference between the female mates of choice and those that are ignored is the amount of soliciting behaviour. Such correlations in the social group may persuade the observer to think it is this aspect of behaviour which is all important. The importance of other behaviour, especially aggressive acts, becomes more obvious if we selectively treat only the lowest-ranking female with oestrogen (Eberhart, Herbert, Keverne & Meller, 1980). Males now direct their attention to this female, although there are no mounts or ejaculations observed, since aggression from the other females now increases considerably towards the low-ranking female. Needless to say, such females avoid males and do not solicit their attention with sexual invitations.

With this simple endocrine manipulation in the social group we reveal how social status can override the effect of endocrine state. The role of oestrogen, although necessary for mating, does not determine which female is mated. This illustrates the importance of behaviour that is not seen, such as overt aggression, but which is nevertheless potentially available in what Hinde has called the 'deep structure' of the group (the underlying principles in terms of which the observed patterning of behavioural interactions can be understood: Hinde, 1976). This only becomes obvious when the lowest-ranking female is selectively treated with oestradiol, a procedure which instead of increasing sexual interactions, increases aggressive interactions. This disruption to social organisation produced by sexual attractiveness occurring out of synchrony may be a plausible explanation for why even tropical species like the Talapoin Monkey exhibit discrete breeding seasons.

Do these findings mean that studies of hormones and behaviour with heterosexual pairs of monkeys reveal nothing of relevance to the field worker? While the concepts relating to female attractiveness and receptivity can be applied to feral troops, implications as to the underlying endocrine determinants of such behaviour may be quite misleading. Hence, field workers who use the term oestrus to describe circumscribed periods of sexual interaction do a disservice to the behavioural complexity of their social groups of monkeys. While gonadal hormones may determine when a female is sexually active, it is the social organisation which determines the sexual inactivity of certain individuals and not necessarily a state of anoestrus. Nevertheless, as we have seen for the male, there may be endocrine correlates of sexual inactivity which reflect that individual's ability to cope, and here I particularly refer to the stress hormones cortisol and prolactin which are high in low-ranking but not high-ranking females

(Keverne, 1979). While we do not yet know what part, if any, these stress hormones might themselves play in behaviour, prolactin in particular has important consequences for reproduction. High levels of prolactin (hyperprolactinaemia) are associated with infertility in monkeys (Bowman *et al.*, 1978) and man (Thorner, McNeilly, Hagan & Besser, 1974). Thus it is interesting to see that both behavioural and endocrine mechanisms again subserve the same end, and social factors can affect reproductive success not only behaviourally, but also by influencing the endocrine state of the individual.

Conclusions

The teasing apart of endocrine, sexual and social variables in mate choice is a difficult task plagued with problems of interpretation. I have reviewed briefly how experiments with heterosexual pairs of monkeys illustrate the importance of gonadal hormones for sexual behaviour. Moreover the action of ovarian hormones on non-behavioural aspects of female attractiveness are in themselves sufficient to account for the changes in behaviour that gonadal hormones provoke in monkeys in the laboratory. The crucial problem is reconciling these facts with what we know about sexual behaviour and mate choice within the framework of a social group. Clearly, gonadal hormones are necessary for sexual behaviour in social groups of monkeys but mate choice is determined primarily by social status. Social status itself has clear effects on the soliciting behaviour of individuals in the group, and while this may play an influential part in determining which females are mated, non-behavioural aspects of female attractiveness cannot be excluded. Indeed, one could argue that in polygynous primate groups where sexual bonding is short lived and mate choice a recurrent event, the pressures are such as to force males' attention to non-behavioural aspects of attractiveness, not so much for the choice of appropriate mates, but as a way of minimising social instability.

Mate choice has to be viewed in a framework that is broader than gonadal hormones and sexual behaviour. Thus we have seen how in a social group of Talapoin Monkeys mate choice and sexual behaviour are the prerogative of the dominant males. Hence, one way, indeed the only way, that high-ranking males can ensure priority over mate choice is to maintain the social hierarchy. This does not necessarily involve permanently high levels of violence and aggression. Social subjugation may be such that males of low rank, even in the absence of high-ranking males, are sufficiently anxious as to reduce their sexual performance, a factor enhanced by the enlargement of a sexual skin handicap in the female.

Among females, we see how treating all of the group with the same amount of oestrogen, which from pair tests studies we know stimulates non-behavioural aspects of attractiveness, does not make all females equally attractive. Females of higher rank are the mates by choice. Even selective oestrogen treatment of only the lowest-ranking female does nothing for her sexual interactions. Males may display increased interest in this female (looks and inspects), but the aggression to her from other females increases considerably. Other studies have also shown how sexual behaviour can be disruptive to social organisation by increased aggressive interactions in males (Richard, 1976; Keverne *et al.*, 1978) and here we see how the same may apply to females, especially if they become attractive out of synchrony. A limited breeding season may be one way of ensuring more synchrony, thereby reducing the potential for aggression. In the real world of feral monkeys, incomplete synchrony is unavoidable, even within a restricted breeding season. However, one could argue that some behavioural disruption, providing it falls within certain constraints and is not destructively violent, produces a necessary and valuable challenge to the social organisation. The social disruptions created by the periodic appearance of sexual behaviour may thus be viewed as providing an integral part of social organisation by strengthening the deep structure (the underlying principles which govern the observed patterning of behavioural interactions) in order to meet up to the potential demands of external challenges.

Without question gonadal hormones are necessary for sexual interactions. Nevertheless the levels of gonadal hormones in monkeys living in social groups do not determine the sexual inactivity of low-ranking individuals. The restrictions on the mate choice of subordinate monkeys are not gonadal, since sexual motivation persists even in their complete absence. This is not, of course, true for other mammals where sexual motivation and behaviour are primarily determined by gonadal hormones (e.g. rat, hamster, cat, Guinea pig, sheep). In such cases the brain and behaviour follow the dictates of the gonad. Nevertheless, it is of biological significance that such co-ordination enhances the reproductive fitness of this species. In monkeys, we see that the social environment may exert a powerful influence on an individual's reproductive capabilities and here too behavioural and endocrine mechanisms (not necessarily gonadal) subserve the same end. However, we now appear to have a shift in emphasis in the reciprocal interaction between the gonads and the brain as we ascend the phylogenetic scale, with the brain primarily influencing activity of the gonad.

Summary

Sexual behaviour in social groups of monkeys is often the prerogative of dominant males. Since dominant males exhibit increased plasma testosterone, the possibility exists that such endocrine changes may in some way reinforce the nature of the hierarchy, e.g. by improving their sexual performance and making them more attractive to females. However, since castration itself has little effect on the sexual interest of males for females and administration of testosterone to subordinate males does not stimulate their sexual behaviour, low levels of plasma testosterone in subordinates is not a plausible explanation for their lack of sexual behaviour.

The hormones cortisol and prolactin also vary according to a monkey's social status, and the profiles of these stress hormones change in different ways to meet behavioural or endocrine challenges depending on social rank. Most important is the finding that behavioural experiences in the social group may have repercussions for a monkey's ability to cope with changing circumstances depending upon whether that individual was of high or low social status. Hence, increases in prolactin and cortisol in subordinate males in the presence of females and in the absence of higher-ranking males would suggest that such males experience more problems in coping with sexual behaviour.

In females too, the social hierarchy has repercussions for behaviour and endocrine status, with low-ranking females not only receiving less sexual behaviour, but failing to release an LH surge when challenged with positive oestrogen feedback. Moreover, although oestrogen stimulates non-behavioural aspects of female attractiveness (odour cues, sexual skin swelling), in the social group this treatment does not render all females equally attractive. Even selective oestrogen treatment of only the lowest-ranking female does not increase the sexual interactions she receives, but it does increase aggression towards her from other females. Hence, although gonadal hormones are essential for sexual interactions their effects on behaviour in the social group are modified by the social organisation. The stress hormones clearly indicate differences in ability to cope with sexual behaviour depending on rank, and in turn have repercussions for reproductive fitness according to social rank.

References

Abbott, D. H. & Hearn, J. P. (1978). Physical, hormonal and behavioural aspects of sexual development in the marmoset monkey, *Callithrix jacchus. Journal of Reproduction and Fertility*, **53**, 155–66.

Baum, M. J., Everitt, B. J., Herbert, J. & Keverne, E. B. (1976). Reduction of sexual interaction in rhesus monkeys by a vaginal action of progesterone. *Nature*, **263**, 606–8.

Baum, M. J., Keverne, E. B., Everitt, B. J., Herbert, J. & de Greef, W. J. (1977). Effects of progesterone and oestradiol on sexual attractivity of female rhesus monkeys. *Physiology & Behaviour*, **18**, 659–70.

Baum, M. J., Slob, A. K., de Jong, F. H. & Westbroek, D. L. (1978). Persistence of sexual behaviour in ovariectomised stumptail macaques following dexamethasone treatment or adrenalectomy. *Hormones & Behaviour*, **11**, 323–47.

Bernstein, I. S. (1976). Dominance, aggression and reproduction in primate societies. *Journal of Theoretical Biology*, **60**, 459–72.

Bernstein, I. S., Rose, R. M. & Gordon, T. P. (1977). Behavioural and hormonal responses of male rhesus monkeys introduced to females in the breeding season and non-breeding seasons. *Animal Behaviour*, **25**, 609–14.

Bowman, L. A., Dilley, S. R. & Keverne, E. B. (1978). Suppression of oestrogen induced LH surges by social subordination in talapoin monkeys. *Nature*, **275**, 56–8.

Carpenter, C. R. (1942). Sexual behaviour of free-ranging rhesus monkeys (*Macaca mulatta*). I. Specimens, procedures and behavioural characteristics of estrus. *Journal of Comparative Psychology*, **33**, 113–42.

Chamove, A. S. & Bowman, R. E. (1978). Rhesus plasma cortisol response at four dominance positions. *Aggressive Behaviour*, **4**, 43–55.

Czaja, J. A. & Bielert, C. (1975). Female rhesus sexual behaviour and distance to a male partner: relation to the stage of the menstrual cycle. *Archives of Sexual Behaviour*, **4**, 583–98.

Dixson, A. F. & Herbert, J. (1977). Gonadal hormones and sexual behaviour in groups of adult talapoin monkeys (*Miopithecus talapoin*). *Hormones & Behaviour*, **8**, 141–54.

Drickamer, L. C. (1974). A ten-year summary of reproductive data for free-ranging *Macaca mulatta*. *Folia primatologica*, **21**, 61–80.

Dunbar, R. I. M. (1980). Determinants and evolutionary consequences of dominance among female gelada baboons. *Behavioral Ecology & Sociobiology*, **7**, 253–65.

Dunbar, R. I. M. & Dunbar, E. P. (1977). Dominance and reproductive success among female gelada baboons. *Nature*, **266**, 351–2.

Eberhart, J. A., Herbert, J., Keverne, E. B. & Meller, R. E. (1980). Some hormonal aspects of primate social behaviour. In *Endocrinology*, pp. 622–5. Australian Academy of Sciences: Melbourne.

Eberhart, J. A. & Keverne, E. B. (1979). Influences of the dominance hierarchy on luteinizing hormone, testosterone and prolactin in male talapoin monkeys. *Journal of Endocrinology*, **83**, 42–3.

Eberhart, J. A., Keverne, E. B. & Meller, R. E. (1980). Social influences on plasma testosterone levels in male talapoin monkeys. *Hormones & Behaviour*, **14**, 247–66.

Everitt, B. J. & Herbert, J. (1975). The effects of implanting testosterone propionate into the central nervous system on the sexual behaviour of adrenalectomised female rhesus monkeys. *Brain Research*, **86**, 109–20.

Everitt, B. J., Herbert, J. & Hamer, J. D. (1972). Sexual receptivity of bilaterally adrenalectomised female rhesus monkeys. *Physiology & Behaviour*, **8**, 409–15.

Hall, K. R. L. (1967). Social interactions of the adult male and adult females of a patas monkey group. In *Social Communication among Primates*, ed. by S. A. Altman, pp. 261–80. University of Chicago Press: Chicago.

Hinde, R. A. (1976). Interactions, relationships and social structure. *Man*, **11**, 1–17.

Keverne, E. B. (1976). Sexual receptivity and attractiveness in the female rhesus monkey. *Advances in the Study of Behaviour*, **7**, 155–200.

Keverne, E. B. (1979). Sexual and aggressive behaviour in social groups of talapoin monkeys. *Ciba Foundation Symposium No. 62, Sex, Hormones & Behaviour*, pp. 271–86. Excerpta Medica: Amsterdam.

Keverne, E. B., Eberhart, J. A. & Meller, R. E. (1982). Dominance and subordination: concepts or physiological states? In *Advanced Views in Primate Biology*, ed. O. Chiarelli, pp. 81–94. Springer-Verlag: Berlin.

Keverne, E. B., Meller, R. E. & Martinez-Arias, A. M. (1978). Dominance, aggression and sexual behaviour in social groups of talapoin monkeys. In *Recent Advances in Primatology*, vol. 1, ed. D. J. Chivers & J. Herbert, pp. 533–48. Academic Press: New York.

Leshner, A. I. & Candland, D. K. (1972). Endocrine effects of grouping and dominance rank in squirrel monkeys. *Physiology and Behaviour*, **8**, 441–5.

Mendoza, S. P., Coe, C. L., Lowe, E. L. & Levine, S. (1979). The physiological response to group formation in adult male squirrel monkeys. *Psychoneuroendocrinology*, **3**, 221–9.

Michael, R. P. (1971). Neuroendocrine factors regulating primate behaviour. In *Frontiers in Neuroendocrinology*, ed. L. Martini & W. F. Ganong, pp. 359–98. Oxford University Press: New York, London, Toronto.

Michael, R. P. & Herbert, J. H. (1963). Menstrual cycle influences grooming behaviour and sexual behaviour in the rhesus monkey. *Science*, **140**, 500–1.

Michael, R. P., Herbert, J. & Welegalla, J. (1967). Ovarian hormones and the sexual behaviour of the male rhesus monkey (*Macaca mulatta*) under laboratory conditions. *Journal of Endocrinology*, **39**, 81–98.

Michael, R. P., Saayman, G. S. & Zumpe, D. (1967). Sexual attractiveness and receptivity in rhesus monkeys. *Nature*, **215**, 554–6.

Michael, R. P., Saayman, G. S. & Zumpe, D. (1968). The suppression of mounting behaviour and ejaculations in male rhesus monkeys (*Macaca mulatta*) by administration of progesterone to their female partners. *Journal of Endocrinology*, **41**, 421–31.

Michael, R. P. & Welegalla, J. (1968). Ovarian hormones and the sexual behaviour of the female rhesus monkey (*Macaca mulatta*) under laboratory conditions. *Journal of Endocrinology*, **41**, 407–20.

Michael, R. P. & Zumpe, D. (1970). Rhythmic changes in the copulatory frequency of rhesus monkeys (*Macaca mulatta*) in relation to the menstrual cycle and a comparison with the human cycle. *Journal of Reproduction and Fertility*, **21**, 199–201.

Phoenix, C. H., Slob, A. K. & Goy, R. W. (1973). Effects of castration and replacement therapy on sexual behaviour of adult male rhesuses. *Journal of Comparative Physiological Psychology*, **84**, 472–81.

Resko, J. A. & Phoenix, C. H. (1972). Sexual behaviour and testosterone concentrations in the plasma of the rhesus monkey before and after castration. *Endocrinology*, **91**, 499–503.

Richard, A. (1976). Patterns of mating in *Propithecus verreauxi verreauxi*. In *Prosimian Behaviour*, ed. R. D. Martin, G. A. Doyle & A. C. Walker, pp. 49–74. Duckworth: London.

Rose, R. M., Bernstein, I. S. & Gordon, T. P. (1975). Consequences of social conflict on plasma testosterone levels in rhesus monkeys. *Psychosomatic Medicine*, **37**, 50–61.

Rose, R. M., Gordon, T. P. & Bernstein, I. S. (1972). Plasma testosterone levels in the male rhesus: influences of sexual and social stimuli. *Science*, **178**, 643–5.

Rose, R. M., Holaday, J. W. & Bernstein, I. S. (1971). Plasma testosterone, dominance rank and aggressive behaviour in male rhesus monkeys. *Nature*, **231**, 366–8.

Sade, D. S., Cushing, K., Cushing, P., Dunaif, J., Figueros, A., Kaplan, J. R., Lauer, C., Rhodes, D. & Schneider, J. (1977). Population dynamics in relation to social structure on Cayo Santiago. *Yearbook of Physical Anthropology*, **20**, 253–62.

Sassenrath, E. N. (1970). Increased adrenal responsiveness related to social stress in rhesus monkeys. *Hormones & Behaviour*, **1**, 283–98.

Scallet, A. C., Suomi, S. J. & Bowman, R. E. (1981). Sex differences in adrenocortical responsiveness to controlled agonistic encounters in rhesus monkeys. *Physiology and Behaviour*, **26**, 385–90.

Steinberger, E. (1971). Hormonal control of mammalian spermatogenesis. *Physiological Reviews*, **51**, 1–22.

Struhsaker, T. T. (1967). Social structure among vervet monkeys (*Cercopithecus aethiops*). *Behaviour*, **29**, 83–121.

Thorner, M. O., McNeilly, A. S., Hagan, C. & Besser, G. M. (1974). Long-term treatment of galactorrhoea and hypogonadism with bromocriptine. *British Medical Journal*, **ii**, 419–22.

Trimble, M. & Herbert, J. (1968). The effect of testosterone or oestradiol upon the sexual or associated behaviour of the adult female rhesus monkey. *Journal of Endocrinology*, **42**, 171–85.

Wilson, M., Plant, T. M. & Michael, R. P. (1972). Androgens and the sexual behaviour of male rhesus monkeys. *Journal of Endocrinology*, **52**, ii.

VII: DECISION RULES

20

Life history tactics and alternative strategies of reproduction

R. I. M. DUNBAR

An animal's reproductive strategy determines its contribution to the species' gene pool, and is hence an important variable on which natural selection operates. In very general terms, we may view a reproductive strategy as a hierarchically organised series of decisions. At the very broadest level, successful reproduction means successfully solving the key problems of survival, mating and rearing (Goss-Custard, Dunbar & Aldrich-Blake, 1972). An animal that does not eat enough, or is not fleet enough to escape a predator, cannot expect to be able to mate; if it does not mate, it cannot expect to rear offspring that will, in their turn, propagate its genes. This last step is crucial, for mere numbers of offspring born is in itself irrelevant: evolution is a consequence of the successful propagation of genetic material into future generations, and genetic material will manifestly not be propagated if any of the offspring born to successive generations of parents themselves fail to reproduce.

The fact that an animal has a number of choices available to it in terms of reproductive strategy inevitably raises the possibility that one strategy may be better than the others in a given set of circumstances or, alternatively, that sets of strategies may be equally advantageous (i.e. net reproductive gains are equilibrated). I have reviewed elsewhere at some length the more specific problem of alternative mating strategies (see Dunbar, 1982a). In this paper, I generalise some of the ideas developed in that paper to reproductive strategies as a whole by combining these ideas with those from the now well developed literature on life-history tactics. As in my paper on mating strategies, I shall limit the discussion to consider only male reproductive strategies.

423

Reproductive decisions

Each of the three general problems introduced above (i.e. survival, mating and rearing) consists of a cluster of decision points about particular problems. Thus, survival consists of finding satisfactory solutions to the problems of: obtaining sufficient quantities of the right kinds of foods so as to remain in energy (or nutritional) balance; avoiding climatic stress; and avoiding being eaten by predators. These in turn consist of complexes of more specific problems (e.g. do I eat this small food item now, or search a bit longer in the hope of finding a bigger one?). Mating consists of a series of decisions about the timing and methods of acquiring mates, the number of mates taken (i.e. 'harem' size) and the bases on which mate choice itself should be made. Rearing similarly consists of decisions about how much investment should be made in offspring, how it should be distributed over time among the members of the same or different litters and whether or not investment should be made in the offspring of other individuals (related or otherwise).

All of these problems are individually very familiar to behavioural biologists. What seems to be appreciated less often is the extent to which they form a complex of interacting problems that must be solved, severally and jointly, if any animal is to contribute to its species' gene pool effectively. Certain decisions may limit the choice at other levels if net reproductive output is to be maximised: thus, deciding to invest heavily in rearing offspring may limit the number of matings that can be achieved per season, or heavy investment in the offspring of other individuals may preclude any possibility of personal reproduction. Consequently, the final strategy selected will be a compromise between the conflicting demands of the various problems with the result that solutions to any one problem may be less than optimal (see also Dunbar, 1982*b*). An animal *could* produce more offspring, but it might then end up by rearing fewer of them because its limited resources were too thinly spread (for many avian examples, see Lack, 1966).

Components of reproduction

I shall develop the argument by setting the problem out as a series of increasingly better approximations to genetic fitness in order to show how the component sub-problems of successful reproduction are related to each other. To highlight this, I formulate the argument in simple mathematical form. This is intended mainly to expose the bones of the argument in the clearest possible way. Arguments of this type would usually be formulated in terms of the 'classic' equations of population genetics or the Lotka-Volterra equation of population growth. In the present context, these are not especially helpful, for they pass over all intermediate levels to present output in terms of its *ultimate* currency, thus making it difficult to see how the component parts inter-relate. Moreover, these classical approaches are necessarily population-oriented (fitness is a property of populations, not of individuals: see Dunbar, 1982c), and this greatly obscures what is happening at the level of the individual. It is in this translation between individual behaviour and the behaviour of populations of genes that sociobiological arguments are most likely to run aground and it is hence imperative that the consequences of choices are viewed at the actual level of decision-making. Only thus can the constraints imposed by decisions at other levels be effectively identified.

Maximising mating success

At a first approximation, the numbers of offspring produced by an individual over a life-time depend on the number of females he can fertilise at any given time (his 'mating rate') and the length of time for which he can sustain this rate (his reproductive lifespan, or what we might term his 'tenure' as a breeding male). Crudely, we can write an expression for R, his life-time reproductive output, as

$$R_1^* = mt \tag{20.1}$$

where R_1^* is an estimator of R, m is his mating rate and t is his tenure. It will be obvious from this formulation that a male could maximise his output R *either* by maximising m (while minimising t) *or* by maximising t (while minimising m). This observation is crucial, for it underlines very sharply the distinction between short-term and long-term reproductive output, between what I have elsewhere (Dunbar, 1982a) termed *instantaneous* and *life-time* reproductive success. This distinction is ignored surprisingly often in studies of reproductive strategies. It will be obvious that a high instantaneous mating rate will not necessarily generate a high life-time output, particularly if, as seems often to be the case, mating rate and tenure are inversely related (Stearns, 1976, reviews some of the data showing that reproductive effort negatively influences life expectancy). Mating success and tenure will tend to be inversely related because high mating rates will generally require the defence of access to large numbers of females, which will invariably result in increasing frequencies of attack from other males (except, perhaps, in populations where females *greatly* outnumber males). As the level of competition for mates rises, so males will in general be less able to withstand repeated attacks for any length of time.

An example here might be male Gelada Baboons: these can pursue mutually exclusive strategies that contrast markedly in initial harem size and expected tenure such that the expected life-time reproductive outputs of the two strategies are more or less in balance (Dunbar, 1983).

Timing of reproductive effort

Equation (20.1) assumes that a male can pursue only one strategy during its life-time. In many cases, males are in fact able to pursue different strategies at different stages of their reproductive lives. Thus, red deer males may pursue 'sneak' strategies while young, but more conventional territorial harem-holding strategies in their prime (Gibson, 1978). In species where males form a dominance hierarchy that determines access to breeding females, each rank may be considered a separate state with its own rank-specific mating rate and tenure. Hence, equation (20.1) may be generalised to the form:

$$R_2^* = \sum_i m_i t_i \tag{20.2}$$

In simplified form, this takes into account the implications of life-history theory on the timing of reproductive effort. (An exceptionally clear-headed review of this area is given by Stearns, 1976.) From the present point of view, two findings in particular are relevant. First, the energetic resources available to an animal at any given moment are limited, so that it must choose between investing these either in reproduction or in growth. Investment in one must be made at the expense of the other (Williams, 1966; Gadgil & Bossert, 1970), and there is some empirical evidence that this is indeed so (summarised by Stearns, 1976, Table 2). As a consequence, we can expect early investment in reproduction to result in reduced growth rates that will, in turn, be reflected either in small size relative to late reproducers in subsequent breeding seasons (e.g. platyfish: Sohn, 1977; sunfish: Gross & Charnov, 1980) or in higher age-specific mortality rates for early breeders (e.g. mountain sheep: Geist, 1971). Secondly, the value of maximum reproductive effort at any given age will depend on the demographic state of the population: early reproduction will be favoured in expanding populations, late reproduction in declining ones because individuals contribute a larger proportion of offspring (genes) to the next generation by doing so (Hirshfield & Tinkle, 1975; Stearns, 1976).

One problem here is that the conventional demographic models tend to work in terms of genetic fitness: consequently, individuals are assumed to sacrifice themselves in the interests of maximising gene representation. Natural selection, however, operates on the behaviour of individuals, and, to the extent that they can decide such issues, individuals may 'prefer' to hedge their bets in order to produce at least some offspring, even though more *copies* of a given *gene* would survive if all carriers tried to pursue the most successful strategy (during the course of which many of them fell by the wayside) (see also Mountford, 1971; Rubenstein, 1982). The implications of this distinction for reproductive strategies have yet to be worked out in any detail, but it will undoubtedly make a considerable difference to predicted outcomes.

These problems aside, it will not be apparent that not only may males be able to equilibrate R by varying m and t, but they may also do so by deciding how long they should remain in any given state, i. Thus, a male may decide to remain middle-ranking throughout its life since it can do so without having to defend its status to any great extent; by so doing, it may be able to gain a higher average rank over its life time than it would otherwise be able to achieve if it competed for higher ranks. Males would thereby be able to balance a low state-specific mating rate against a high state-specific probability of tenure. Hausfater (1975) suggests that *Papio cynocephalus* baboons might behave in this way.

Maximising birth rate

Although a male may mate with a great many females, he will not necessarily thereby gain many offspring. There are at least two reasons for this. First, too hasty a courtship may not result in fertilisation, particularly if courtship is necessary to stimulate ovulation. Secondly, females may be differentially fertile, so that choice of mating partner may become important if the number of offspring born is to be maximised. Thus, mating females in the pre-ovulatory period will be of little value in terms of fertilisations, even though a male may have uninterrupted access to the female during this phase of her ovarian cycle, and may therefore be able to mate with her at very high rates.

We can easily incorporate this into equation (2) by adding a function, b_i, defined as the mean fecundibility of females mated in state i (i.e. the mean number of offspring born per mating):

$$R_3^* = \Sigma \, b_i(m_i t_i) \tag{20.3}$$

Thus males, potentially at least, have a further option on strategy choice in so far as they can be more or less selective in their choice of females to mate. Males may again be able to equilibrate output by balancing female quality against numbers mated to yield identical net reproductive output in terms of numbers of offspring born over a life-time.

An example of this is given by toads where the number of eggs a female can lay is a function of her size (see for example Davies & Halliday, 1977). Males could, in principle at least, choose to mate either with a few large (but heavily competed for) females or many small (less desirable) ones. There is some suggestion that something comparable might be operating among humans: males may choose between courting (socially) highly desirable females (with limited chances of success) or courting less attractive (but more easily 'conquered') females (see Duck & Miell, this volume). Presumably, males who opt to court highly desirable females take longer to obtain a mate because they are likely to suffer more refusals and can therefore expect a shorter reproductive lifespan. If the overt qualities of attractiveness have consequences for successful reproduction, then males may be selecting for mate 'quality' in order to maximise reproductive gain (though, in this case, the latter may be mediated through pair-bond stability or the likelihood of breeding equally 'attractive' offspring, to name but two of the more obvious possibilities). The same may apply equally to animals (male monkeys *are* selective about which females they mate with: Kaufman, 1965; Taub, 1980). Further aspects of this problem are discussed in greater detail by Wittenberger (this volume).

For convenience, we can subsume a number of different effects of female quality under this single variable, and this could include the contribution the female makes to rearing.

Maximising rearing rate

As noted earlier, the number of young born is less important than the number of offspring that survive to breed. As is well understood, animals may, at least in some circumstances, be able to influence the chances of their offspring maturing to breed by investing more or less parental care in them. We should thus add a further refinement to equation (20.3) by including a component representing the effects of male parental care on an offspring's survival and chances of breeding. If we denote this by c_x, the probability that a given amount of parental investment, x, will result in one offspring reaching breeding age, we obtain:

$$R_4^* = c_x \sum_i (b_i m_i t_i) \tag{20.4}$$

I define c_x as a probability of maturing in order to incorporate all possible forms of parental investment, both direct and indirect, into a single function. Furthermore, c_x should strictly be interpreted in terms of the amount of *male* parental care provided *given* the species' characteristic quantities of care already provided by the female (incorporated into the variable *b*); *c* may thus be interpreted as the *increment* in the probability of an infant maturing consequent on a given amount of paternal care.

Again, given that the amount of time/energy available for paternal care is limited it is obvious that the numbers of offspring reared to maturity can be maximised either by investing a lot of care in a small number of young, or by investing negligible quantities of care into many young. Examples of this are too numerous to be worth mentioning. More importantly, it should be noted that decisions about rearing strategy may place major restrictions on a male's freedom of choice at other decision points. In the extreme case, a decision to make a heavy commitment to parental care may so limit a male's options on mating frequency as to force him to be monogamous.

Maximising fitness

In the final analysis, it is, of course, genetic fitness that is maximised during evolution, and although reproductive output and fitness will often be at least monotonically related, it has been widely appreciated ever since the publication of Hamilton's (1964) seminal papers that an animal can behave so as to maximise the genetic fitness of a character by promoting reproduction in related individuals without necessarily reproducing itself. Thus, an animal's (absolute) contribution to the species' gene pool, *F*, can be written as:

$$F = f(R_4^*) + r_a(hf[R_4^a]) \tag{20.5}$$

where *f* transforms numbers of offspring (as determined by equation (20.4)) into fitness units (numbers of genes) and *h* is a scalar specifying the proportion of the reproductive output (R_4^a) of a relative, *a* (devalued by the degree of relatedness, Hamilton's *r*), that is acquired by the individual expending energy to assist that relative's reproduction.

Two points require comment. First, *F* is not conventional fitness in the population-genetic sense (commonly designated as ω) since genetic fitness is strictly speaking a measure of the frequency of a given gene relative to that of other alleles for that character in the population. Secondly, the relative's contribution to an individual's inclusive fitness is qualified by the scalar *h* (where $0 < h < 1$). It is important to remember that the fitness component due to the relative is *not* some proportion of his *total* reproductive output, but rather only a proportion of the *increment* in output that the kin gains as a direct result of the subject's intervention:

everything else the subject gets anyway irrespective of whether or not he helps that relative. The actual gain will, of course, be very much smaller than the relative's total output, and the difference will have to be substantial if aiding a relative is to be worthwhile (unless the cost of doing so in terms of lost reproduction is trivial).

Considering equation (20.5), we can again see that, in principle at least, an animal can maximise its genetic contribution either by maximising the component due to its own reproduction (so-called 'personal fitness'), while minimising the gain from assisting relatives, *or* by maximising the gain from relatives while minimising personal reproduction. As Hamilton pointed out, the point of equilibrium is determined by the difference between r (the degree of relatedness) and the ratio of the benefits to the costs.

The relative contribution of the two components may be contrasted by considering the difference between them when both relative and subject pursue the same breeding strategy. In order that a total commitment of all resources to a relative's reproductive effort be worthwhile,

$$r_a(h \cdot R_4^a) \geqslant R_4^* \tag{20.6}$$

since f is a constant in both equations and $f(R_4^*) = 0$ for non-breeders and $r_a(fh[R_4^a]) = 0$ for non-helpers. (Inequality (20.6) merely rewrites Hamilton's (1964) classic equation in more specific form in terms of actual reproductive output rather than in terms of generalised cost functions.) Since h is small and $r < 0.5$, the ratio $\cdot R^*/R^a$ will have to be large for inequality (20.6) to hold: it will only pay an animal to be a non-breeding helper if it is unable to breed itself (at least for the time being). In fact, it will rarely pay an animal to give up its own prospects of future reproduction *entirely* in order to help rear the offspring of relatives unless it cannot expect to breed itself. Conversely, animals will in general be willing to assist relatives only if the loss to their own reproductive success in doing so is negligible. There is some evidence to suggest that Rhesus Monkeys, for example, may be willing to give coalitionary support to relatives only when the likelihood of winning is high (Datta, 1981).

Reproductive strategies

Fig. 20.1 summarises the sequence of decisions and options open to a male in 'determining' its reproductive strategy, listed in descending order of logical priority. Animals need not 'make' such decisions in the indicated order, though doing so may constrain options higher up the chain.

With the exception of the first decision, the successive decisions are completely inter-related so that what is lost on the roundabout can be made up on the swings at a later stage. In theory, with a bifurcating decision process, there are 2^5 different permutations of reproductive strategy. Because certain decisions limit options at other decision nodes, not all of these possible strategy routes will be admissible (if reproductive output is to be maximised in the end). Obviously, there will be a single *absolutely* best strategy (no paternal care, large litter size, optimal mate quality, early start to breeding, many mates). However, within the context of a given species, individuals will be constrained both by the ecological niche that they occupy and by frequency-dependent feedback consequences that will render certain combinations of decisions impossible to sustain from a purely practical point of view. Instead, individuals will have to compromise on individually optimal decisions to find a 'best overall route'.

Fig. 20.1. Decision network summarising the relationships between the various decision options, arranged in descending order of logical status. Arrows indicate main choice routes; broken arrows indicate less likely, but possible, routes.

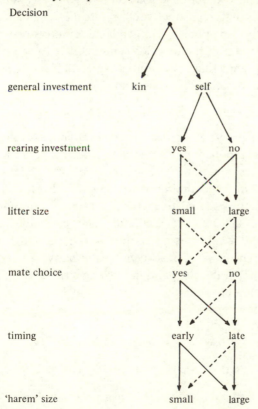

Two other points should be noted concerning the specific shape of the distributions characterising any given variable.

First, in most cases these will tend to be logistic in form, partly because of frequency-dependent feedback consequences and partly because they are cumulative density functions for what will often be normal distributions. The probability of fertilising a female, for example, will be a cumulative function of the probability that she will ovulate on any given day during the period that the male is mating with her. Since this will usually be normally distributed around the mean cycle length, the cumulative function will be logistic in form. Consequently, males will rapidly reach a point at which continued investment in a particular female will yield diminishing returns in terms of certainty of fertilisation, and at that point he would do better to seek another mate.

Secondly, all the variables in Fig. 20.1 are in reality continuous, even though for pedagogical convenience I have considered them as bifurcating choice-points. This raises the prospect of very fine quantitative adjustments between variable sets aimed at optimising net output. Thus, an animal need not 'decide' to invest *all* of its reproductive effort into its own or a relative's reproduction: instead, it can apportion its available resources between the two in order to get the best of both worlds. This is likely to be especially important in terms of adjusting losses on variables that affect personal reproduction (see also Wittenberger, this volume).

Summary

In this paper, I have examined male reproductive strategies by considering how the component parts interact to determine an animal's contribution to its species' gene pool. Five main components are considered, namely the number of matings, timing of reproductive effort, number of births, number of offspring reared to maturity and contributions to the reproductive outputs of kin. In most cases, individuals can trade losses on one component for additional gains on another in order to maximise net contribution to the gene pool. Consequently, alternative reproductive strategies that yield comparable net gains in the long term by emphasising different components are possible.

References

Datta, S. B. (1981). *Dynamics of Dominance Among Free-Ranging Rhesus Females*. Ph.D. thesis, University of Cambridge.

Davies, N. B. & Halliday, T. R. (1977). Optimal mate selection in the toad *Bufo bufo*. *Nature*, **269**, 56–8.

Dunbar, R. I. M. (1982a). Intraspecific variations in mating strategy. In *Perspectives in*

Ethology, vol. **5**, ed. P. P. G. Bateson & P. H. Klopfer, pp. 385–431. Plenum Press: New York.

Dunbar, R. I. M. (1982*b*). Social systems as optimal strategy sets. In *Adaptation, Population and Environment: Design of Evolution*, ed. J. B. Calhoun. Praeger: New York.

Dunbar, R. I. M. (1982*c*). Adaptation, fitness and the evolutionary tautology. In *Current Problems in Sociobiology*, ed. The King's College Sociobiology Group, pp. 9–35. Cambridge University Press: Cambridge.

Dunbar, R. I. M. (1983). *Reproductive Decisions: An Economic Analysis of Gelada Baboon Reproductive Strategies*. Harvard University Press: Cambridge, Mass.

Gadgil, M. & Bossert, W. H. (1970). Life historical consequences of natural selection. *American Naturalist*, **104**, 1–24.

Gibson, R. M. (1978). *Behavioural Factors Affecting Reproductive Success in Red Deer Stags*. Ph.D. thesis, University of Sussex.

Geist, V. (1971). *Mountain Sheep*. University of Chicago Press: Chicago.

Goss-Custard, J. D., Dunbar, R. I. M. & Aldrich-Blake, F. P. G. (1972). Survival, mating and rearing strategies in the evolution of primate social structure. *Folia Primatologica*, **17**, 1–19.

Gross, M. T. & Charnov, E. L. (1980). Alternative male life histories in bluegill sunfish. *Proceedings of the National Academy of Sciences of the USA*, **77**, 6937–40.

Hamilton, W. D. (1964). The genetical evolution of social behaviour. *Journal of Theoretical Biology*, **7**, 1–52.

Hausfater, G. (1975). *Dominance and Reproduction in Baboons* (Papio cynocephalus). Karger: Basel.

Hirshfield, M. F. & Tinkle, D. W. (1975). Natural selection and the evolution of reproductive effort. *Proceedings of the National Academy of Sciences of the USA*, **72**, 2227–31.

Kaufman, J. H. (1965). A three-year study of mating behavior in a freeranging band of rhesus monkeys. *Ecology*, **40**, 500–12.

Lack, D. (1966). *Population Studies of Birds*. Clarendon Press: Oxford.

Mountford, M. D. (1971). Population survival in a variable environment. *Theoretical Population Biology*, **32**, 75–9.

Rubenstein, D. I. (1982). Risk, uncertainty and evolutionary strategies. In *Current Problems in Sociobiology*, ed. The King's College Sociobiology Group, pp. 91–111. Cambridge University Press: Cambridge.

Sohn, J. J. (1977). Socially induced inhibition of genetically determined maturation in the platyfish, *Xiphophorus maculatus*. *Science*, **195**, 199–201.

Stearns, S. C. (1976). Life-history tactics: a review of ideas. *Quarterly Review of Biology*, **51**, 3–47.

Taub, D. M. (1980). Female choice and mating strategies among wild Barbary macaques (*Macaca sylvana* L.). In *The Macaques: Studies in Ecology, Behavior and Evolution*, ed. D. Lindburg, pp. 287–344. Van Nostrand: New York.

Williams, G. C. (1966). *Adaptation and Natural Selection*. Princeton University Press: Princeton, N.J.

21

Tactics of mate choice

JAMES F. WITTENBERGER

Long-standing interest in sexual selection theory has generated a strong and continuing interest in the mating process. The two major components of this process, mate competition and mate choice, have consequently been viewed in many studies as alternative (or complementary) means by which sexual selection takes place. While such a view is certainly legitimate for furthering our understanding of sexual selection, it is not wholly appropriate for understanding the mating process itself. The appropriate view for a behavioural biologist concerned with the evolutionary origins of mating tactics is to treat mate competition and mate choice as means by which individuals strive to enhance their inclusive fitness.

These two views of the mating process are by no means the same. Sexual selectionists are concerned primarily with the translation of mate competition and mate choice into selective forces (e.g. O'Donald, 1980; Lande, 1981) and with the impact of those forces on male traits (or, in the rare cases of sex role reversal, female traits) (e.g. see Halliday, 1978; Thornhill, 1979; Morse, 1980; Wittenberger, 1981a). Behavioural biologists, on the other hand, are mainly concerned with how particular tactics of mate competition and mate choice affect inclusive fitness. They are concerned with such questions as optimal outbreeding (Bateson, this volume), why males should either patrol or advertise for females (Alcock, 1975; Campanella, 1975; Otte & Joern, 1975; Wells, 1977; Mangan, 1979; Howard, 1980), why males display on dispersed mating stations or on leks (Hjorth, 1970; Alexander, 1975; Wittenberger, 1978; Borgia, 1979; Bradbury, 1981), why males establish territories or dominance hierarchies (Geist, 1974; Wittenberger, 1979, 1980), or why males compete for particular classes of females (Dunbar, this volume). Clearly, these two approaches lead to quite different studies of essentially the same phenomena.

While a great many studies have focused on tactics of mate competition and why they evolve (see Wittenberger, 1981*a*), relatively few studies have focused on the tactics of mate choice. Indeed, mate choice has typically been viewed as an essentially non-tactical acceptance or rejection of prospective mates who happen to present themselves to the choosing individuals, rather than as a potentially complex set of tactics that are designed to find the most suitable mate available given existing constraints.

Mate choice may not be as simple a process as many authors seem to imply. It may entail a series of tactical choices during both information-gathering and decision-making phases. Choosing individuals must acquire information about one or more prospective mates before they make any choices, and they can employ any of several tactics to that end. Once they have obtained the necessary information, choosing individuals must make their actual choices of mates. This decision-making process may often be based on multiple criteria (e.g. see Burley, 1981), and when it is, a variety of methods might be employed to weight the importance of each.

The information-gathering and decision-making processes involved in mate choice have not been addressed from this perspective. To date most research on female mate choice has been concerned with identifying the criteria used by females to choose mates. Little attention has been given to the information-gathering process or to the ways that females might weight the importance of each choice criterion when more than one is involved. An exception is the theoretical work of Janetos (1980), who modelled several female choice tactics based on a single male characteristic, namely male fitness. This work lays some important groundwork for analysing mate choice tactics, but it falls short of analysing mate choices based on multiple criteria. My purpose here is to approach the problem from a new direction, with the intent of providing some new ideas and of raising some new issues with regard to mate-choice tactics.

The discussion that follows presumes that only females choose mates selectively, but this presumption is made for the sake of convenience. Males also are likely to choose mates selectively under some circumstances (see Wittenberger, 1979, 1981*a*), and in those cases the discussion below can be applied equally well to them.

Information gathering

In mating contexts information gathering cannot be wholly separated from decision-making. Presumably, mate choice is an iterative procedure: females first obtain information about a prospective mate, then make a decision about that prospect, and then repeat the procedure with a new prospect until a mate is chosen. Three types of decisions can be made during each iteration. A female can reject the male as unsuitable, accept the male as her mate, or defer a decision until information about additional males has been obtained. The following sections discuss several ways that females might perform this iterative procedure.

Threshold-criterion tactic

The simplest procedure a female could adopt is to choose the first male encountered who meets some minimum specifications. These specifications would presumably be based on the male's species identity, his physiological readiness to mate, and perhaps his mated status. A simpler procedure would be to mate completely indiscriminately, but that is never biologically feasible because the costs stemming from hybridisation and prolonged delay prior to mating are always high (at least for females).

The threshold-criterion tactic should be adopted when the cost of comparing several prospective mates outweighs any benefits to be gained by such a tactic. This condition is most likely to be met when the cost of comparing several prospective mates is relatively high and/or the benefit of choosing from among several prospects is relatively low.

The cost of comparing several prospective mates could be high for several reasons. One reason may be that the time required for making such comparisons has a crucial impact on reproductive success. The reproductive season may be very short, early breeding may be markedly more successful than later breeding, or rapid production of multiple clutches may be essential for achieving high fitness. The mate comparison process itself may or may not be time-consuming, depending on how long it takes to find each prospective mate and on how easy or difficult it is to assess the suitability of each one reliably. When the comparison process is time-consuming, mate choice based on comparisons of several prospective mates may be a costly procedure or may be constrained by limitations imposed by a female's memory capabilities (see Janetos, 1980).

A second potential cost has to do with the risks entailed by seeking additional mating prospects. If mortality rate or the hazards of entering unfamiliar terrain are high, the risks may be substantial. In social species females may be unable to seek other mating prospects without leaving their social groups, which may be a hazardous or otherwise costly proposition (e.g. through loss of previously established social or kinship ties). This may be one reason (though probably not the only one) why females of harem polygynous mammals accept whichever male is victorious in controlling access to the female group.

The benefits derived from comparing several prospective mates would be low if males do not vary much in quality. This condition is possible only if additive genetic variance for secondary sexual characteristics is low among males (see Maynard Smith, 1978), if males do not differ much in their ability to provide females with nourishment during courtship, if males do not differ much with respect to their parental propensities and capabilities, and if the degree of outbreeding attained by particular mating choices is unimportant with regard to female fitness.

The conditions for low benefit are relatively stringent and are probably not often met. For instance, recent genetic models suggest that additive genetic variance is probably always substantial for polygenic traits (Lande, 1976). Males of some invertebrates and vertebrates provide females with significant amounts of food through courtship feeding, and they are likely to differ with respect to the size of prey provided or the rate at which prey are provided due to variations in male size or foraging ability (e.g. see Thornhill, 1976; Nisbet, 1973, 1977). Males of many vertebrates provide parental care, and their parental capabilities often vary due to differences in size (Perrone, 1978; Downhower & Brown, 1980), age (Nelson, 1966), experience (Nelson, 1966; Davis, 1976; Brooke, 1978; Ollason & Dunnet, 1978), and perhaps mate compatibility (as evidenced by termination of long-term pair bonds following nest failure in seabirds (see Richdale, 1957; Coulson, 1966, 1972; Mills, 1973). Finally, there is increasing evidence that maintenance of outbreeding is an important consideration in female (and possibly male) mating choices (see Wittenberger, 1981a; Bateson, this volume).

A more-refined version of the threshold criterion tactic can occur if additional standards are imposed during the mate-choice process. In addition to species identity, male readiness to mate, and male mated status, females may require that a suitable mate be healthy, not deformed or injured, older than some minimum age, persistent in courtship to a specified degree, aggressive during courtship within specified bounds, etc. Many standards could be imposed, but as more standards are added, the difficulty, and hence the cost, of finding a suitable mate increases. The cut-off point should be determined by the incremental benefit and cost entailed by imposing each additional standard, or, in more theoretical terms, the improved accuracy to which females can estimate the fitness outcomes entailed by choosing particular male prospects that result from relying on additional standards for making their assessments. Presumably, lower standards for each criterion (and, hence, fewer rejections due to each criterion) allow more standards to be imposed.

Basing choices on threshold criteria would be most suitable for qualitative characteristics such as species identity and presence/absence of deformities. It would also be suitable when traits are difficult or costly to assess quantitatively, in some cases when multiple criteria are used for choosing mates (see later section), and when primary consideration is given to territory or habitat attributes rather than to male attributes (e.g. as in polygynous birds). Factors that favour use of a mate-comparison tactic instead of the threshold-criterion tactic include female gregariousness, male nuptial feeding, and occurrence of male parental care. In these cases males are likely to vary greatly in quality, which would make the benefits derivable from a comparison tactic relatively high (see also Janetos, 1980).

Sequential-comparison tactic

A second approach to choosing mates is to compare prospective mates sequentially and then choose from among the two most recent candidates according to some set of rules. For instance, a female might continue the information-gathering process as long as the ith male is better than the $(i-1)^{th}$ male and then choose either the ith or $(i-1)^{th}$ male once that condition no longer holds. The ith male should be chosen unless the $(i-1)^{th}$ male was nearby and had been assessed rather recently, in which case the female would probably risk little by returning to him.

Sequential comparison involves an alternation of mate assessment (i.e. information gathering) and decision making as each new prospect is found, with a minimum of at least two prospects being assessed before a choice is made. The sequence is: assess male 1; assess male 2; accept male 2 (or male 1) or else defer a decision to the next iteration; assess male 3 if the decision was deferred; accept male 3 (or male 2) or else defer a decision to the next iteration; etc. Rejection comes about automatically through repeated deferrals of a decision.

Conditions that might favour a sequential comparison tactic will be discussed in the next section.

Pool-comparison tactic

An alternative to the sequential comparison tactic is to spend a fixed amount of time assessing as many prospective mates as possible or making an assessment of some predetermined number of prospective mates before making a choice. Once this information-gathering phase is completed, the best male is chosen from the pool of candidates previously evaluated.

The pool-comparison tactic differs from the sequential comparison tactic in that all information about prospective mates is gathered before any decisions are made rather than iterating successive information-gathering/decision-making steps. This tactic is equivalent to the best-of-n-males tactic modelled by Janetos (1980).

The sequential-comparison and pool-comparison tactics are alternative ways of evaluating the relative quality of prospective mates. Both tactics involve trade-offs, and these trade-offs determine when each should be most advantageous.

An important advantage of the sequential-comparison tactic is that it minimises the chances that another female will choose the best male under consideration before a choice is made. A major disadvantage is that the tactic greatly reduces a female's chances of making the best possible choice. Once a female encounters an above-average male, she is very likely to encounter a poorer male next. A female may also be unlucky enough to encounter a very poor male immediately after she has encountered a slightly better but still low-quality male. This latter problem could be circumvented by using a set of minimum specifications to weed out the poorest prospects, but even so, the sequential comparison tactic greatly limits the number of prospective mates that will be considered. Hence, it carries substantial risk that a suboptimal or less-than-best-feasible choice will be made.

The pool comparison tactic has just the opposite characteristics. It greatly enhances a female's chances of finding the best possible mate, but it also entails greater risk that other females will choose the best males first. This risk can be reduced by spending less time on the information-gathering phase, but then the female's range of choices becomes more limited. In the extreme, when only two males are compared, the pool-comparison tactic takes on the same characteristics as the sequential-comparison tactic. Clearly, some intermediate number of mating prospects would be the optimal number to evaluate. The theoretical work by Janetos (1980) suggests that females should ordinarily not compare more than five or six males before making a choice.

Some sort of comparison tactic should evolve when the costs of comparing several males do not exceed the potential benefits. This condition is most likely to be met when: the time required to assess several prospective mates is not greatly detrimental to female fitness; male quality varies substantially with respect to quantitative characters; and other constraints, such as variations in habitat quality or limitations imposed by social organisation (e.g. male guarding behaviour, affinities with other females) or female memory capabilities, do not preclude mate choices based on male traits (cf. Weatherhead & Robertson, 1979; Searcy & Yasukawa, 1981; Wittenberger, 1981*b*).

Given that some comparison tactic is advantageous, the above considerations allow one to predict when each should be most appropriate. The sequential-comparison tactic should be advantageous when males are widely dispersed relative to female locomotory abilities, when assessment of the relevant male traits is time-consuming, or when the mating period is relatively short and synchronous. That is, sequential comparison should be advantageous when the risks of being pre-empted by another female are high. The pool-comparison tactic should be advantageous when males are clumped (on leks, in colonies, or in social groups), when male traits are fairly easy to assess, or when information can be gathered before any females begin to choose mates (e.g. during prior years or non-breeding seasons within stable social groups or during prior years in sedentary populations or in migratory populations with high site fidelity).

Decision making

The actual criteria used by females to choose mates are still not clearly known for most species. What is presently known has been adequately reviewed by Trivers (1972), Halliday (1978), and Wittenberger (1981*a*) and will not be discussed further here. The present discussion is concerned instead with how females go about making their choices.

The decision-making process is straightforward when mate choice is based on only a single criterion or on a set of standards that most males meet. In those cases females can accept or reject males according to single criteria, and weighting of multiple criteria is unnecessary. The interesting questions arise when mate choices are based on multiple criteria which most males do not satisfy equally well. In such circumstances females could base their choices on some sort of priority system or by weighting various combinations of traits in a way that best enhances their inclusive fitness.

Priority systems

In a priority system females successively narrow their options in a hierarchical manner. The criteria used for making mate choices are ranked in priority. Females first screen prospective mates according to the criterion that is given highest priority. They then screen the subset of remaining males according to the criterion that is given next highest priority. This process continues until the choice is narrowed to one male or until all criteria have been considered.

Such a screening process would be most appropriate when females are using the pool-comparison tactic to choose mates. Females could first choose a subset of prospective mates who are rated as the best males according to a high-priority criterion. This could be done for quantitative characters by rank ordering males and then narrowing further evaluation to those who are above average or in some top bracket. Females could then further narrow their prospects by repeating the process with respect to successive criteria until the field is reduced to one male. Such a process would require that females retain a considerable amount of information about prospective mates, unless all prospective mates remain in close proximity to one another during the screening process.

If females adopt the threshold-criterion tactic, no priority system is necessary initially. Females could screen each male encountered with respect to the various criteria being used and choose the first one who satisfies them all. However, if no suitable mate has been found after an initial screening process, the female might be forced to change her standards according to some priority system to improve her chances. She could do that either by discarding one or more criteria or by lowering her standards for one or more criteria. This sort of situation could arise if males vary greatly in their ability to satisfy female standards from one mating period to the next, if females use a set of high standards when many unmated males are available and then lower their standards as mate availability decreases (which would result in different females using different standards), or if females can afford to spend only a limited amount of time seeking mates and are forced to lower their standards as time runs out (the 'last-chance' option described by Janetos, 1980).

If females adopt the sequential-comparison tactic, a priority system would not be appropriate. An initial screening of suitable mates may occur, but comparison of successive mates would presumably be based on some combination of quantitative characters as described in the next section.

Weighting systems

The alternative to a priority system is to rate males according to a combination of traits. This could be done by devising some sort of index to rank males. Females presumably do not consciously compute indices of male quality, but they may seek males with particular combinations of traits ('Gestalts') that are weighted unconsciously according to their fitness consequences. Such a decision-making procedure could easily result in strikingly different males being adjudged as equivalent in quality because different combinations of traits could lead to similar fitness outcomes.

Decision-making based on weighting of male traits would be appropriate mainly when choices are based on multiple quantitative characters. It would therefore be most relevant to the two comparison tactics described above.

Weighting male traits would lessen the amount of information that females would have to retain about each prospective mate. Females would only have to remember some sort of rank value or quality index (or the degree of match between a particular male's traits and the female's search image) and not a whole series of assessments based on each of the various relevant criteria. Further, individual females could rate males in different ways by weighting criteria differently (cf. Burley, 1981). This would enable females to fine-tune their choices in light of their individual requirements or characteristics. Such fine-tuning would not be as feasible when a priority system is used for screening prospective mates.

The possibility for fine-tuning raises some questions about whether and how females take their own phenotypic characteristics into account when choosing mates. As an example, a female bird in poor physiological condition during the laying period may give more weight to a male's ability to feed her during courtship and less to other aspects of male quality, while a female in good physiological condition during the laying period may given more weight to other aspects of a male's quality and less to his courtship feeding ability. Female experience may also play an important role here. Females may discover idiosyncratic weaknesses in their pheno-types during previous breeding attempts and may compensate for them by choosing complementary mates who are particularly strong with respect to those traits. This kind of choice pattern could contribute to the higher reproductive success often exhibited by experienced individuals.

The existence of fine-tuning would obviously hamper attempts to identify the criteria that females use to choose mates, especially if the poasibility for fine-tuning has not even been considered during the study.

Discussion

The above analysis has been made largely in the abstract, and with good reason. Up to now, virtually no one has been concerned with the tactics involved in gathering information about prospective mates and in making choices based on multiple criteria. Nearly all research on mate choice to date has been concerned instead with why females are usually more choosy than males (Bateman, 1948; Trivers, 1972), why males might sometimes choose males as well as or instead of females (Jenni, 1974; Maynard Smith, 1977; Wittenberger, 1979, 1981a) or the identity of criteria used for making mate choices (Trivers, 1972; Halliday, 1978;

Wittenberger, 1981*a*). A notable exception is the work of Janetos (1980), which has been referred to earlier.

Studying the tactics of mate choice has considerable theoretical value. One way to demonstrate that females actually choose from among the available males, which is often debatable (see Halliday, this volume), is to show that specific tactics are employed to that end. In many species the origin of the mating system cannot be understood adequately until female mate-choice patterns have been clarified. This is particularly true for lek species (see Alexander, 1975; Borgia, 1979; Wittenberger, 1979) and certain polygynous birds (see Weatherhead & Robertson, 1979; Heisler, 1981; Yasukawa, 1981). When individual females fine-tune their choices according to their own phenotypic characteristics, the way that females make their choices must be taken into account before the criteria used by them can be identified. Tactics used by females to choose mates may represent an important component of social organisation, just as tactics used by males to compete for mates do. Finally, the tactics discussed here are not limited to mating contexts. Similar tactics could be employed for choosing habitats, breeding territories, colony locations, or nest sites. In all cases the individuals involved must gather information and then make decisions based upon that information, often in light of multiple-choice criteria. Hence, research on the tactics of mate choice could shed light on these other processes, and vice versa.

The tactics of mate choice have rarely been studied partly because they are difficult to investigate. Data must be based on continuous surveillance of individually known females throughout the mating process, and operational criteria must be devised to distinguish between the various types of mate-choice tactics that are possible. Neither task is easy, but neither is impossible either. Continuous surveillance of females is possible by radio tracking and, in some cases, by prolonged observation at mating stations (e.g. at leks) or in laboratory populations. Alternative tactics of mate choice can be distinguished by the mating patterns observed. For instance, when the threshold-criterion tactic is being used, at least some females should choose the first male they encounter, rejected males should be rejected by all females (unless different individuals use different standards), and rejected males should be separable from accepted males by clear-cut differences. When the sequential-comparison tactic is used, females should always choose the most recent or the immediately preceding male visited. In contrast, when the pool-comparison tactic is used, females should often choose males encountered earlier in the mating process.

What is needed next is more careful observation of the exact sequence of events that takes place during the mating process. Special focus should be placed on the sequence in which males are visited and on the particular male that is chosen. This will necessarily entail continuous observation of individually known females throughout the mating process. Hopefully, the discussion presented here will provide a useful framework for undertaking studies of this sort.

Summary

Mate choice may involve more than a non-tactical acceptance or rejection of prospective mates. Tactical behaviour may be necessary during both information-gathering and decision-making phases of the mating process. For instance, females could choose the first male who meets minimum specifications (the threshold-criterion tactic). They could sequentially compare males until the most recent male encountered is inferior to the previous male encountered and then choose either of those two males (the sequential-comparison tactic). Finally, females could assess a whole series of males before making any decisions and then choose the best male from among those who were assessed (the pool-comparison tactic). The different tactics are likely to evolve under different circumstances, and the advantages and disadvantages of each allow one to predict when each should be adopted.

Decision making should be a straightforward procedure when choices are based on a single criterion, but it can become complicated if choices are based on multiple criteria. In the latter circumstance decisions may be made by ranking the various criteria in some sort of priority system or by weighting the various criteria to obtain an index or search image of mate suitability. The latter procedure could lead to further complexity if individual females weight criteria differently in the light of their particular requirements or phenotypic characteristics in order to find a mate with complementary characteristics.

I thank Patrick Bateson for his encouragement and for making several helpful comments on the manuscript.

References

Alcock, J. (1975). Territorial behaviour by males of *Philanthus multimaculatus* (Hymenoptera: Sphecidae) with a review of territoriality in male sphecids. *Animal Behaviour*, **23**, 889–95.

Alexander, R. D. (1975). Natural selection and specialized chorusing behavior in acoustical insects. In *Insects, Science, and Society*, ed. D. Pimentel, pp. 35–77. Academic Press: New York.

Bateman, A. J. (1948). Intrasexual selection in *Drosophila. Heredity*, **2**, 349–68.

Borgia, G. (1979). Sexual selection and the evolution of mating systems. In *Sexual Selection and Reproductive Competition in Insects*, ed. M. S. Blum & N. A. Blum, pp. 19–80. Academic Press: New York.

Bradbury, J. W. (1981). The evolution of leks. In *Natural Selection and Social Behavior*, ed. R. D. Alexander & D. Tinkle, pp. 138–69. New York: Chiron Press.

Brooke, M. de L. (1978). Some factors affecting the laying date, incubation and breeding success of the Manx shearwater, *Puffinus puffinus. Journal of Animal Ecology*, **47**, 477–95.

Burley, N. (1981). Mate choice by multiple criteria in a monogamous species. *American Naturalist*, **117**, 515–28.

Companella, P. J. (1975). The evolution of mating systems in temperate zone dragonflies (Odonata: Anisoptera). II. *Libellula luctuosa* (Burmeister). *Behaviour*, **54**, 278–310.

Coulson, J. C. (1966). The influence of the pair-bond and age on the breeding biology of the kittiwake gull *Rissa tridactyla. Journal of Animal Ecology*, **35**, 269–79.

Coulson, J. C. (1972). The significance of the pair-bond in the kittiwake. In *Proceedings of the 15th International Ornithological Congress*, pp. 424–33.

Davis, J. W. F. (1976). Breeding success and experience in the arctic skua, *Stercorarius parasiticus* (L.). *Journal of Animal Ecology*, **45**, 531–6.

Downhower, J. F. & Brown, L. (1980). Mate preferences of female mottled sculpins, *Cottus bairdi. Animal Behaviour*, **28**, 728–34.

Geist, V. (1974). On the relationship of social evolution and ecology in ungulates. *American Zoologist*, **14**, 205–20.

Halliday, T. R. (1978). Sexual selection and mate choice. In *Behavioural Ecology: an Evolutionary Approach*, ed. J. R. Krebs & N. B. Davies, pp. 180–213. Sinauer Associates: Sunderland, Massachusetts.

Heisler, I. L. (1981). Offspring quality and the polygyny threshold: a new model for the "sexy son" hypothesis. *American Naturalist*, **117**, 316–28.

Hjorth, I. (1970). Reproductive behaviour in Tetraonidae, with special reference to males. *Viltrevy*, **7**, 183–596.

Howard, R. D. (1980). Mating behaviour and mating success in woodfrogs, *Rana sylvatica. Animal Behaviour*, **28**, 705–16.

Janetos, A. C. (1980). Strategies of female mate choice: a theoretical analysis. *Behavioral Ecology and Sociobiology*, **7**, 107–12.

Jenni, D. A. (1974). Evolution of polyandry in birds. *American Zoologist*, **14**, 129–44.

Lande, R. (1976). The maintenance of genetic variability by mutation in a polygenic character with linked loci. *Genetics Research*, **26**, 221–35.

Lande, R. (1981). Rapid speciation by sexual selection on polygenic characters. *Proceedings of the National Academy of Sciences of the USA*, **78**, 3721–5.

Mangan, R. L. (1979). Reproductive behavior of the cactus fly, *Odontoloxozus longicornis*. Male territoriality and female guarding as adaptive strategies. *Behavioral Ecology and Sociobiology*, **4**, 265–78.

Maynard Smith, J. (1977). Parental investment: a prospective analysis. *Animal Behaviour*, **25**, 1–9.

Maynard Smith, J. (1978). *The Evolution of Sex*. Cambridge University Press: Cambridge, England.

Mills, J. A. (1973). The influence of age and pair-bond on the breeding biology of the red-billed gull, *Larus novaehollandiae scopulinus. Journal of Animal Ecology*, **42**, 147–62.

Morse, D. H. (1980). *Behavioral Mechanisms in Ecology*. Harvard University Press: Cambridge, Massachusetts.

Nelson, J. B. (1966). The breeding biology of the gannet *Sula bassana* on the Bass Rock, Scotland. *Ibis*, **108**, 584–626.

Nisbet, I. C. T. (1973). Courtship-feeding, egg-size and breeding success in common terns. *Nature*, **241**, 141–2.

Nisbet, I. C. T. (1977). Courtship-feeding and clutch-size in common terns. In *Evolutionary Ecology*, ed. B. Stonehouse & C. M. Perrins, pp. 101–9. Macmillan: London.

O'Donald, P. (1980). *Genetic Models of Sexual Selection*. Cambridge University Press: Cambridge, England.

Ollason, J. C. & Dunnet, G. C. (1978). Age, experience and other factors affecting the breeding success of the fulmar, *Fulmarus glacialis*, in Orkney. *Journal of Animal Ecology*, **47**, 961–76.

Otte, D. & Joern, A. (1975). Insect territoriality and its evolution: population studies of desert grasshoppers on creosote bushes. *Journal of Animal Ecology*, **44**, 29–54.

Perrone, M., Jr. (1978). Mate size and breeding success in a monogamous cichlid fish. *Environmental Biology of Fish*, **3**, 193–201.

Richdale, L. E. (1957). *A Population Study of Penguins*. Clarendon Press: Oxford.

Searcy, W. A. & Yasukawa, K. (1981). Does the "sexy son" hypothesis apply to mate choice in red-winged blackbirds? *American Naturalist*, **117**, 343–8.

Thornhill, R. (1976). Sexual selection and paternal investment in insects. *American Naturalist*, **110**, 153–63.

Thornhill, R. (1979). Male and female sexual selection and the evolution of making strategies in insects. In *Sexual Selection and Reproductive Competition in Insects*, ed. M. S. Blum & N. A. Blum, pp. 81–121. Academic Press: New York.

Trivers, R. L. (1972). Parental investment and sexual selection. In *Sexual Selection and the Descent of Man, 1871–1971*, ed. B. Campbell, pp. 136–79. Aldine: Chicago.

Weatherhead, P. J. & Robertson, R. J. (1979). Offspring quality and the polygyny threshold: "the sexy son hypothesis." *American Naturalist*, **113**, 201–8.

Wells, K. D. (1977). The social behaviour of anuran amphibians. *Animal Behaviour*, **25**, 666–93.

Wittenberger, J. F. (1978). The evolution of mating systems in grouse. *Condor*, **80**, 126–37.

Wittenberger, J. F. (1979). The evolution of mating systems in birds and mammals. In *Handbook of Behavioral Neurobiology*, vol. **3**, *Social Behavior and Communication*, ed. P. Marler & J. Vandenbergh, pp. 271–349. Plenum Press: New York.

Wittenberger, J. F. (1980). Group size and polygamy in social mammals. *American Naturalist*, **115**, 197–222.

Wittenberger, J. F. (1981a). *Animal Social Behavior*. Duxbury Press: Boston.

Wittenberger, J. F. (1981b). Male quality and polygyny: the "sexy son" hypothesis revisited. *American Naturalist*, **117**, 329–42.

Yasukawa, K. (1981). Male quality and female choice of mate in the red-winged blackbird (*Agelaius phoeniceus*). *Ecology*, **62**, 922–9.

INDEX

adaptive cue hypothesis, 127–34; in changing populations, 130–1; cues for female choice, 132; demography, (components) 131–2, (consequences) 133; and fitness, 127–8, 130–1, (costs and benefits) 131; male viability, 127, 128–31, 133–4; measurement of, 129–31; models, 128–31; in stable populations, 128–30

advertisement, 142–4; calls, 183, 189, 196, 200–1; costs and benefits, 142–4; phenotypes, 141–4

age, 363, 370; arrival dates at colony, 362, 363, 370, (of females and males) 371–2; cue for female choice, 124, 132; divorce rate, 365, 366; duration of pair bond, 366, 368; indication by plumage, 16; kin preference, 263n, 264n; and parental care, 438; and productivity, 333, 334–7; scent signal information, 219; survival rate, 365; see also experience; longevity

albatrosses: *Diomedea bulleri*, *Diomedea exultans*, *Diomedea immutabilis*, *Diomedea irrorata*, 343; divorce rates, *D. irrorata*, 350–1; foraging efficiency, *D. immutabilis*, 43; pair bonds, 333, 343, 350

alternative strategies, xiv; behavioural variability, 191–2; choice by females, 192–5, 201; in explosive breeders and prolonged breeders, 184–7; functions, 190–1; in male, of survival, mating and rearing, (maximising mating success) 425–6, (maximising birth rate) 427–9, (maximising fitness) 430, (network of decisions) 431–2; in mate-locating behaviour, 187–90; of reproduction, 423–32

androgens; acquisition of preference, 396–7; action at cellular level, 393; and behaviour, 393, 395; in blood plasma, 392, 394, 396, 401; expression of mate choice, 394–6; and hypothalamic areas, 393; metabolism of, 393; receptiveness in females, 413; scent gland control, 219, 220; secondary sexual characters, 390;

sperm production and transport, 393; synchrony between partners, 397–402; target cells in brain, 393; see also individual androgens

androstenedione, 391

anuran amphibians, male–male competition and mate choice, 181–20

Argus Pheasant *Argusianus argus*, 16

aromatase activity, 391, 392, 400–1

Asellus spp., males: choice for fecundity, 5, 177; guard of female, 161

Asellus aquaticus, 5

assortative mating (positive assortment), 240–2, 311; among ecotypes, 8; genetic variation, 240, 311; genic covariance, 73, 79; and local adaptations, 236–7, 246; mate choice and reproductive fitness in Snow Geese, 279–95; offspring fitness, 240–2; for quality, 152; recognition of phenotype, 240; in rodents 311; for size, 156, 194, 201–3, (and male density) 202–3; and speciation, 240; species-recognition mechanism, 290–1; see also disassortative mating

attractiveness: of females, 174, 377, 378, 379–80, 408; in feral troops of monkeys, 414; levels between couples, 380; loss of, and compensatory behaviour, 412; of males, 409; non-behavioural, 410–11, 413, 416; and ovarian hormones, 410–11, 416; and pheromones, 411, and testosterone levels in males, 408; see also advertisement

auditory stimuli, 316

babblers *Turdoides* spp., pair bonds and mate replacements, 346–7

Barbet Bird *Trachyphonus d'arnaudii*, monogamy, 37

bats: dispersion in leks, 116–17; female copying, 125; male dispersion, 112; male dominance, 118; measurement of adaptive cues in, 129; position effect in female choice, 121, 122; predation by, 4

Beagles: oestrus and behaviour, 389–90

beetles: mate choice and wasps, *Chauliognathus pennsylvanicus*, 20; monogamy in, 40; rare male effect, flour beetle, ladybird, 242

behaviour: compensatory, for loss of attraction, 412; and deep structure of social group, 414, 416; dominance hierarchies, (defined by aggression) 409, 414, 415, 416, (among females) 407, 413–414, 416, (among males) 407–14, (*see also* status); effects on hormone secretion, 407–9; evolution of, 59–60; female receptiveness, 413; and hormones, 390, 391–3, 395, 397–402, 407–14; of inbred mice, 324; and interspecific barriers, 311, 314–15; littering frequency, 218; male density, 192, 193; nest soliciting, 398–9; synchronous, 397–402, 414, 416; synchrony between partners, 397–402; testosterone and, 407–9; variability in mating systems, 191–2, 203–4; *see also* cross-fostering

Bicoloured Antbird *Gymnopithys bicolor*, pair bonds, 348

birds: mate choice in, 389–406; re-mating in, 331–60

Bird of Paradise *Paradisaea decora*, mating system, 14–15

birth rate, maximisation of, 427–8

Blackbird: pair bond persistence, *Turdus merula*, 342, 348; territorial resources, *Agelaius phoeniceus*, 7, 12, 13

Blackcock: male dispersion in leks, 112

boobies: foraging efficiency, of Red-footed Booby, 43; pair bond persistence of *Sula dactylatra*, 344; productivity of *S. dactylatra*, 344; *see also* Gannet

brain: androgen metabolism, 393; hormone action on, 399–402; neuroendocrine system, 392, 401; testosterone action, 393, 397

Budgerigar *Melopsittacus undulatus*: monogamy, 37; pair bond duration, 43

butterflies: display and sperm supply, *Pieris protodice*, 5, 233; female solicitation, *P. protodice*, 25; male choice by size, *P. protodice* 5; size and mating success, 234.

buxom redhead hypothesis, 291, 293

calls: *see* vocal signals

cattle egret, 44

Chimpanzee *Pan troglodytes*: inbreeding avoidance, 263; mate complementarity, 8

choice of mate: *see* mate choice

Chough, white-winged *Concorax melanorhampus*, pair bonds and mate replacements, 346–7

cimcid bugs, 44

clumping of males in leks, 111–14

cockatoos: *Cacatua leadbeateri*, 342, 347; *Cacatua roseicapilla*, 342, 347; *Cacatua tenuirostris*, 344; *Calyptorrhynchus funereous*, 334–350

Coke's Hartebeest *Alcelaphus cokii*, mother-son monogamy, 40–1

cockroach *Nauphoeta cinerea*, male status, 7

coloniality costs and benefits, 216

colonies: fidelity to, 362–3, 370; survival rates, 363; *see also* nest sites; territories; warrens

compatibility, 8–9, 235, 257; in birds, 339–40, 350, 354, 375; in Kittiwakes during egg incubation, 367

competition, 211; and choice, 3, 11–14, 20; inclusive fitness effect, 237; intensity of and parental investment, 13, 167

competition between females, 2, 12, 13, 214; benefits and costs, 168; intensity of, and parental investment, 167; for males, 167, 170–2; for male quality, 168–72, 173–4; for paternal investment, 167, 172; risks, 168, 171; for resources, 167–8, 173–4

competition between larvae, 145, 245; heritable fitness, 90

competition between males, 181–92, 215–16; fitness of offspring, 233; on leks, 14–15, 118; male mating success, 233; parental investment, 160–1; passive female choice, 233; plumage, 305; rare male effect, 245; by sexual advertisement, 141–4; size assortative mating 202–3; size dependent mating, 202–3; social displays, 305; sperm, 27–8; vocal signals *q.v.*; *see also* male–male competition

Corella *Cacatua tenuirostris*, 344

Cormorant, Flightless *Nannopterum harrisi*: divorce rate, 353, 354; pair bond persistence, 342

cortisol, 409, 414–15, 417

cotingids, male dispersion in leks, 112

courtship: dating choice, 378; evolution of, 382–3; hormone effects, 390, (androgen) 393; (synchrony between partners) 397–402, (testosterone) 400; intensity of, 10, (fitness indicator) 233, (sperm supply) 5, 233; love levels in, 383; matching hypothesis, 378–9; negotiation of, 382–3; partner familiarity, 339;

courtship (*cont.*)
  partner fidelity, 42–3; and physical
  attractiveness, 377, 378, 379–80, (level
  of, between couples) 380; scent release,
  220; stimulus-value-role-theory, 379–80;
  value systems, 380; *see also* displays by
  males; vocal signals
courtship behaviour, functions of, 24–5
courtship feeding, 5–6; egg size, 334;
  fecundity of female, 6; as male quality,
  168, 438; pair bond strength, 6
cousins: first-, preference for, 269, 275,
  (result of inbreeding with) 271–2; third-,
  preference for, 269
crickets, 112; competitive female choice,
  Anabrus simplex, 12, 13, 173; male
  choice for fecundity, *A. simplex*, 5, 13,
  176–7
cross-fostering: behaviour, social and
  sexual, 312, 315; broadening of species
  identity, 312; differences between sexes,
  315; feeding specialisation, 241;
  interspecific barriers, 311, 314–15; male
  plumage preferences, 302; mating
  preferences, 301–2, 315, 317, 323;
  olfactory preferences, 323–4; preference
  for familiarity, 320–3, (siblings) 323–4;
  sibling recognition, 321–3, 324; species
  preferences, 312, 314; strain preferences,
  323–4; *see also* experience, early;
  imprinting
Crustacea; monogamy, 40
cuckoldry, 40; avoidance in anuran
  amphibians, 204; likelihood of, 177; by
  satellite males, 192
cues: adaptive cue hypothesis, 127–34;
  attractiveness *q.v.*; behavioural,
  (individual interest) 304–5, (social
  displays) 303–5; olfactory; species
  isolation, 315; passive female attraction
  to, 142; plumage, 303–5; vocal,
  195–201; *see also under* age; experience;
  phenotypes; size
cues in leks: adaptive cue hypothesis,
  127–34; age, 124, 132; arbitrary cue
  hypothesis, 126–7; dominance of males,
  123–4, 132–3; phenotypes of males,
  124–6; position effects, 15, 121–3, 145;
  vigour of display, 124–5, 132

Darwin, Charles Robert: epigamic
  characters, (evolution of) 53–8,
  (intersexual selection) 10, (sexual
  selection) 53, 71; sexual selection, 55,
  102, (inter- and intra-) 3, 10, 11, 13, 53,
  279, (versus natural selection) 68–71
decisions: mate choice tactics, 436–7,

441–3; reproductive strategies, 423, 424,
  430–2
Deer, Red: measurement of adaptive cues,
  129; reproductive strategies, 426
demes, 319
demography, in sociobiology, 33
Desert Woodlouse *Hemilepistus* sp., 46;
  monogamy and brood care, 41; partner
  fidelity and latent pair bond, 43
diethylstilboestrol, 400
5α-dihydrotestosterone: in blood plasma,
  392; effect on mate choice, 394–5;
  secondary sexual characters, 391
disassortative mating (negative
  assortment), 240, 242, 311; and offspring
  fitness, 242
dispersal, 298; of birds from natal area, 8,
  241; of males in leks, 109, 111–15, 134,
  275; of mice, 319; of migrant birds, 348,
  349; and outbreeding, 237, 262–3;
  probability, 272
displays by males, 10–11, 14–16:
  androgens, 399–400; evolution of, 60;
  leks, (costs) 130, (habitats for) 111, 112,
  (intrasexual) 14–15, 118, (vigour of) 15,
  124, 132; mate assessment, 390; social,
  297, 298, 303; spawning of females, 25;
  species recognition, 299–300; strain
  recognition, 304–5; vigour of, 10, (and
  sperm supply) 5, 233
disruptive selection, and fitness heritability,
  231
divorce, 332, 364; and age, 365, 366, 368;
  breeding failure, 353–4, 367, 369–70,
  373; in migrant, nomadic and resident
  bird species, 342–4, 347, 350–1, 353–4;
  as mate choice, 354; in migratory
  passerines, 349; and pair status, 366,
  367, 368; past duration of pair bond,
  366, 369
domestic chicks *Gallus gallus*, kin
  recognition, 263
dominance, 7, 11, 14, 62, 261; behavioural
  and reproductive success in rabbits, 213;
  in breeding groups of rabbits, 213; in
  female monkeys, 407, (and male sexual
  attention) 413–14; in female rabbits, and
  warren occupation, 212–14, 218; in
  female sticklebacks, 171; and gonadal
  hormones in male monkeys, 407–10;
  hierarchy, 426–7; in human married
  couples, 381; male hierarchy, 27, (as
  index of assessment by female) 133;
  male, in leks, 118, 120, 123–4, 132, 134,
  191; in male Mallard social displays,
  303; in male monkeys, and sexual
  behaviour, 407–17; in male rabbits, 213,

dominance (*cont.*)
215; in nest site selection, 372; in
rabbits, and scent marking, 219–20
Dove, Ring *Streptopelia risoria:* hormone
action and courtship behaviour, 25, 393,
397–402; male mate choice, 177
Drosophila melanogaster Fruit Fly:
artificial selection on female choice, 90;
competition between larvae, 145, 245;
courtship of yellow mutants, 5; female
preferences and genotype, 64–5; fitness,
(components of) 231–3, (heritability of)
228–31; rare male effect, 55, 242–6;
sexual difference in fitness variances, 93
duck: American Black Duck, 300;
hybridisation, *Anas platyrhynchos*,
300–1; innate preferences, *A.
platyrhynchos*, 301, 303; Kaspar Hauser
females, *A. platyrhynchos*, 301–2; life
pattern, *A. platyrhynchos*, 297–9; pair
bond, *Calidris alpina*, 343; pair bond
maintenance, *Anas ferina, Anas fuligula*,
348; pair bond persistence, *Tadorna
tachiodes, Tadorna tadorna*, 343, 344,
349; plumage of male and choice, *A.
platyrhynchos*, 11, 305, 306; sexual
selection, *A. platyrhynchos*, 305–6; social
displays, *Anas* spp., 299, 303; winter
pairing, *Athya* spp., 340

eggs: age of parent, (clutch size) 334, (egg
size) 334, (hatching success) 336;
courtship feeding, (clutch weight) 6, (egg
size) 334; double clutching, 172, 173;
size of parent, and egg number, 292–3;
Elephant Seal *Mirounga angustirostris*,
intrasexual selection, 11, 13, 20
emancipation, female: male paternal care,
172–3; from ovarian hormone
influences, 413
endocrines and monkey sexual
behaviour, 407–20
energetics: mating behaviour, 185–7
epigamic characters, 11, 14, 16, 28, 103–4,
105, 120, 169; evolution of, 53–8;
intersexual selection, 10; sexual
selection, 53, 71
European Rabbit, mate choice in, 211–23
evolution: adaptive cue hypothesis, 127;
of behaviour, 59–60; conflict between
sexes, 158–60; diversity of outcomes,
86–7; dynamic modelling strategies,
71–88; female preferences, 56–9; of
fitness, 429; freedom from control of
oestrus, 413; and genetic variability,
288–9; genetical models, 67–8, 73–88,
(male character) 74–88, (preferences)

60–4, 75–8; maladaptive, 89; male
characteristics, 53, 58; mate-comparison
tactics, 440–1; and monogamy, 46–7;
natural selection versus sexual selection,
79–81; Panglossian view, 88; of paternal
care, 174; of polyandry, 172–4; primary
sexual characters, 69–70; and
recombination, 239; reproductive
strategies, 423; runaway sexual selection,
57–9, 72–3, 83, 84; secondary sexual
characters, 69–70; sexual reproduction,
260; species differences, 184–7;
trajectories and equilibria, (stable) 82,
(unstable) 83, 84
evolutionarily stable strategies (ESS):
degree, of monogamy, 44;
discrimination, 151–2, (both sexes)
152–6, 165–7, (one sex) 151–2; mate
choice, 150–2; mate location, 187;
random mating, 151, (mate quality) 151;
sexual advertisement, 142–5; sexual
conflict and mating decisions, 156–7;
versus dynamic models, 72
experience: display performance, 124;
early, (biological function of) 320,
(mating preferences) 264–5, (*see also
under* age; cross-fostering; imprinting);
kin recognition, 263; and parental care,
438; and productivity, 334–7; and
reproductive success, 339, 443

Fairy Prion *Pachystila turtur*, pair bond
persistence, 344
fecundity, xiv, 5, 6, 9, 13, 101, 129, 132,
292–3; of female, and male mate choice,
177; of females in maximising birth rate,
427–8, (and food supplied) 6; male
choice for, 5; related to similarity
between spouses, 261; variability in,
sources, 176; and weight of adult female,
232
female–female competition, 172–4, 177; in
Gallinula chloropus, 170; in Three-spined
Stickleback, 171; in wild birds, 171
fertility, xiv, 5, 10, 71, 101, 232, 292–3;
female choice for, 5; of male or female
Yellow-eyed Penguin, 336; of mate and
male mating success, 93, 94, (in *Rana
catasbeiana*) 95, 96, 106; potential,
assessment of by possible mate, 390
fidelity: to family, 352; to mate, 36, 37,
42–3, 46, 305, 341, 351, 352, (*see also*
pair bond, duration); to site, 121–2, 281,
286, 349–50, 351, 353, 370–1, 374
finches: assortative mating, Darwin's
Medium-billed Finch, 241; optimal
discrepancy hypothesis, *Taeniopygia*

finches (*cont.*)
guttata, 267, 270; pair bonds, *Fringella
coelebs, Pyrrhula pyrrhula*, 37, 348; *P.
pyrrhula*, 44; *T. guttata*, 44
fishes: assortative mating among ecotypes,
Gasterosteus aculeatus, 8; brood care,
Apistogramma spp., *Tilapia mariae*, 40;
choice for size, *Cottus bairdi*, 5, 6, 13,
19, 177, 201; female choice, competitive
in *G. aculeatus*, 171–2, (male colour) 10,
54–5, (nest) 6; male courtship, *Chromis
cyanea*, 25; monogamy, chaetodonts,
*Opistognathus aurifrons, Serranus
tigrinus*, 35, 40, 46; pair bond duration,
Apistogramma spp., 43; partner fidelity,
T. mariae, 37; polyandry *Ceratius* spp.,
36, 42; rare-male effect, Guppy, 242;
solitary reproduction, *Rivulus
marmoratus, Serranus subligarius*, 35;
spawning, *C. cyanea, C. bairdi*, 13, 22;
territorial resources, *Pseudolabrus
celidotus*, 6; timing of reproduction,
Platyfish, Sunfish, 426
fitness: components of, 95, 231–3, (and
mutations) 232; contributions by
relatives, 429–30; Darwinian selection,
71; decline and inbreeding, 238;
deleterious mutations, 230–1; energy of
vocal calls, 198; in evolution, 429;
female choice of qualities of, 438; and
female mating strategies, 17–18; genetic
equilibrium, 91; genetic variance for,
91–2; and good genes, 193–4;
heritability of, 9, 90, 92, 194, 228–31,
(mutations) 229–30; of individuals,
(mate choice tactics) 435, (mate
competition tactics) 435; male mating
success, 228, 232; maximisation of,
429–30; and monogamy, 37; mutant
strategies, 149; mutation dominance,
230; natural selection, 75; non-random
mating, 228; and nutrition, 233;
Panglossian view, 88; population
equilibria, 84; and tactics, 435; tallying
of, (by descendents) 89, (by
productivity) 89; variance in relative
fitness 92, (calculation method) 92n; *see
also* offspring, fitness
fitness variance, analysis of: mathematical
guides, 94; and selection, 93–4, 100–2
flukes *Diplozon* spp., monogamy, 36
Fly, Hanging *Hylobittacus apicalis*,
courtship feeding, 5
friendship choice: negotiation of, 383, 385;
personality, 383–5; personal appearance,
384; social activities, 384–5
frogs: calls and species identification,

*Eleutherodactylus coquii, Hyla cinerea,
Hyla gratiosa, Physalaemus pustulosus*, 4,
10, 22–3, 124, 183, 188–9, 196; call
preferences, *Hyla versicolor*, 199; calling
sites, *Centrolenella fleischmanni, H.
versicolor*, treefrogs, 184, 198; choruses,
Hyla regilla, 10, 198–9; competitive
female choice, *Dendrobates auratus*, 173;
displays, costs of, *P. pustulosus*, 130;
female mate choice, *Hyla rosenbergi*,
treefrogs, 195; hybrid mating risks, *H.
cinerea*, 22–3, 196; male calls, *H.
gratiosa, Hyla squirella, P. pustulosus,
Rana sylvatica*, 22, 189; male choice for
size, *R. sylvatica*, 177; male density and
sex ratio, *Hyla crucifer, H. rosenbergi,
H. versicolor, Rana catasbeiana, Rana
clamitans, R. sylvatica, Rana temporaria*,
185; male dispersion in leks, *H.
versicolor*, 112; mate location, *Hyla
chrysoscelis, H. cinerea, H. crucifer,
Hyla ebraccata, Hyla microcephala, Hyla
minuta, H. regilla, Hyla squirella, Hyla
versicolor, R. catasbeiana, R. clamitans,
R. temporaria*, 188–9; mating success, *P.
pustulosus*, 124; mating system, *R.
catasbeiana*, 191–2; natural and sexual
selection intensities, *R. catasbeiana*,
95–6, 97; non-random mating, *H.
cinerea, Hyla crucifer, Hyla marmota, H.
versicolor, R. catasbeiana, R. clamitans,
R. sylvatica, Triprion petasatus*, 202;
resource-based territories, *R.
catesbeiana, R. clamitans*, 6–7, 184, 195;
size and mating success, *P. pustulosus*,
124; size assortative mating, *R.
temporaria*, 202; weight loss, *R.
clamitans*, 186, 191
Fulmar, Northern, *Fulmaris glacialis*, 344

Galah *Cacatua roseicapilla*, 342, 347
Gammarus spp., male investment, 161
Gammarus pulex, non-random mating, 283
Gannet *Sula bassana:* pair bond
persistence, 344; productivity and age,
334–6; *see also* boobies
geese: assortative mating, *Anser
caerulescens*, 241, 279, 281–91, 291–3;
breeding success and partner familiarity,
Anser brachyrhynchus, Anser rossii, 339,
340; early experiences and mating
preferences, *Branta canadensis*, 265;
evolution and mate choice, *A.
caerulescens*, 289–90; mate choice, *A.
caerulescens*, 289–90; mating
preferences, *B. canadensis*, 265;
outbreeding, *A. caerulescens*, 263; pair

geese (*cont.*)
  bonds in migratory geese, 349; pair
  bond duration in Greylag Geese, 42;
  pair formation, *A. caerulescens*, 281;
  partner familiarity and breeding success,
  A. brachyrhynchus, *A. rosssii*, 339, 340;
  partner fidelity, *Anser canagicus*, 43;
  productivity and size, *A. caerulescens*,
  292–3
gene complexes, co-adapted: epistasis and
  fitness, 235–6
gene pools: contributions to, 216, (by
  relatives) 429–30; reproductive
  strategies, 423, 424
genes: good, *see* good genes; hitch-hiking
  q.v.; for mating preferences, 319
genetic equilibrium, 81–3, 86; and fitness,
  91
genetic polymorphism, rare male effect, 55
glucocorticoid synthesis, 391
good genes, 67; female choice, 145–6;
  fitness, 193–4; genetic variation, 193–4;
  handicap theory, 9–10, 144; male
  quality, 168; mate choice, 105, (for
  phenotypic expression of) 9–10; sexual
  selection, 90–1, (Panglossian view) 88
Green Anoles *Anolis carolinensis*, male
  displays and ovarian development, 25
grouse, 15–16; copulation interference in
  Black Grouse, Sage Grouse, 119; female
  copying, Prairie Grouse, 125; male
  dispersion in leks, 112; measurement of
  adaptive cues, Sage Grouse, 129;
  position effect in female choice, Sage
  Grouse, 121, 122; strategies in leks, Sage
  Grouse, 110, 117, 118; territory
  acquisition in leks, *Pedioecetus
  phasianellus*, 15
Guinea Pig *Cavia porcellus*, effects of early
  experience to stimuli, 312, 313
gulls, 44; divorce rate, *Larus
  novaehollandiae*, 350; mate feeding and
  fidelity, *Larus novaehollandiae scopulinus*,
  6; nest site quality, *Larus ridibundus*,
  339; pair bonds, *Larus argentalus*, *Larus
  glaucescens*, *L. novaehollandiae*, 344,
  350; productivity, *L. novaehollandiae*,
  333–4

hamster *Mesocricetus auratus*, interspecific
  cross-fostering, 314, 315
handicap theory, 9–10, 127, 144–5, 146–7
Hardy-Weinberg equilibrium, 311
harems, 12, 34, 45, 172; reproductive
  strategies, 424, 426; victorious male
  acceptance, 437
Hawaiian Bird *Neomorpha acutirostris*,
  natural selection, 69

Hermit Hummingbirds, 124, measurement
  of adaptive cues, 129
heterozygotes: and inbreeding, 235; mating
  preferences, 319; mating success, 229
hierarchy: in adult female rabbits, 214,
  217; in adult male rabbits, 213;
  dominance, 132–3, 426–7, (in breeding
  groups of rabbits) 213–14; of male
  dominance, 27; in social groups of
  monkeys, 407–10, 413, 415, 417
hitch-hiking genes: in optimal outbreeding,
  260; preference and preferred characters,
  60–2; and runaway process, 61
homozygotes: assortative mating, 311;
  fitness decline, 238; inbreeding, 235;
  maintenance, (parthenogenesis) 236,
  (self-fertilization) 236; mating success,
  229
Honey Bee, monogamy, 44
hormonal mechanism of mate choice in
  birds, 389–406
hormones: acquisition of preference,
  396–7; and behaviour, 390, 391, 393,
  395; expression of mate choice, 394–6;
  female perception of, 389; levels of,
  affected by social structure, 407–8;
  maintenance of hierarchies, 415; mate
  assessment, 390, 391; mate
  indentification, 391; mechanisms of
  action, 391–3; ovarian, and sexual
  interactions, 410–13; receptive
  behaviour, 413, (in feral monkeys) 414;
  secondary sexual characters, 390, 391;
  sexual imprinting, 391, 393–4; and status
  in hierarchies, 407–10; stress, 217, 409,
  410, 414–415, 417, (in dominant and
  subordinate males) 409; synchrony
  between partners, 397–402: *see also
  individual hormones;* neuroendocrine
  system
House Martin *Delichon urbica:* pair bond
  persistence, 343; productivity and age of
  female, 334
humans: costs of outbreeding, 261–2; early
  experiences and mating preferences,
  264–5; mate choice, 377–85, (and
  reproductive gain) 428; monogamy, 34,
  38–9, 42, 44, 46
hybridisation, 300–1

Ibis, 349
imprinting: habituation and fine tuning,
  270–1; hormones, 391, 393–6; and
  innate preferences, 301; mate choice,
  265; and odour, 317–18; in optimal
  discrepancy hypothesis, 265; and pair
  bond, 36; plumage colour, 283, 288,
  289; and speciation, 273; species

imprinting (*cont.*)
  recognition, 290–1; and strain
  discrimination, 304–5; *see also*
  cross-fostering; experience, early
inbreeding: balance with outbreeding, 239,
  257–62, 273–4, (optimal) 273–4; and
  behaviour, 324 benefits of, 8, 235–7, 239,
  (offspring fitness) 235–6; coefficient of,
  235; and common ancestry, 234;
  evolutionary potential, 239; fitness
  decline, 237–8; genetic recombinations,
  235, 238–9; inclusive fitness effect, 237,
  (skewed sex ratios) 237; non-random
  mating, 234–40; offspring fitness, 157; in
  optimal discrepancy mechanism, 271–2;
  and outbreeding balance, 320; restriction
  in environment, 263; sexual conflicts,
  156–7; species sub-divisions, 234
inbreeding costs, 8, 238, 239, 257–62;
  avoidance, xi, 150; genetic effects, 234–5,
  259, 260–1; and offspring fitness, 247;
  and outbreeding costs, balance, 239,
  257–62, 273–4;
inbreeding depression, 237–8, 239, 261, 280
Indigo Birds, display and reproductive
  success, 124–5
interpersonal process, xiii; of behavioural
  adjustment in human courtship and
  mate choice, 382–3, 385; of negotiations
  in human mate choice, 377–85

Jacana, American *Jacana spinosa*,
  competitive female choice, 173
Japanese Quail *Coturnix coturnix:*
  assortative mating, 240–1; fostering and
  sexual preferences, 323; hormones, and
  courtship behaviour, in acquisition of
  preference, 394–7; optimal discrepancy
  hypothesis, 265–71; optimal
  outbreeding, 8, 265–71; sexual
  imprinting, 265, 393, 396

Kaspar Hauser females, 301–2
keeping company, 333, 347, 350–1, 354
Kestrel, Greater *Falco rupicoloides*, 342
kin: contributions to fitness, 429–30; early
  experiences and mating preferences,
  264–5; inbreeding and outbreeding, 260;
  optimal outbreeding, 262–4; preferences
  among, optimal discrepancy hypothesis,
  265–71; recognition, 320, (by olfaction)
  324, *see also under* olfactory
  experiences); similarities and assortative
  mating, 311; *see also* siblings
kin selection, 8, 260, 263, 265, 267, 269–72,
  273, 275, 301
Kittiwakes: divorce, *Rissa tridactyla*, 365,
  366, 367, 370, 371, 373; life pattern, *R.*

tridactyla, 361–3; mate choice, *R.*
tridactyla, 361–76; mortality rates, *R.*
tridactyla, 365, 367, 371, 372;
  non-random mating, *R. tridactyla*, 283
pair bonds, Black-legged Kittiwake, 350,
  (and productivity, *R. tridactyla*) 8–9,
  367–70, 372

Ladybird, Two spot, rare male effect, 242
Lark Bunting *Calamospiza melanocorys:*
  monogamy and polygamy, 35; territorial
  resources, 7
leks, 14–16, 109–35; adaptive cue
  hypothesis, 127–34; of anurans, 124,
  182, 184, 191; arbitrary cue hypothesis,
  126–7; benefits, (to females) 126–8, (to
  males) 109–10; binary, 114, 117;
  copulation interferences, 110, 119, 123;
  costs, (to females) 126–8, (to males)
  109–10, 128, 130; cues in female choice,
  120–6, 132; displays by males, 14–15,
  111–12, 118, 124–5, 130, 132; female
  mate choice, (between leks) 101, 111–18,
  (within leks) 14–15, 109, 118–26, 145;
  interstitial, 115, 116; male dispersion,
  111–13, (and female choice) 111–12,
  (female preference model) 113, 114–18,
  (hotspot-model) 113–114, 116, 117–18,
  (size of female home range) 114, 115,
  116, 117; male interactions, 15, 118–20,
  123; male mating success, 110; and mate
  choice, 109–38; origins of, 191, 444;
  pool-comparison tactic, 441; satellite,
  15, 114, 117; selection on female choice,
  76–7, 89–90; size of, (female preference)
  115–16, (male mating frequency) 115;
  spacings between, 116–17
lemmings *Dicrostonys groenland, Lemmus*
  trimucronatus, interspecific
  cross-fostering, 312, 314, 315
Lesser Sheathbill *Chionis minor*, pair bond,
  342
life history tactics and alternative strategies
  of reproduction, 423–33;
linkage disequilibria, 61–2, 63–4, 79
Lion, African, polygamy, 42
location of mates: *see* mate location
longevity, 331; reproductive decline, 333;
  and re-uniting, 340–1; survival of
  partner, 340–1; *see also* age
Lotka-Volterra equation, 425
lyrebirds *Menura superba*, plumage of, 16

magpies: nest site quality and productivity,
  Gymnorhina tibicen, 337–8; territory
  quality, *Pica pica*, 339
male-male competition, x, 27, 141–4,
  159, 161, 162, 233, 435; in anuran

male–male competition (*cont.*)
amphibians, 181–210; calling, 195–204, (female response to) 205; combat, 103–5; display, 124–5; in leks, 335–6, 364; and rare-male effect, 245; scramble, 143, 182, 194, 205; strategy, 204; territorial defence, 15, 118–19, 142, 159, 162, 195, 204, 205, 346, 353, 364

Mallard, mate choice in, 297–309

manakins: copulation interference, Golden-headed manakin, White-bearded Manakin, 119; female choice in leks, *Chiroxiphia linearis*, 118; male dispersion in leks, 112; position effect in female choice, White-bearded Manakin, 15

marmots: intersexual conflict, Yellow-bellied Marmot, 218–19; monogamy and brood care, Hoary Marmot, Yellow-bellied Marmot, 40

marriage: personality characteristics, 378, 380–1, (complementarity) 381, (negotiation of roles) 381–2

mate choice, 443–4; active, 141–5; assortative mating and reproductive fitness in Geese, 279–95; benefits, 4–9, 141; in birds, 389–406; buxom redhead hypothesis, 291, 293; for complementarity, 8–9; conflict between sexes *q.v.*; costs, 9–10, 141; (of discrimination), 148; (major gene effects), 146–9, (gene drift) 146–7, (genetic variance) 148–9, (mistakes) 148, (mutant strategies) 149, (polygenic effects) 149–50; criteria for, 4–11, (immediate benefits) 5–6, (predictors of benefits) 6–11; date of return to colony, 363, 371–2; dating, and self-esteem, 379; discriminate, (both sexes) 152–6, 165–7, (one sex) 151–2; in European rabbit, 211–23; evolutionary consequences, questions to consider, 280; hormonal mechanisms 389–406; in humans, 377–86; and idealisation, 382; and impression of self, (physical attraction) 377, (self-esteem) 377–8; indiscriminate, both sexes, 151; keeping company, 333, 347, 350–1, 354, (in Kittiwake Gull) 361–76; in leks, 109–38; and life style of species, 341, 345–51; and male–male competition in anuran amphibians, 181–210; in Mallard, 297–309; and mate replacement, 345–8; pairing zones, 155, 157; passive attraction, 141–5; and personality, 381; problems in demonstration of, 19–28; random mating, 150; in role-reversed species,

167–79; single allele effect, 264; study of, 3–32; tactics, 435–47

mate choice by females: active, 145–6; costs, 149–50; criteria used, 443–4; decisions, 436–7, 441–3, (fine-tuning) 443, 444, (mate-comparison) 437, (multiple criteria) 441–3, (weighting systems) 442–3, (sequential-comparison) 439, (threshold-criterion) 437–9; demonstration of, by tactics, 444; evolutionary predictions, 84–7; fitness outcomes, 438; handicap theory, 144–5; high fertility, 5; individual interest by male, 304–5; innate model of male, 301–2, 303; intrasexual competition, 211 (dominance hierarchies) 214; leks, between or in, 15, 76–7, 89–90, 109–18, 118–20, 120–6; and major genes, 146–9; of male character, polygenic models, 73–8, 85; and male combat, 102–4; male density, 194; male sampling, 201; mediation of rare male effect, 243–4; multiple mutations, 149–50, (environmental noise) 150; passive, 141–5, (male mating success) 233; preferences, 53–6, (analysis of theory) 63–4, (evolution of) 56–9, 60, 62, (models) 60–4, (genetic differences) 64–5; (genetics of) 60–2, (rare male effect) 55–6, (rate of selection) 63, (relative expression of) 59–60, (response to stimuli) 59; in role-reversed species, 167–74; runaway sexual selection, 73, 83, 84; sexual motivation, 23–7, 411–12; sexual selection by 53–66; size dependent, 6, 13, 19, 22–3, 124, 132, 201, (*see also* assortative mating, size); species discrimination, (male calls) 192–3, (temperature effects) 196, 201

mate choice by males, 436, 443; attractiveness of female, 379, (non-behavioural) 410–12, 413; for high fecundity, 5, 13; innate factors in, 301; matching hypothesis, 378–9; ovarian hormones of female, 410–13, 414; in role-reversed species, 175–7; and self-esteem, 378–9; and social status, 407–10, 415; species discrimination, 304–5

mate-comparison tactics, 437–41; benefits, 438, 439; costs, 437; evolution of, 440–1

mate location by females: male calls, 4, 10, 183–4, 187, (properties of) 196–201; passive attraction, 141–5

mate location by males, 185, 189; and breeding season lengths, 182–91; models of, 187–90; and male density, 192, 193

mate quality and mating decisions, 141–66
mating decisions, and mate quality, 141–66
mating, non-random, and offspring fitness, 227–55
mating preferences: genes for, 319; innate abilities, 301–2, 303 optimal discrepancy hypothesis, 320, 265–71, (fine tuning) 265–6, 269, 270–1, 273; purposes of, 319–20; *see also* cross-fostering; experience, early; imprinting; mate choice by females, preferences preferences
memory, 18; latent pair bonds, 43–4; mate comparisons, 437, 443
mice: cross-fostering, *Mus musculus, Onychomys torridus, Peromyscus leucopus, Peromyscus maniculatus,* 312, 314–5, 322–4; effects of early exposure to stimuli, *Acomys cahirinus,* 313, 324; inbreeding and variation, *Mus domesticus,* 262; mating preferences, 315–24; optimal discrepancy hypothesis, fine tuning preferences, *M. musculus,* 273; *Peromyscus* spp., 324
migration, 319, 348–9
models: assortative mating, 85; dynamic, (evolution by sexual selection) 71–80, (polygenic) 73–88, (runaway sexual selection) 72–3, 83, 84, (versus short-cut methods) 72; and evolution, 67–8, 73–88, (of behaviour) 59–60, (of paternal care) 174–5, (of preferences) 60–4, 75–8; (*see also* evolutionary stable strategies, ESS); female mating strategies, 17–18, (choice thresholds) 17, 152–3, 165; female preference, 54; hormone action and mate choice, 401; hybrid disadvantage, 157; leks, (adaptive cues) 128–31, (cues in female choice) 125–6, (despotic) 114, (female preferences) 114–18, (hotspots) 113–14, 117–18, (position effect) 122–3; limitations of, 71–2; major gene, 146–9; maladaptation, 89; male competition, 56; mate choice, 17–19, 149; optimal discrepancy hypothesis, 265, 266; optimal discrepancy mechanism, 271–2; optimum mating decision, 150–2; polygenic inheritance, (evolutionary predictions) 84–7, (genic covariance between sexes) 79, 80, (geographic variation) 86, (male character and female preference) 77–8, (trait heritability) 78; preferential mating, 56, 60–4; rare male effect, 55, 244–6; recombination and evolution, 239; sexual conflict, gaming models, 158–60,

175; sexual reproduction in variable environment, 258–9
monkeys: dominance hierarchies, *Papio cynocephalus,* 27; female androgens, Stumptail Macaques, 413; hormone effects, *Macaca mulatta, Miopithecus talapoin,* 408–15; male status and mating success, *Papio anubis,* 27; marmosets, 38; mating and status, *M. mulatta, P. anubis,* 27, 407, 408; motivation and ovulation, baboons, 26; reproductive strategies, Gelada Baboons, 426; sexual behaviour, endocrines and, 407–20; status and mating, *M. mulatta, P. anubis,* 27, 407, 408; support to kin, *M. mulatta,* 430; timing of reproductive effort, *P. cynocephalus,* 427
monogamy, xii, 33–47, 55, 297–8, 331, 345; bases for occurrence, 45; behaviour suggestive for, 37–9, 45–6; brood care, 39–41; concepts of, 33–6; continuity, 41–4; degree of, 44–5; discrepant uses of term, 34–6, 41–2; effect of female choice, 55; emotional bond, 38; and evolution, 46–7; fidelity of partner, 42–4, 46; and gametic contribution ratio, 35–6; in Mallard, 297, 298; as mating system, 33–5, 37, 39, 45; parental care commitment, 429; in resident species, 345, 347; as social unit, 34–5, 38–9, 45; sociobiological versus sociographical views, 33, 34, 36, 38–9, 41, 45; *see also* pair bonds
Moorhen *Gallinula chloropus,* female mate choice, 6, 12, 13, 170–2
mortality rates: Kittiwakes, 365, 372; of migratory Passerines, 340–1; and nest site quality, 339, 364; and re-pairing, 306
moths: local adaptations, 237; *Panaxia dominula,* dissassortative mating, 242

Nash equilibrium, 143, 159
Natal Robin *Cossypha natalensis,* pair bond persistence, 342, 348
natural selection: Darwinian, 68–9; fitness, 75: individual behaviour, 427; polygenic models, male character, 74, 75; primary sexual characters, 69; reproductive strategies, 423; secondary sexual characters, 69; and sexual selection, 57, 68–71, 79–81, 86, 279–80, (analysis of intensities) 95–7; of site fidelity, 353
negative assortment: *see* disassortative mating
nest sites: change of, at re-mating, 370–1; quality, 195, 337–9, (breeding

nest sites (*cont.*)
performance) 364, 374, (female
selectivity) 171–2, (mortality) 339, 364,
(productivity 337–8, 339; spacing of, and
brood survival, 298; *see also* colonies;
territories; warrens
neuroendocrine system: influence of
environment on, 392; synchrony
between partners, 401
newt: courtship, *Notophthalmus viridescens,
Triturus vulgaris, Triturus* spp., 19–20,
21, 22, 23–4, 233; display rate and
sperm supply, 5
non-random mating: alternative
hypotheses, (gene flow) 286–8, (sexual
selection) 282–4; benefits, 227; body
size, 291–3; costs, 227; frequency
dependent mating, 242–7; inbreeding
and outbreeding, 234–40; pattern of,
reflection of immigration, 286–8;
plumage colour, 281–91; off spring
fitness, 227–55; variation in mating
success, 227–34, (and fitness) 228–31; *see
also* assortative mating
nutrition: and egg formation, 335–6; and
egg laying, 298; of female, and male
quality, 168; from protein in
spermatophores, 12; seminal feeding,
233; *see also* courtship feeding

odour: kin recognition, 264, 313, 316,
317–18, 320–4; male status, 7
oestradiol: receptiveness in females, 413; in
subordinate females, 414
oestradiol-β, 392, 400; formation of, 400–1
oestrogens: behaviour in males, 400;
female motivation, 411–12; female
non-behavioural attractiveness, 410–12,
413; formation of, 391, 392; secretion
of, stimulus for, 25; and subordinate
females, 414; synchrony between
partners, 400–2; mate choice, (by males)
410, (by females) 26, 389–90
offspring fitness: assortative mating,
240–2; components, 232, 235–7;
disassortative mating, 242; epistasis,
235–6; heritability of, 229; inbreeding,
157; local adaptations, 236–7; male
quality, 160; mate choice, 229, 254–5;
and non-random mating, 227–55;
warren usage to size ratio, 218
offspring parental care in monogamy,
39–40
offspring phenotype prediction, 77–9
offspring survival, 428–9; and parental
care, 71
olfactory experiences: early exposure to,

313; and imprinting, 317–18; scent
marking, 219–20; sexual preferences,
316, 317–18, 320–1; sibling recognition,
264, 321–3, 324; species isolation, 315;
strain preferences, 323–4
optimal discrepancy hypothesis, 265–71,
280, 320; fine tuning of preferences,
265–6, 269, 270–1, 273; imprinting, 265;
stimulus cage experiments, 268–70
optimal discrepancy mechanism, 271–2;
protection against inbreeding, 271–2;
rate of inbreeding, 271–2
optimal outbreeding, 257–77; kin
recognition, 262–4; optimal discrepancy
hypothesis, 265–71; and rare-male effect,
242; risks and offspring number, 237;
spatial separation of sexes, 262–3
outbreeding, 435; balance with inbreeding,
239, 257–62, 263, 273–4, (multiple
optima) 262, (optimal) 257, 258;
benefits, 237–9; evolutionary potential,
239; maintenance, 438
outbreeding costs, 257, 258–62; breakage
of co-adapted gene complexes, 259–60;
excessive, avoidance, 150; genetic,
261–2; and inbreeding costs, balance,
239, 257–62, 273–4; infection by
pathogens, 259, 262; loss of
advantageous genes, 259; and offspring
fitness, 247; mate mismatching, 259,
262; optimal, 257–75, (mechanisms) 261;
in polygynous species, 259, 260; risks of
environment change, 259, 262, 263
outbreeding depression, 261, 280
Oystercatcher *Haematopus ostralegus*:
assortative mating, feeding
specialisation, 241, pair bond
persistence, 344, 350

pair bonds: autumnal, 340; duration, 41–4,
46, 281, 298–9, 305, 332, 342–4, 345,
366, 368, (and divorce) 285, 366, 369,
(and egg laying date) 335; equivalents
of, 36–7; and freedom of action, 36;
incompatibility within, and breeding
failure, 367, 369–70, 372; keeping
company, 333, 347, 350–1, 354; latent,
43–4; in long breeding seasons, 340; of
migrant species, 343, 348–9, (passerine)
343, 349; motivations for, 37; of
nomadic species, 343–4, 349–51, 353–4;
of resident species, 342, 345–8, 352; of
seasonal breeders, 352–3; skewed sex
ratios, 298; *see also* fidelity; re-mating
parental care, 438; by males, evolution of,
174–5, (and female emancipation)
172–3; mate complementarity, 8;

parental care (*cont.*)
offspring survival, 71; productivity,
428–9; as quality of males, 168; as
resource, 167, 173
parental investment, 141, 424, 428–9; costs
and benefits, 100–1; definition of, 167;
degree of, and mate choice, 13, 167; in
fitness, 101–2; by Mallard, 299; and
sexual selection, 160–1
Pelican, Brown *Pelecanus occidentalis*,
productivity, 334
penguin: age, chick-raising and, *Pygoscelis
adeliae*, 336–7; age of parent and
hatching success, *Eudyptes chrysolophus*,
Megadyptes antipodes, 336; chick-raising
and age, *P. adeliae*, 336–7; divorce rate,
Eudyptula minor, *M. antipodes*, *P.
adeliae*, 351, 352–4; hatching success
and age of parent, *E. chrysolophus*, *M.
antipodes*, 336; pair bond, Emperor
Penguin, *E. minor*, *M. antipodes*, *P.
adeliae*, 43, 333, 343, 350; pair bond
persistence, *Eudyptes chrysocome*, 343;
parent, age/weight and hatching success,
E. chrysolophus, *M. antipodes*, *P.
adeliae*, 336–7; parental behaviour, *P.
adeliae*, 351, 352; weight of parents and
hatching success, *E. chrysolophus*, 336
personality: and friendship choice, 383–5;
in marriage, 378, 380–1; negotiation of
roles, 381–2
phenotypes: as cues, 124–6; expression of
good genes, 9–10; of male quality,
variation in, 169; of mate and chosen
mate, 280, 377–8, 443, 444; of offspring
and parents, 77–9; rare-male effect, 55;
sexual advertisment, 141–4
Pigeon, Feral *Columba livia:* pair bond
persistence, 342; male mate choice, 177
Platyfish, timing of reproduction, 426
plumage colour: genetic basis of, 288–9,
(and imprinting) 283–5, 288, 289; colour
assortative mating, 279, 281–5;
elaborate, evolution of, 14–15, 16;
female choice, 11, 14, 16, 302, 305, 306;
genetical relatedness, 268
polyandry, xi, 27, 35, 36, 42; conditions
possibly leading to, 172–3, 177; and
sex-role reversal, 174; *see also*
polygamy; polygyny
polygamy, 12, 34, 35, 41, 42, 44, 331n; and
female choice, 55; in Long-billed Marsh
Wren, 7; Potential, 44; *see also*
polyandry; polygyny
polygenic inheritance models: *see under*
models
polygyny, 34, 35, 55; in lek species, 12; in

male Yellow-bellied Marmot, 218–19; in
primate, 415; in Red-winged Blackbird,
172; *see also* polyandry, polygamy
pool-comparison tactic, 439–40; conditions
favourable for, 441; detection
experimentally, 444; disadvantages, 440;
multiple criteria, 442
populations: common ancestry of, 234;
deleterious mutations in, 230–1; density
of, (and aggression) 214, (and breeding
group size) 212, 213, (of males and sex
ratio) 185; equilibria, 81–4, 86, (and
fitness) 84, 91–2, (and maladaptive
structures) 88–9, (and starting position)
83; evolution, (natural versus sexual
selection) 81–4, (predictions) 84–7;
extinction of, 84; fitness heritability,
228–31; genetic variance, maintenance
of, 168–9; histories of, and mating
patterns, 227; mutation selection
balance, 230–1; optimal discrepancy
mechanism, 271–2; rare-male effect, 55
position effects and female choice in leks,
15–16, 121–3, 145
positive assortment: *see* assortative mating
Prairie Chickens leks: copulation
interference, 119; male dispersion 112
predation, 4, 7, 212, 218; and display
activities, 130; of late egg clutches, 335;
protection against, (by clumping in leks)
111, 112, (by coloniality) 216, (number
of eggs) 6, (warren quality) 218
productivity, factors affecting: age, 333,
334–7; body size, 292–3; mate retention,
367; nest site quality, 364, 337–9; pair
bond duration, 332–4, 351–2; status of
female parent, 215–17; warren quality
218; *see also* reproductive output
progesterone: female attractiveness,
410–11, 412; secretion of, stimulus for,
25
prolactin, 409, 414, 415, 417; and
infertility, 415
promiscuity, 41–2; definitions of, 35, 36; in
Mallard, 298–9

quality, 3, 141, 150–6, 157–8; and body
weight, 171; of breeding sites, 6–7,
171–2, 195, 216, 217–18, 337–9, 364;
thresholds of, 154–5; *see also* fitness
quality of females, and mate choice, 175–6
quality of males, 171, 299, 305, 211–12;
advertisement of, 169–70, (*see also* vocal
signals); female assessment of, 299, 305;
and mate choice, 152, 155–6; offspring
fitness, 160–1; variance in and female
competition, 168–72

Rabbit, European *Oryctolagus cuniculus:*
    intrasexual competition, 211, 213–14;
    reproductive success, 214–17;
    scent-marking, 219–20; social
    organisation, 212–13
rare male effect: as artefact, 246;
    assessment of, 243–4; causes of 55–6, 63;
    competition between males, (mating
    ability) 245, (within a strain) 245–6; and
    outbreeding, 242
rat: interspecific cross-fostering, *Baiomys
    taylori, Rattus norvegicus,* 312, 314, 315
ravens: mate-replacement, *Corvus
    coronoides,* 345–6; pair bonds, *C.
    coronoides, Corvus mellori,* 342, 344, 345,
    350; partner familiarity, *Corvus* spp., 339
Red Deer: *see* Deer, Red
relatives: *see* kin
re-mating: in birds, 331–60; causes,
    (divorce) 365, 367, (mortality) 306,
    364–5, 367; change of nest site, 370–2;
    terminology, 332; *see also* re-pairing;
    re-uniting
re-pairing, in birds, 332; *see also*
    re-mating; re-uniting
reproductive fitness, assortative mating and
    mate choice in Snow Geese, 279–95
reproductive output, 425–30; aided by
    relatives, 429–30; birthrate
    maximisation, 427–8; energetic
    resources, 426; fitness, 429–30; parental
    investment, 428–9; timing of effort
    426–7; *see also* productivity
reproductive strategies: birth rate
    maximisation, 427–8; components of,
    424–5; decisions, 423, 424, (network of)
    430–2, (mating success) 423, 424,
    (maximisation of) 425–6; rearing, 423,
    424, (maximisation of) 428–9; survival,
    423, 424; timing of effort, 424, 426–7,
    432, (energetic resources) 426,
    (population demography) 426–7
resources, 6–7; in colonies, 216; energetic,
    in reproductive output, 216, 424, 426; of
    males and female choice, 234; as
    parental investment, 167, 168, 169;
    scarcity of, and competition, 167–8,
    173–4; territorial, 172, 184, 194, 195; *see
    also* nest site, quality; warrens, qualities
    of
re-uniting, 342–4, 353; advantages, 332–40;
    and breeding success, 351–2, 369, 373;
    and life style of species, 341, 345–51;
    and longevity, 340–1; *see also* re-mating;
    re-pairing
Robins, pair bond persistence, *Cossypha
    natalensis, Erithacus rubecula,* 342, 348

rodents, early experience and sexual
    preference in, 311–27
role-reversed species: female mate choice,
    167–74; male mate choice, 175–7
Ruff: copulation interference in leks, 119;
    mating system, *Philomachus pugnax,* 15;
    position in leks, effect on female choice,
    122; strategies in leks, 110, 117
runaway sexual selection, 57–9, 60, 72–3,
    83, 84, 126–7; call loudness, 199, 200;
    checks to, 58; mating success and
    offspring fitness, 228; origin and
    cessation, 87–8

sandpiper: copulation interference in leks,
    Buff-breasted Sandpiper, 119; double
    clutching, *Actitis macularia,* 172; pair
    bond persistence, *Calidris alpina,
    Calidris mauri, Micropalama himantopus,*
    343
satellite males, 188–93, 195, 212, 213, 215,
    216; in leks, 15, 114, 117
scent marking, 219–20; *see also* olfactory
    experiences
selection, analysis of: and analysis of
    fitness variance, 100–2; correlated
    responses, 99; and evolution, 98–100; on
    males and females, intensities of, 93–4;
    natural and sexual, intensities of, 95–7
selection, multivariate, 97–8
selection differentials, 95, 97, 98
self-esteem: matching hypothesis, 378–9;
    mate choice, 377–8
sequential-comparison tactic, 439–40;
    advantages and disadvantages, 440;
    conditions favourable for, 441; detection
    experimentally, 444
sex-limited characters, 73n
sex ratio, 93, 153, 156, 168, 266, 286;
    asymmetry, 158; female-biased, 237; in
    leks, 112; male-biased, 185; operational,
    44, 160, (in anuran amphibians) 185, (at
    breeding site) 205; (in Kittiwake
    breeding colonies), 371–2; skewed, 172,
    237, 298; in Variegated Tinamou, 174
sexual behaviour, 4, 18; display in birds,
    124, 303, 397–9; effects of rearing
    disturbances in early life of rodents,
    312–16; in monkeys, endocrines and,
    407–20; in North American Red-spotted
    Newt, 23–4
sexual conflict: *see* conflict between sexes
sexual preference, and early experience in
    rodents, 311–27
sexual selection: assortative mating, 73, 79,
    85; Darwinian, 3, 10, 11, 13, 53–5, 58,
    68–71, 102, 279; dynamic models of

sexual selection (*cont.*)
evolution by, 56–9, 60–4, 71–88;
extinction of population, 84; by female
choice, 53–66; female mate choice,
102–4; and fitness, 71; inter- and intra-,
3, 10, 11–14, 53; in leks, 76–7, 89–90,
109–10; maladaptation, 88–9; male
characteristics, 53, 55, 71; male combat,
102–4; male investment, 160; male
mating success, 71; and natural
selection, 57, 68–71, 79–83, 86, 279–80;
Panglossian view, 88–9; and parental
investment, 160–1; partitioning, 102;
polygenic models of male character,
74–88; runaway process, 57–9, 60,
126–7, (dynamic models) 72–3, 83, 84;
theories of, and mating process, 435

sexy son hypothesis 10, 89

shag *Phalacrocorax aristotelis*, nest site
quality and breeding success, 339

shearwater: divorce rate, *Puffinus puffinus*,
353; pair bond persistence, *Puffinus
griseus*, *P. puffinus*, 344

Sheep, Mountain, timing of reproduction,
426

Shrike, Yellow-billed *Corvinella corvina*,
346–7

shrimps *Hymenocera* spp., monogamy, 37

siblings: colour and mate choice, 284–5;
early experiences and mating
preferences, 301, 323–4; recognition by
olfaction, 324; *see also* kin

size: assortative mating for, 194, 201–3,
292; cue for choice, 5, 6, 13, 19, 124,
132, 201; dependent mating, 201–2, 203;
and egg number, 292–3, 428; heritability
of, 292; of males and mating success,
234, 245; mate location, 187–8, 191; and
parental care, 438; and vocal calls,
189–90, 191, 196; *see also* weight

skua: colour morphs and selection,
Stercorarius parasiticus, 280, 286; pair
bond persistence, *Stercorarius skua*, 344;
productivity, *S. parasiticus*, 333–4;
selection, *S. parasiticus*, 280, 286

Skylark *Alanda arvensis*, pair bond
persistence, 342, 348

Snow Geese, assortative mating, mate
choice and reproductive fitness, 279–95

Song-thrush *Turdus philomelos*, pair bond
persistence, 342

sparrow: assortative mating,
White-crowned Sparrow, 241;
monogamy and brood care, *Passerculus
sandwichensis*, 41; pair bond persistence
Melopsiza melodia, *Spizella pusilla*, 343;
Treesparrow, 44

speciation; and assortative mating, 240;
sexual imprinting, 273; sexual selection,
87

species reproductive barriers: and
behaviour, 311, 314–15; and
cross-fostering, 311, 314–15; differential
dispersal of young, 8; maintenance of,
315; olfactory cues 315; vocal signals,
22, 181, 196

sponges *Euplectella* spp., 36

status, female: and access to males, 407;
and aggression, 413–4; dominance
hierarchies, 214, (aggression) 216; and
metabolic rate, 216–17; and oestrogen
treatment, 414, 416; reproductive
success, 214–17; sexual attention
received, 413

status, male: and access to females,
213–14; dominance hierarchies, 213,
(aggression) 215–16; female choice, 7,
11, (leks) 123–4, 132–3; hormone levels,
407–10; maintenance of hierarchies, 415;
lek size and mating frequency, 115;
mating success, 7, 27; social displays,
303; scent marking, 219–20

Stellar's Jay *Cyanoccita stelleri*, pair bonds,
348

stimulus-value-role theory, 379–80

Sunfish, timing of reproduction, 426

survival, 331; and advertisment, 143–4;
migratory passerines, 340–1; and nest
spacing, 298; of offspring, 71, 218,
428–9; and parental care, 71; of partner
and re-uniting, 340–1; reproductive
strategies, 423, 424; status of female
parent, 215

swallow: brood care, *Riparia riparia*, 40;
monogamy, *R. riparia*, 40; pair bond
persistence, *Hirundo neoxena*, 343, 349;
Woodswallows, 349

swan: pair bonds, 333, 349, (*Cygnus olor*)
342; partner fidelity, 37

swift *Apus apus*, pair bond persistence,
343

tactics, life history and alternative
strategies of reproduction, 423–33; of
mate choice, 435–47

target cells: androgen metabolism, 393;
aromatase activity, 391, 400;
diethylstilboestrol, 400; oestradiol
formation, 400–1; oestrogen formation,
391, 392; oestrogen receptors, 400

Temminck's Stint *Calidris temminickii*,
double clutching, 172

Tern, common *Sterna hirundo*, courtship
feeding, 6

territories: and breeding groups, 212;
defence, (by female rabbit) 212, 218, (by
male) 15, 205, 336, 346, 353, 364; lek,
15–16, (male dominance) 118, 123–4;
mating systems, 182, 184, 188–9; of
migrant species, 348; of nomadic species,
349–50; quality of, 6–7, 172, 195,
(mortality rates) 339, (productivity) 335,
337–8, 339; of resident species, 345–8,
352; resources, 172, 184, 194, 195; scent
marking of, 219–20; *see also* colonies;
nest sites; warrens
testosterone: aggression between males,
408–9: brain mechanisms, 397; courtship
behaviour, 400; hypothalamic areas,
393; levels of, affected by social
structure, 407–8; mate preferences, 395,
397; precursor of androgens, 391;
receptiveness in females, 413; scent
gland activity, 219, 220; and sexual
activity, 407–9, (of dominant males) 407,
409, (of subordinate males) 408–9;
spermatogenesis, 409–10
threshold-criterion tactic, 437–9: costs and
benefits, 437, 438; detection
experimentally, 444; multiple criteria,
439, 442
timing, of reproductive effort, 424, 426–7,
432
Tinamou, Variegated *Crypturellus
variegatus*, competitive female choice,
174
tit: fitness heritability, *Parus major*, 231;
optimal discrepancy hypothesis, *P.
major*, 270; pair bond persistence, *P.
major, Parus palustris*, 342;
productivity, *P. major*, 334; territory
quality, *P. major*, 388–9
toad: androgen effects, *Xenopus laevis*,
390; calls, *Bufo calamita*, 197, 199,
200–1; male density and sex ratio, *Bufo
americanus, Bufo typhonius*, 185; mate
location, *Bufo bufo, B. calamita, Bufo
cognatus, Bufo houstonensis, Bufo
speciosus, Bufo valliceps, Bufo
woodhouseii*, 182–3, 186, 188–90; mating
system, *B. calamita, Bufo canoris*, 192;
non-random mating, *B. americanus, B.
bufo, B. calamita, Bufo quercinus, Bufo
terrestris, B. typhonius*, 202; sex ratio
and male density, *B. americanus, B.*

typhonius, 185; size assortative mating,
B. bufo, 194, 202–3; weight loss, *B. bufo,
B. calamita*, 186, 191

Uganda Kob, position effect in lek, 15,
121–2

vocal signals, anurans: advertisement calls,
14, 183, 189, 196, 200–1; auditory
limitations, 199–201, 205; body size,
189–90, 191, 196; call groups, 190, 191;
choruses, 184, 197, 198–9; encounter
calls, 183; energy content, 198–9; female
mate choice, 195–201; and male density,
192, 193; mate location, 188–91, 192;
pitch and female discrimination, 196–8,
(temperature effects) 196; sites of calling,
197–8; species identification, 192–3;
species isolating mechanisms, 22, 181,
196; synthetic, 181, 183, 189, 190, 197,
198–9; temperature effects, 196, 201, 205
vole: interspecific cross-fostering, *Microtus
canicaudus, Microtus montanus*, 314

Wagtail, White *Motacilla alba*, pair bond
maintenance, 348
warbler: brood care, *Acrocephalus
palustris*, 40; pair bond maintenance,
*Acrocephalus orientalis, Phylloscopus
trochipodes*, 348; pair bond persistence,
Dendroica discolor, 343
warrens, 212; evolution of, 217; qualities
of, 216, 217–18
wasps, 20; rare-male effect, 243–4,
(parasitic wasp) 242
weight of female, and mate choice, 12, 177,
(and mate quality) 171; loss of, and
energetics, 186, 191; of parent, (and
fledglings) 337, (and hatching success)
336
wren: age of female and productivity,
Malurus splendens, 334; mate
replacements, *Malurus* spp., 346–7; pair
bond, *Malurus* spp., *M. splendens*, 342,
346–7; pair bond persistence,
Troglodytes aedon, 343; productivity and
age of female, *M. splendens*, 334

Zebra, steppe *Equus quagga*, polygamy, 34,
42